ORTHOPEDIC CLINICS OF NORTH AMERICA

www.orthopedic.theclinics.com

Musculoskeletal Disorders

October 2022 • Volume 53 • Number 4

ii

ELSEVIER

1600 John F. Kennedy Boulevard • Suite 1800 • Philadelphia, Pennsylvania, 19103-2899.

http://www.orthopedic.theclinics.com

ORTHOPEDIC CLINICS OF NORTH AMERICA Volume 53, Number 4
October 2022 ISSN 0030-5898, ISBN-13: 978-0-323-96195-0

Editor: Megan Ashdown
Developmental Editor: Ann Gielou Posedio

Orthopedic Clinics of North America (ISSN 0030-5898) is published quarterly by Elsevier Inc., 360 Park Avenue South, New York, NY 10010-1710. Months of issue are January, April, July, and October. Business and Editorial Offices: 1600 John F. Kennedy Blvd., Suite 1800, Philadelphia, PA 19103-2899. Customer Service Office: 3251 Riverport Lane, Maryland Heights, MO 63043. Periodicals postage paid at New York, NY and additional mailing offices. Subscription prices are $354.00 per year for (US individuals), $1,033.00 per year for (US institutions), $420.00 per year (Canadian individuals), $1,064.00 per year (Canadian institutions), $486.00 per year (international individuals), $1,064.00 per year (international institutions), $100.00 per year (US students), $100.00 per year for (Canadian students), $220.00 per year for (international students). Foreign air speed delivery is included in all *Clinics* subscription prices. All prices are subject to change without notice. **POSTMASTER:** Send change of address to *Orthopedic Clinics of North America*, **Elsevier Health Sciences Division, Subscription Customer Service, 3251 Riverport Lane, Maryland Heights, MO 63043. Customer Service (orders, claims, online, change of address): Elsevier Health Sciences Division, Subscription Customer Service, 3251 Riverport Lane, Maryland Heights, MO 63043. Tel: 1-800-654-2452 (U.S. and Canada); 314-447-8871 (outside U.S. and Canada). Fax: 314-447-8029. E-mail:** journalscustomerservice-usa@elsevier.com **(for print support);** journalsonlinesupport-usa@elsevier.com **(for online support).**

Reprints. For copies of 100 or more, of articles in this publication, please contact the Commercial Reprints Department, Elsevier Inc., 360 Park Avenue South, New York, NY 10010-1710. Tel.: 212-633-3874; Fax: 212-633-3820; E-mail: reprints@elsevier.com.

Orthopedic Clinics of North America is covered in *MEDLINE/PubMed (Index Medicus), Cinahl, Excerpta Medica*, and *Cumulative Index to Nursing and Allied Health Literature*.

EDITORIAL BOARD

CONTRIBUTORS

EDITOR

FREDERICK M. AZAR, MD
The University of Tennessee Health Science Center, Campbell Clinic Department of Orthopaedic Surgery and Biomedical Engineering, Memphis, TN, USA

AUTHORS

KEVIN ABBRUZZESE, PhD
Senior Engineer, Department of Orthopaedic Surgery, Stryker, Mahwah, New Jersey, USA

MOHAMMAD S. ABDELAAL, MD
Rothman Orthopaedic Institute, Thomas Jefferson University, Philadelphia, Pennsylvania, USA

OKE A. ANAKWENZE, MD, MBA
Chief of Shoulder Surgery, Department of Orthopedic Surgery, Duke University Medical Center, Durham, North Carolina, USA

PAIGE ANDERSON, PharmD, MBA
FAJR Scientific, Resident Research Partnership, Northville, Michigan, USA; Cedarville University, Cedarville, Ohio, USA

KENDALL ANIGIAN, MD
Resident Physician, Department of Orthopaedic Surgery, UT Southwestern, Dallas, Texas, USA

MOHAMED E. AWAD, MD, MBA
FAJR Scientific, Resident Research Partnership, Northville, Michigan, USA; NorthStar Anesthesia, Detroit Medical Center, Detroit, Michigan, USA; Michigan State University College of Osteopathic Medicine, East Lansing, Michigan, USA

C. LOWRY BARNES, MD
Department of Orthopaedic Surgery, University of Arkansas for Medical Sciences, Little Rock, Arkansas, USA

AMIT K. BHANDUTIA, MD
Attending, LSU-Orthopaedics, New Orleans, Louisiana, USA

KIER M. BLEVINS, MD, MBS
Resident, Department of Orthopedic Surgery, Duke University Medical Center, Durham, North Carolina, USA

JAYSSON T. BROOKS, MD
Assistant Professor, Department of Orthopaedic Surgery, Scottish Rite for Children/UT Southwestern, Dallas, Texas, USA

BENNET A. BUTLER, MD
Department of Orthopaedic Surgery, Northwestern University Feinberg School of Medicine, Chicago, Illinois, USA

ZACKARY O. BYRD, MD
Orthopaedic Attending, Department of Orthopaedic Surgery, Joint Implant Surgeons, New Albany, Ohio, USA

COLIN K. CANTRELL, MD
Department of Orthopaedic Surgery, Northwestern University Feinberg School of Medicine, Chicago, Illinois, USA

ZHONGMING CHEN, MD
Research Fellow, Rubin Institute for Advanced Orthopedics, Sinai Hospital of Baltimore, Baltimore, Maryland, USA

WILLIAM O. COOPER, MD, MPH
Center for Patient and Professional Advocacy, Department of Pediatrics, Vanderbilt University Medical Center, Nashville, Tennessee, USA

PETER D'AMORE, MD
Resident, LSU-Orthopaedics, New Orleans, Louisiana, USA

MATTHEW DARLOW, MD
Resident, LSU-Orthopaedics, New Orleans,
Louisiana, USA

ANNABELLE P. DAVEY, MD
University of Connecticut, Farmington,
Connecticut, USA

DANG-HUY DO, MD
Department of Orthopaedic Surgery, The
University of Texas Southwestern Medical
Center, Dallas, Texas, USA

HENRY DOMENICO, MS
Vanderbilt University Medical Center, Center
for Patient and Professional Advocacy,
Nashville, Tennessee, USA

ALI S. ESSEILI, BS
FAJR Scientific, Resident Research
Partnership, Northville, Michigan, USA;
University of Michigan, Dearborn, Michigan,
USA

BRENDAN J. FARLEY, MD
FAJR Scientific, Resident Research
Partnership, Northville, Michigan, USA;
Resident, Department of Orthopaedic
Surgery, West Virginia University,
Morgantown, West Virginia, USA

DOMINIC M. FARRONATO, BS
Rothman Orthopaedic Institute, Thomas
Jefferson University, Philadelphia,
Pennsylvania, USA

MITCHELL B. GALLOWAY, MS
Vanderbilt University Medical Center, Center
for Patient and Professional Advocacy,
Nashville, Tennessee, USA

DONALD S. GARBUZ, MD, FRCSC
Department of Orthopaedics, University of
British Columbia, Vancouver, British
Columbia, Canada

BORNA GUEVEL, MA, MB, BChir, MRCS
Department of Orthopedic Sports Medicine,
Boston Children's Hospital, Boston,
Massachusetts, USA

EMILY L. HAMPP, PhD
Principal Engineer, Department of
Orthopaedic Surgery, Stryker, Mahwah, New
Jersey, USA

BENAJMIN C. HAWTHORNE, BS
University of Connecticut, Farmington,
Connecticut, USA

BENTON HEYWORTH, MD
Department of Orthopedic Sports Medicine,
Boston Children's Hospital, Boston,
Massachusetts, USA

JUSTIN HRUSKA, MD
NorthStar Anesthesia, Department of
Anesthesiology, Detroit Medical Center,
Wayne State University, Detroit, Michigan,
USA

MEGAN JOHNSON, MD
Assistant Professor, Department of
Orthopaedic Surgery, Scottish Rite for
Children/UT Southwestern, Dallas, Texas, USA

NYSSA KANTOREK, BS
Medical Student, UT Southwestern School of
Medicine, Dallas, Texas, USA

YVES J. KENFACK, BS
Medical Student, UT Southwestern School of
Medicine, Dallas, Texas, USA

MININDER KOCHER, MD, MPH
Department of Orthopedic Sports Medicine,
Boston Children's Hospital, Boston,
Massachusetts, USA

JOHN E. KUHN, MD, MS
Department of Orthopaedic Surgery,
Vanderbilt University Medical Center,
Nashville, Tennessee, USA

JASON S. LONG, MD, MBA
Resident, Department of Orthopedic Surgery,
Duke University Medical Center, Durham,
North Carolina, USA

MICHAEL R. MANCINI, MD
University of Connecticut, Farmington,
Connecticut, USA

BASSAM A. MASRI, MD, FRCSC
Department of Orthopaedics, University of
British Columbia, Vancouver, British
Columbia, Canada

AUGUSTUS D. MAZZOCCA, MS, MD
Massachusetts General Hospital, Boston,
Massachusetts, USA

SIMON C. MEARS, MD, PhD
Department of Orthopaedic Surgery,
University of Arkansas for Medical Sciences,
Little Rock, Arkansas, USA

LUCY E. MEYER, MD
Resident, Department of Orthopedic Surgery,
Duke University Medical Center, Durham,
North Carolina, USA

MICHAEL A. MONT, MD
Orthopaedic Attending, Rubin Institute
for Advanced Orthopedics, Sinai Hospital
of Baltimore, Baltimore, Maryland,
USA; Department of Orthopaedic
Surgery, Northwell Orthopaedics, Lenox
Hill Hospital, New York, New York,
USA

ROTEM MOSHKOVITZ
Department of Orthopaedics, University of
British Columbia, Vancouver, British
Columbia, Canada

GAMAL MOSTAFA, MD, FACS, FRCS
Wayne State University, School of Medicine,
Detroit, Michigan, USA

MICHAEL E. NEUFELD, MD, FRCSC
Department of Orthopaedics, University of
British Columbia, Vancouver, British
Columbia, Canada

CHRISTINE PARK, BA
Department of Orthopedic Surgery, Duke
University Medical Center, Durham, North
Carolina, USA

JAVAD PARVIZI, MD, FRCS
Rothman Orthopaedic Institute, Thomas
Jefferson University, Philadelphia,
Pennsylvania, USA

ALEXANDRA V. PAUL, MD
Resident, Department of Orthopedic Surgery,
Duke University Medical Center, Durham,
North Carolina, USA

MATTHEW C. PEARL, MD
Department of Orthopaedic Surgery,
Lenox Hill Hospital, Northwell Orthopedic
Institute, New York, New York,
USA

JOSHUA D. PEZZULO, BS
Rothman Orthopaedic Institute, Thomas
Jefferson University, Philadelphia,
Pennsylvania, USA

JAMES W. PICHERT, PhD
Vanderbilt University Medical Center, Center
for Patient and Professional Advocacy,
Nashville, Tennessee, USA

NATHAN REDLICH, MD
Resident, LSU-Orthopaedics, New Orleans,
Louisiana, USA

ANDREW REES, BS
Department of Orthopaedic Surgery,
Vanderbilt University Medical Center,
Nashville, Tennessee, USA

JOHN ROATEN, MD
Department of Orthopedic Sports Medicine,
Boston Children's Hospital, Boston,
Massachusetts, USA

KHALED J. SALEH, MD, MSc, FRCS(C),
MHCM, CPE
FAJR Scientific, Resident Research
Partnership, Northville, Michigan, USA;
Michigan State University College of
Osteopathic Medicine, East Lansing,
Michigan, USA; Department of Surgery, John
D. Dingell VA Medical Center, Detroit,
Michigan, USA

SHUMAILA SARFANI, MD
Department of Orthopaedic Surgery,
Vanderbilt University Medical Center,
Nashville, Tennessee, USA

STEFAN SARKOVICH, BS
Research Assistant, LSU-Orthopaedics, New
Orleans, Louisiana, USA

LAURA SCHOLL, MS
Principal Engineer, Department of
Orthopaedic Surgery, Stryker, Mahwah, New
Jersey, USA

GILES R. SCUDERI, MD, FACS, FAAOS
Department of Orthopaedic Surgery, Lenox
Hill Hospital, Northwell Orthopedic Institute,
New York, New York, USA

GERARD A. SHERIDAN, MD, FRCSI
Department of Orthopaedics, University of
British Columbia, Vancouver, British
Columbia, Canada

RYAN SMITH, MD
Orthopaedic Attending, Department of
Orthopaedic Surgery, Orthopaedic Institute of
Ohio, Lima, Ohio, USA

JEFFREY B. STAMBOUGH, MD
Department of Orthopaedic Surgery,
University of Arkansas for Medical Sciences,
Little Rock, Arkansas, USA

BENJAMIN M. STRONACH, MD
Department of Orthopaedic Surgery,
University of Arkansas for Medical Sciences,
Little Rock, Arkansas, USA

JOSHUA JIAN SUN, MD
Department of Orthopaedic Surgery, The
University of Texas Southwestern Medical
Center, Dallas, Texas, USA

SARA J. SUSTICH, BS
Department of Orthopaedic Surgery,
University of Arkansas for Medical Sciences,
Little Rock, Arkansas, USA

RYAN M. SUTTON, MD
Rothman Orthopaedic Institute, Thomas
Jefferson University, Philadelphia,
Pennsylvania, USA

PATRIK SUWAK, DO
Resident, LSU-Orthopaedics, New Orleans,
Louisiana, USA

BREANN TISANO, MD
Resident Physician, Department of
Orthopaedic Surgery, UT Southwestern,
Dallas, Texas, USA

MAXWELL T. TRUDEAU, BS
University of Connecticut, Farmington,
Connecticut, USA

COLIN L. UYEKI, BA
Frank H. Netter School of Medicine,
Quinnipiac University, North Haven,
Connecticut, USA

ALEXANDRA L. VALENTINO, BS
Research Study Manager, Department of
Orthopaedic Surgery, Stryker, Mahwah,
New Jersey, USA

JUSTIN VICKERY, MD
Department of Orthopaedic Surgery,
Vanderbilt University Medical Center,
Nashville, Tennessee, USA

IAN J. WELLINGTON, MD
University of Connecticut, Farmington,
Connecticut, USA

JESTIN WILLIAMS, MD
Resident, LSU-Orthopaedics, New Orleans,
Louisiana, USA

DANE K. WUKICH, MD
Department of Orthopaedic Surgery, The
University of Texas Southwestern Medical
Center, Dallas, Texas, USA

STEVEN YACOVELLI, MD
Rothman Orthopaedic Institute, Thomas
Jefferson University, Philadelphia,
Pennsylvania, USA

CONTENTS

Knee and Hip Reconstruction

> Pharmacogenomic testing, together with the early detection of drug–drug–gene interactions (DDGI) before initiating opioids, can improve the selection of dosage and reduce the risk of adverse drug interactions and therapeutic failures following Total Joint Arthroplasty. The variants of CYP genes can mediate DDGI. Orthopedic surgeons should become familiar with the genetic aspect of opioid use and abuse, as well as the influence of the patient genetic makeup in opioid selection and response, and polymorphic variants in pain modulation.

> Knee pain is among the most common complaints that an orthopedic surgeon may see in practice. It is often worked up with X-rays and MRI, leading to a myriad of potential diagnoses ranging from minimal edema patterns to various types of osteonecrosis. Similarities in certain causes can pose diagnostic challenges. The purpose of this review was to present the 3 types of osteonecrosis observed in the knee as well as additional causes to consider to help aid in the diagnosis and treatment.

> There are many soft tissue structures around the hip joint that may serve as a source of pain in both the native and prosthetic hip. In this review, the role of the gluteal, piriformis, iliopsoas, and rectus femoris musculotendinous units in the etiology of pathology around the hip joint will be discussed. Management options ranging from tailored physical therapy regimens to local steroid infiltration along with more invasive open and arthroscopic surgical techniques will be reviewed for each pathological entity. While not all conditions are well understood, advancements have been made in the management of each of these often challenging cases in both the native and prosthetic hip settings. This review explores these advancing treatment methods which will supplement the practice of any hip surgeon who is presented with problematic tendinopathy around both the native and prosthetic hip joint.

We aimed to assess the prevalence of acetabular retroversion (AR) in patients undergoing total hip replacement (THA) based on age. We retrospectively compared preoperative anteroposterior pelvic radiographs of patients younger than 40 years of age who underwent THA with the age- and body mass index-matched control of 40 years and older patients. Retroversion was determined based on the presence of cross-over sign, ischial spine sign, posterior wall sign, and elephant's ear sign with data stratified based on presence of dysplasia.

This study compared differences in (1) task duration; (2) biometric parameters (ie, caloric energy expenditure, heart rate); and (3) subjective measures of mental as well as physical demand of robotic-assisted total hip arthroplasty (THA) and manual THA. A total of 12 THAs were performed on 6 cadaveric specimens by two surgeons using a wearable technology to track biometric parameters and taking a questionnaire to compare the physical and mental demands. The results of our study suggest that as compared with manual techniques, robotic assistance for THA may reduce mental and physical fatigue.

Sickle cell disease (SCD) is a hemoglobinopathy that commonly has musculoskeletal effects including osteonecrosis of major joints (most often the hip) and medullary infarcts with resultant pain, functional limitations, and decreased quality of life. Patients with SCD may require surgical intervention, including total hip arthroplasty, frequently at a young age. The underlying pathologic process of SCD creates unique medical and surgical challenges that place these patients at increased risk of complications. This necessitates a multidisciplinary approach for providing surgical care to patients with SCD.

Trauma

Insufficiency fractures of the pelvis and acetabulum are occurring at increasing rates. Osteoporosis is the most prevalent risk fracture. Diagnosis begins with plain radiographs followed by advanced imaging with computed tomography and/or MRI. Pelvic ring fragility injuries are classified by the Fragility fractures of the pelvis system. Elderly acetabular fractures may be classified by the Letournel system. Management of these injuries is primarily nonoperative with early immobilization when allowed by fracture characteristics. When warranted, percutaneous fixation and open reduction internal fixation are options for both. Both acute and delayed total hip arthroplasty are options for acetabular fractures.

Pediatrics

Osteochondritis dissecans of the knee in pediatric and adolescent patients remains an incompletely understood entity, with multiple theories proposed for its underlying cause and variable treatment modalities. In addition to the importance of history and examination, treatment is primarily guided by lesion stability, which can be determined by MRI and arthroscopic findings. Other important factors that can influence healing include patient skeletal maturity, lesion location, and the size of the lesion. The purpose of this article is to review the most current epidemiology, classification, and pathoanatomy of the disease and discuss the different treatment options.

The current childhood obesity epidemic, affecting approximately 20% of American children and adolescents, is accompanied by unique orthopedic manifestations. The growing musculoskeletal system is susceptible to the endocrine effects of obesity, resulting in decreased bone mass and quality. As a result, obese children are at increased risk of musculoskeletal injury, fracture, and lower extremity deformities. The efficacy of nonoperative treatment such as casting or bracing may be limited by body habitus and surgical treatment is accompanied by increased risk of perioperative complications.

Shoulder and Elbow

Failed rotator cuff repairs present a complex issue for treating surgeons. Many methods of management exist for this pathology including revision repair with biologic augmentation, repairs with allograft, tendon transfers, superior capsular reconstruction, balloon arthroplasty, bursal acromial reconstruction, and reverse total shoulder arthroplasty. This review discusses the current literature associated with these management options.

Perioperative management for patients undergoing shoulder arthroplasty has evolved significantly over the years to reduce overt complications and improve patient outcomes. The groundwork for perioperative care encompasses initial patient selection and education strategies for achieving successful outcome. Multimodal pain management strategies have advanced patient care with the increased use of new regional/local anesthetics. In addition, complications resulting from blood loss and transfusions have been curtailed with the use of synthetic antifibrinolytic agents. It remains critical for shoulder arthroplasty surgeons to optimize patients during the perioperative period through various modalities to maximize functional progression, outcomes, and patient's satisfaction following shoulder arthroplasty.

Foot and Ankle

Introduction: Unsolicited patient complaints (UPCs) about surgeons correlate with surgical complications and malpractice claims. Analysis of UPCs in orthopedics is limited. Methods: Patient complaint reports recorded at 36 medical centers between January 1, 2015 and December 31, 2018 were coded using a previously validated coding algorithm Patient Advocacy Reporting System. Results: A total of 33,174 physicians had 4 consecutive years of data across the 36 participating medical centers and met other inclusion criteria. Conclusions: Orthopedists with high numbers of UPCs may benefit from being made aware of their elevated risk status in ways that invite reflection on underlying causes.

This review article examines contemporary methods and assesses radiographic outcomes and postoperative complications following the modified Lapidus procedure. A systematic review demonstrated significant improvements in intermetatarsal angle, hallux valgus angle, and tibial sesamoid position. We are updating a modified Lapidus technique for achieving triplanar correction of hallux valgus. Two cases of hallux valgus, one primary and one recurrent, are presented. As demonstrated in the systematic review, outcomes of Lapidus procedures create future opportunities. Surprisingly, only 78% of the studies assessed for this review reported on the hallux valgus angle and only 33% reported on tibial sesamoid position.

Spine

Degenerative cervical myelopathy is most commonly caused by cervical spondylosis, with a predominant elderly population, and is the most common cause of spinal cord impairment. Patients typically present with gait dysfunction, hand impairment, and/or the presence of long tract signs: clonus, Hoffman sign, Babinski sign, or inverted radial reflexes. One of the key surgical strategies is deciding an approach, which is based on patient characteristics and cause of pathologic condition. Without operative intervention, there is a high rate of neurological decline. Most surgeons recommended surgical treatment given the favorable outcomes and well understood natural history of disease.

Lumbar spinal stenosis is a prevalent condition with varied presentation. Most common in older populations, symptoms typically include back, buttock, and posterior thigh pain. Diagnosis is typically based on physical examination and clinical history, but confirmed on imaging studies. Nonsurgical management includes nonsteroidal anti-inflammatories, physical therapy, and epidural injections. If nonoperative management fails or patient presentation involves worsening symptoms, surgical intervention, most commonly in the form of a laminectomy, may be indicated. Recent literature has demonstrated improved pain and functional outcomes with surgery compared with conservative treatment in the middle to long term.

MUSCULOSKELETAL DISORDERS

PREFACE

Musculoskeletal disorders are conditions that affect the muscles, bones, and joints, with a multitude of diagnoses and approaches to treatment. The reviews in this issue cover the current findings and recommendations in the literature for appropriate and efficient management for optimal patient outcomes.

Pain management for disorders of the hip and knee is a common concern for orthopedists as well as their patients. This issue includes reviews on pharmacogenomic testing for drug-drug–gene interactions prior to initiating opioids, knee osteonecrosis diagnosis and treatment, soft-tissue structure pathologic conditions of the hip, and premature hip osteoarthritis in younger patients caused by acetabular retroversion. And, in current technology, we include a report of robotic assistance for total hip arthroplasty (THA) that can reduce both mental and physical fatigue in surgeons when compared with manual techniques.

Sickle cell disease (SCD) frequently affects the musculoskeletal system, including periarticular osteonecrosis of major joints, most commonly the hip, and major infarcts that result in pain, limit function, and decrease quality of life. A multidisciplinary approach for providing surgical care is necessary for patients with SCD undergoing THA who are at increased risk for complications and may require surgery at a young age.

The trauma section includes a review of management options for insufficiency fractures of the pelvis and acetabulum, which are becoming a more prevalent concern with increasing age, with the most prevalent risk factor being osteoporosis. Pelvic and acetabular fractures carry significant morbidity and mortality for the elderly population. This review presents management options for pelvic ring injuries and acetabular fractures in elderly patients.

In pediatric and adolescent patients, osteochondritis dissecans is not completely understood. We include a review of the most current epidemiology, classification, and pathoanatomy of the disease that also discusses different treatment options. Also affecting pediatric patients is the obesity epidemic, which can lead to an increased risk of musculoskeletal injury, fracture, and lower-extremity deformities. The limited efficacy of nonoperative treatments, such as casting and bracing, due to body habitus and the increased risks of perioperative complications from surgical treatment are discussed.

In the shoulder and elbow section, the complex issue of failed rotator cuff repairs and current management options are reviewed. Reverse shoulder arthroplasty and various modalities used during the perioperative period that maximize functional progression, reduce overt complications, and improve patient outcomes over the years are presented.

Unsolicited patient complaints (UPCs) about surgeons correlate with surgical complications and malpractice claims. After finding limited analysis of these complaints, a large national patient complaint database was used to evaluate differences in the number and distribution of UPCs between orthopedic surgeons, other surgeons, and nonsurgeons, describe the distribution of UPCs among orthopedic subspecialties, and assess clinical characteristics that may be associated with UPCs.

Also included in the foot and ankle section is a review of radiographic outcomes and postoperative complications after a modified Lapidus procedure for hallux valgus, noting significant improvements in intermetatarsal angle, hallux valgus angle, and tibial sesamoid position. The authors present an updated modified Lapidus technique for achieving triplanar correction of hallux valgus.

The spine section discusses the typical presentations and operative interventions of degenerative cervical myelopathy, which is often caused by cervical spondylosis and causes spinal impairment in a predominantly elderly population. Also included is a discussion of the diagnosis of lumbar spinal stenosis and the improved mid- to long-term pain and functional outcomes with surgery when compared with conservative treatment.

We thank the authors for their contributions to clinical knowledge that will guide orthopedists in treating patients with musculoskeletal disorders around the world.

Frederick M. Azar, MD
The University of Tennessee Health Science Center
Campbell Clinic Department of Orthopaedic
Surgery and Biomedical Engineering
Memphis, TN, USA

E-mail address:
fazar@campbellclinic.com

Orthop Clin N Am 53 (2022) xv
https://doi.org/10.1016/j.ocl.2022.07.001
0030-5898/22/© 2022 Published by Elsevier Inc.

Knee and Hip Reconstruction

Opioid-Related Genetic Polymorphisms of Cytochrome P450 Enzymes after Total Joint Arthroplasty

A Focus on Drug–Drug–Gene Interaction with Commonly Coprescribed Medications

Brendan J. Farley, MD[a,b,1],
Mohamed E. Awad, M.D, MBA[a,c,d,1],
Paige Anderson, PharmD, MBA[a,e,1], Ali S. Esseili, BS[a,f,1],
Justin Hruska, MD[c,g], Gamal Mostafa, MD, FACS, FRCS[h],
Khaled J. Saleh, MD, MSc, FRCS(C), MHCM, CPE[a,d,i,1,*]

KEYWORDS

- Total joint arthroplasty • Pharmacogenomics • Drug–drug–gene interaction • Opioid • Pain

KEY POINTS

- CYP2D6 poor metabolizers experience suboptimal pain relief, require higher doses of codeine, and be at significant risk of adverse events of other coadministered medications primarily metabolized by CYP2D6 such as beta-blockers (metoprolol), selective serotonin reuptake inhibitors (SSRIs) (citalopram, escitalopram, fluoxetine, fluvoxamine, paroxetine, or sertraline), and amitriptyline.
- Patients with CYP3A4 *1 G/*1G variant consumed significantly less fentanyl than those with either the 1/*1 group or the *1/*1G group ($P < .05$) to achieve a a similar degree of pain control.
- Patients with the AA genotype of CYP2B6 undergoing anesthesia with propofol may have decreased clearance of the drug as compared with patients with the GG genotyT.
- CYP2B6 *6 is associated with decreased clearance of ketamine as compared with CYP2B6 *1.
- CYP2C9*3 requires reducing the dose of warfarin when prescribed with simvastatin to avoid the risk of bleeding.

B.J. Farley and M.E. Awad equally contributed to the work and are considered first authors.
[a] FAJR Scientific, Resident Research Partnership, 9308 Hickory Ridge Rd, Suite 301, Northville, MI, 48167, USA;
[b] Department of Orthopaedic Surgery, West Virginia University, 6040 University Town Centre Dr Drive, Morgantown, WV 26501, USA; [c] NorthStar Anesthesia, Detroit Medical Center, 4201 St Antoine Street, Detroit, MI 48201, USA; [d] Michigan State University College of Osteopathic Medicine, 965 Wilson Rd, East Lansing, MI 48824, USA; [e] Cedarville University, 251 N Main St, Cedarville, OH 45314, USA; [f] University of Michigan, 4901 Evergreen Rd, Dearborn, MI 48128, USA; [g] Department of Anesthesiology, Wayne State University- Detroit Medical Center, 4201 St Antoine Street, Detroit, MI, 48201, USA; [h] Wayne State University, School of Medicine, 3990 John R St, Detroit, MI 48201, USA; [i] Department of Surgery, John D. Dingell VA Medical Center, 4646 John R St, Detroit, MI 48201, USA.
[1] The contents do not represent the views of the U.S. Department of Veterans Affairs or the United States Government
* Corresponding author. Department of Surgery, John D. Dingell VA Medical Center, 4646 John R St, Detroit, MI 48201, USA.
E-mail address: kjsaleh@gmail.com

INTRODUCTION

The increased usage of opioids for the treatment of pain has led to several unanticipated consequences for individual patients and for society at large.[1] The United States uses an estimated 27,400,000 g of hydrocodone annually compared with 3237 g for Great Britain, France, and Italy combined.[1,2] With nontherapeutic opioid use in the United States exceeding $50 million annually[3] and contributing to one death every 19 minutes,[4] the opioid epidemic constitutes both a medical, as well a fiscal dilemma for our nation.

Opioid dependency is a multi-pillar system, constituted by one's sex, ethnicity, age, psychosocial health, environment, comorbidities, other medications, and genetic polymorphism.[5] Total joint arthroplasties (TJA) is largely indicated by postoperative pain.[6] Patients have shown to have higher expectations of relief from pain when compared with improvements in functional ability following arthroplasty.[7,8]

Pharmacodynamic and pharmacokinetic variability from person to person explains the inconsistency in individual efficacy of opioid medications, as well as the potential for adverse drug responses.[5,9] Failure of appropriate postoperative pain management following a total joint arthroplasty, primarily due to pharmacogenomic variability from patient to patient, can govern the difference between efficacious, salubrious pain control, versus therapeutic failure or deleterious drug responses. This propagates the necessity to produce an individually tailored approach to postoperative pain control.[9]

With the exception of morphine, oxymorphone, and hydromorphone, opioid metabolism is primarily mediated by the cytochrome P450 (CYP450) enzyme system located in the liver.[10] This enzyme system is extensively involved in the metabolism of drugs, as well as other chemicals, foods, toxins, or various xenobiotics that are ingested into the body.[11] Although more than 30 CYP450 isoenzymes have been identified, this article focuses on CYP2D6, CYP2C9, CYP2B6, and CYP3A4 in terms of their role in opioid therapeutic response—whose presence and activity level are dependent on a multitude of factors including age, sex, race, ethnic background, tobacco use, concomitant medication use (inducers, inhibitors), opioid receptor expression and distribution.[12] Genetic polymorphism is a term for the variation of structure of genes, which includes structural changes such as deletion, duplication, and translocation.[13] A single-nucleotide polymorphism (SNP) is the most common altered gene form.[14] Depending on genetic expression, patients can be stratified based on their ability to metabolize medications.[15] Genetic polymorphisms play a major role for the function of CYPs 2D6, 2C19, 2C9, 2B6, and 3A4, and lead to distinct pharmacogenetic phenotypes termed as poor, intermediate, and ultrarapid metabolizers.[16] Normal metabolizers respond as expected, experiencing appropriate therapeutic efficacy with minimal to no adverse effects. Poor metabolizers (PM), extensive metabolizers (EM), or nonmetabolizers (NM) may experience suboptimal pain relief and have higher risk of adverse drug reactions.[16]

Genetic variability in the presence and concentration of CYP enzymes determines the plasma concentrations of opioid medications. This is directly proportional to the analgesic effects, as well as adverse opioid reactions, such as ileus, urinary retention, delirium, myoclonus, seizures, and respiratory depression, to said medications.

Pharmacogenomic variability is regulated by a multitude of drug-metabolizing enzymes (CYP450, uridine diphosphate glucuronosyltransferase [UGT], catechol-O-methyl-transferase [COMT]), transporters (P-glycoprotein transporter ABCB1, and organic anion transporter proteins [Solute Carrier (SLC) transporters]) and receptors (Mu-opioid receptors [OPRM1] and kappa-opioid receptors [OPRK1]).[9] The existing pharmacogenomic guidelines for drug–gene interactions have highlighted the interaction between CYP450 enzymes and prescribed medications. However, the impact of different CYP genetic polymorphisms on these interactions has yet to be delineated.[5] The current article is a natural continuation of our previously published article. In this current article, we primarily focus on CYP450 polymorphisms involving commonly prescribed drugs and prior opioid use. In efforts to mitigate the current opioid epidemic striking modern medicine, it is hoped that this investigation will highlight the necessity for pharmacogenomic testing as part of practicing physicians' postoperative pain management repertoire following total joint arthroplasty.

METHODS

We conducted a search on DrugStats database for the 50 most commonly prescribed medications in the United States within the period 1st quarter of 2021. Table 1 This database is a standardized version of publicly available data provided by the US Government.[17] This database is updated yearly and includes more than 3 billion outpatient prescription fills per year. In addition, we used the PharmGKB database to perform a detailed search for the metabolic pathways and relevant genetic polymorphisms of both opioids and the commonly prescribed

Table 1
Genetic variant annotations for the most common 50 prescribed drugs in 2021

Brand Name	Generic Name	Route	Drug Category	Pharmacologic Class	Substrate to	Inducer to	Inhibitor to	Pharmacogenomic Variant
Lortab	Hydrocodone/ Acetaminophen	Oral	Analgesic	Opioid/NSAIDs	CYP3A4, CYP2D6	NA	NA	OPRM1 (rs1799971)
Deltasone	Prednisone	Oral	Inflammation	Corticosteroid	CYP3A4, ABCB1	CYP3A4, CYP2C19	ABCB1	ABCB1 (rs1045642)
Neurontin	Gabapentin	Oral	Central Nervous System	Anticonvulsant and Neuropathic Pain	NA	NA	NA	NA
Ultram	Tramadol	Oral	Central Nervous System	Opioid Analgesic	CYP3A4, CYP2D6	NA	CYP2D6	NA
Xanax	Alprazolam	Oral	Central Nervous System	Anxiolytics	CYP3A4, CYP2C9	NA	NA	NA
Mobic	Meloxicam	Oral	Inflammation	NSAIDs	CYP3A4, CYP2C8, CYP2C9	NA	CYP2C8, CYP2C9	CYP2C9*1*2*3
Cymbalta	Duloxetine	Oral	Central Nervous System	Antidepressant and Neuropathic Pain	CYP2D6, CYP1A2	NA	CYP2D6	CYP2C19*1, CYP2C19*2, CYP2C19*3
Flexeril	Cyclobenzaprine	Oral	Musculoskeletal System	Skeletal Muscle Relaxant	CYP3A4, CYP2D6m CYP1A2	NA	NA	NA
Medrol	Methylprednisolone	Oral	Inflammation	Corticosteroid	CYP3A4, ABCB1	NA	CYP3A4	ABCB1 (rs1045642)

drugs in patients with TJA.[18] The relevant polymorphisms are highlighted in the subsequent sections later in discussion, as well as in Table 2: Pharmacogenomic Interactions Between Top 50 Prescribed Drugs and Pain Medications.

RESULTS
CTYP2D6
CYP2D6 is actively involved in the metabolism of commonly prescribed opioids including codeine, oxycodone, hydrocodone, and tramadol.[10] More than 80 documented variants of CYP2D6 have been identified.[19] The CYP2D6*1/*1 allele is the most common form and considered a "fully functional" normal genotype, also known as wild type. It is also phenotypically referred to as an extensive drug metabolizer (EM) while CYP2D6*4 is nonfunctioning variant and considered CYP2D6-deficient. CYP2D6*4 carriers can be either fully nonfunctioning (*4/*4) or have partially enzymatic activity (*1/*4), depending on the allele designation. These are phenotypically referred to as nonmetabolizers and poor metabolizers (PM), respectively. In addition, there are number of nonfunctioning variants (*2XN, *3, *5, *6, *9, *10, *17, *29, *41) in different ethnicities.[19]

Opioids and CYP2D6
CYP2D6 *4/*4 + *3/*4 are associated with decreased peak plasma concentrations of oxymorphone and noroxymorphone, as well as oxymorphone/oxycodone ratios in patients with cancer when treated with oxycodone as compared with CYP2D6 *1/*1 + *2/*2. In other words, CYP2D6 PM has lower oxymorphone and noroxymorphone serum concentrations and oxymorphone to oxycodone ratios than EM and UM.[20] VanderVaart et al.[21] reported that women with CYP2D6 *4/*4 + *4/*5 experienced less analgesic effect of codeine for postpartum pain management as compared with CYP2D6 *1/*1. Susce and colleagues[22] demonstrate that patients with CYP2D6 *4/*6 allele are highly susceptible to opioid intolerance especially to oxycodone and tramadol after hip surgeries. These individuals may experience almost no pain relief with significant opioid adverse events. However, individuals with the combined allele of *4 or *3 nonfunction allele along with either nonfunctional (*3, *4, *5, *6) or reduced function allele (*9, *10, *17, *29, *41), may have less metabolism/clearance of codeine and tramadol. This would achieve pain relief but with significant adverse events.[23]

CYP2D6 polymorphism is associated with the increasing risk of opioid adverse effects. In a study of 64 normal volunteers, patients with CYP2D6 *1/*2XN had an increased risk of adverse drug reactions when treated with codeine, hydrocodone, or oxycodone in healthy individuals as compared with CYP2D6 *1/*1.[24] Refractory cardiac arrest,[25] renal impairment, and respiratory insufficiency[26] were observed and likely susceptible in patients with CYP2D6 *1/*1XN who were treated with tramadol, as compared with CYP2D6 *1/*1.

CYP2D6 *1/*1 is associated with the inhibition of codeine metabolism when coadministered with acetaminophen and levomepromazine in patients with back pain. Codeine to morphine metabolism was significantly inhibited by levomepromazine in *1/*1 patients but not in *1/*4 patients.[27]

Cardiovascular medications and CYP2D6
Despite its low incidence, cardiac complication is considered a leading cause of mortality after TJA.[28,29] The 30-day cardiac-related mortality after TKA and THA was reported as 0.18% and 0.35%, respectively.[30] In addition, 2% of patients with TJA experienced cardiac morbidity which may extend the length of admission by average 11 days postoperatively.[31,32] American College of Cardiology/American Heart Association guidelines on perioperative cardiovascular evaluation and care for noncardiac surgeries recommended perioperative administration of beta-blockers to prevent myocardial ischemia and infarction postoperatively.[33] Moreover, Van Klei and colleagues reported that the discontinuation of beta-blocker prescription during the first week postoperatively in patients with TJA was significantly associated with myocardial infraction (odds ratio (OR): 2.0, 95% confidence interval (CI): 1.1–3.9) and death (OR: 2.0, 95% CI: 1.0–3.9).[34]

Patients with CYP2D6 *4 have a higher risk of severe bradycardia with metoprolol prescription as compared with CYP2D6 *1.[35] While patients with variant *1/*1 may have increased metabolism and clearance of metoprolol and less efficacy for heart rate reduction as compared with individuals with *1 or more reduced functional allele (*9, *10, *17, *29, *41) or nonfunctional (*3, *4, *5, *6) allele. Those individuals may also experience increased metabolism/clearance of codeine and tramadol with decreased, but not absent risk for side effects, as compared with patients with nonfunctional or reduced function alleles.[36–38] While individuals with reduced functional allele (*10,*17 or 42*) in combination with a reduced function (*9, *10, *17, *29, *41) or nonfunctional (*3, *4, *5, *6) may have decreased metabolism/clearance

Table 2
Pharmacogenomic interactions between top 50 prescribed drugs and pain medications

Gene	Variant	Drug	Genotype	Evidence	Type	Phenotype Effect	References
CYP2D6							
		Codeine	*1/*2XN	NA	Toxicity/ADR	Increased risk of refractory cardiac arrest, renal impairment, respiratory insufficiency	Manchikanti, L., et al,[2] 2012
		Oxycodone	*1/*2XN	NA	Toxicity/ADR	Increased risk refractory cardiac arrest, renal impairment, respiratory insufficiency	Manchikanti, L., et al,[2] 2012
		Hydrocodone	*1/*2XN	NA	Toxicity/ADR	Increased risk refractory cardiac arrest, renal impairment, respiratory insufficiency	Manchikanti et al,[2] 2012
		Citalopram	*4/*4	NA	Metabolism	Impaired metabolism, increased risk of side effects including tachycardia and agitation	Zineh et al,[23] 2004
		Escitalopram	*4/*4	NA	Metabolism	Impaired metabolism, increased risk of side effects including tachycardia and agitation	Zineh et al,[23] 2004
		Fluoxetine	*4/*4	NA	Metabolism	Impaired metabolism, increased risk of side effects including tachycardia and agitation	Zineh et al, 2004[23]
		Fluvoxamine	*4/*4	NA	Metabolism	Impaired metabolism, increased risk of side effects including tachycardia and agitation	Zineh et al,[23] 2004
		Paroxetine	*4/*4	NA	Metabolism	Impaired metabolism, increased risk of side effects including tachycardia and agitation	Zineh et al,[23] 2004
		Sertraline	*4/*4	NA	Metabolism	Impaired metabolism, increased risk of side effects	Zineh et al,[23] 2004

(continued on next page)

Table 2
(continued)

Gene	Variant	Drug	Genotype	Evidence	Type	Phenotype Effect	References
		Venlafaxine	*4/*4	NA	Metabolism	Impaired metabolism, increased risk of side effects including tachycardia and agitation	Zineh et al,[23] 2004
CYP2C9	*1, *2, *3						
		Diclofenac	*3/*3	2A	Toxicity/ADR	Increased risk of GI bleeding	Robert, and Pelletier,[14] 2018; Ventola,[15] 2011
		Ibuprofen	*3/*3	2A	Toxicity/ADR	Increased risk of GI bleeding	Robert, and Pelletier,[14] 2018; Ventola,[15] 2011
		Naproxen	*3/*3	2A	Toxicity/ADR	Increased risk of GI bleeding	Robert, and Pelletier,[14] 2018; Ventola,[15] 2011
		Piroxicam	*3/*3	2A	Toxicity/ADR	Increased risk of GI bleeding	Robert, and Pelletier,[14] 2018; Ventola,[15] 2011
		Celecoxib	*3/*3	2A	Dosage	Poorly metabolized	Zanger and M. Schwab,[16] 2013
CYP2B6	rs2279343	Ketamine	*1/*1	3	Metabolism	Rapidly Metabolized	Susce et al,[22] 2006
		Methadone	*1/*1	3	Toxicity/ADR	Increased pain tolerance and threshold	Zineh et al,[23] 2004
			*1/*1	3	Metabolism	Rapidly Metabolized	de Leon et al,[24] 2003
CYP3A4	rs2246709	Fentanyl	GG	3	Dosage	Requires less dose of fentanyl	Hansen et al,[3] 2011
		Methadone	GG	3	Toxicity/ADR	More severe side effects and opioid withdrawal symptoms in heroin dependent	Manchikanti et al,[2] 2012

of metoprolol, and better efficacy in reducing the heart rate as compared with patients with *1/*1 genotype.[38–40] In addition, Takekuma and colleagues demonstrates that cardiac patients with the CYP2D6 *1/*4 genotype may have decreased clearance of carvedilol as compared with patients with the *1/*1 genotype.[41]

Preoperative pharmacogenomics testing, as well as cardiology evaluation for patients at risk, may ultimately reduce the likelihood of adverse events or therapeutic failure of both b-blockers and opioids after TJA.

Selective serotonin reuptake inhibitors and CYP2D6

Patients with CYP2D6*4/*4 may require a lower dose of citalopram, escitalopram, fluoxetine, fluvoxamine, paroxetine, or sertraline as compared with patients with CYP2D6*1/*1).[42] Patients with the *1/*1 genotype may have increased metabolism/clearance of venlafaxine as well as increased risk of higher venlafaxine dose tolerance. In addition, these patients have decreased, but not absent risk for side effects as compared with patients with nonfunctional (*3, *4, *5, *6) and reduced functional alleles (*10, *41).[43] Wijnen and colleagues demonstrate that CYP2D6 *4/*4 is associated with tachycardia and agitation when treated with 225 mg/d venlafaxine.[44]

Antidepressants/anxiolytics and CYP2D6

TJR patients seem to have higher rates of clinically significant symptoms of depression were noted in 50% and 24% of patients before discharge and before surgery, respectively.[45,46] The effect of amitriptyline in managing depression, anxiety, and neuropathic pain is well documented and established in clinical use.[47]

Patients with 2 functional CYP2D6 alleles *1/*1 and who are using amitriptyline may have less nortriptyline plasma levels and more clearance of amitriptyline. Additionally, they would have decreased, but not absent, the risk for side effects as compared with patients with CYP2D6 nonfunctional alleles (*3, *4, *5, *6) or reduced function alleles. These patients would also have decreased metabolism of amitriptyline as compared with patients with the duplication of a functional CYP2D6 gene.[48] However, CYP2D6 *4/*4 is associated with high risk of amitriptyline toxicity.[49]

Conclusion and clinical application for the TJA setting

Patients identified as CYP2D6 poor metabolizer (PM) such as *4/*4 may not optimally experience pain relief and requires higher doses of codeine. The patient may also be at significant risk of adverse events from other coadministrated medications primarily metabolized by CYP2D6 such as beta-blockers (metoprolol), selective serotonin reuptake inhibitors (SSRIs) (citalopram, escitalopram, fluoxetine, fluvoxamine, paroxetine or sertraline), and amitriptyline.

CYP2C9

CYP2C9 metabolism primarily involves nonsteroidal antiinflammatory drugs (NSAIDs) and aspirin, though it is also the system that metabolizes phenytoin and warfarin.[50]

Nonsteroidal antiinflammatory drugs and CYP2C9

Nonsteroidal antiinflammatory drugs are one of the most common over-the-counter prescribed drugs. NSAIDs are recommended as a part of multimodal pain management protocol after TJA.[51] Recent meta-analysis of 8 studies concluded that perioperative administration of selective COX-2 inhibitors might be effective in reducing postoperative pain and opioid consumption after TKA. Their postoperative continuation did not increase the risk of bleeding.[52]

CYP2C9 *1/*1 is associated with increased metabolism of diclofenac in healthy individuals as compared with CYP2C9 *1/*3.[53] Allele C of CYP2C9 (rs1057910) is associated with the increased risk of gastrointestinal bleeding when treated with antiinflammatory agents, nonsteroids, celecoxib, diclofenac, ibuprofen, naproxen or piroxicam as compared with allele A.[54] CYP2C9 *1/*2 is associated with increased metabolism of celecoxib and decreased maximum plasma concentration in healthy individuals as compared with CYP2C9 *1/*1.[55]

Cardiovascular medications and CYP2C9

Patients with CYP2C9 *1/*1 may achieve less blood pressure control with losartan treatment. Results show that healthy individuals with the CYP2C9 *1/*1 genotype may have increased metabolism of losartan as compared with patients with *1/*3, *1/*5, *1/*6, *5/*6, *5/*8, or *1/*13 genotype.[56] Addepalli and colleagues demonstrate that patients with the *1/*1 variant may require a higher dose of warfarin for VTE prevention and management as compared with patients with *1/*3 CYP2C9 alleles.[57] The same fully functional genotype may have decreased risk of over-anticoagulation when warfarin is used in the management of atrial fibrillation[58] or thyrotoxicosis[59] as compared with patients with CYP2C9*2, *3, *5, *6 or *11. Furthermore, patients with CYP2C9*1/*1 are associated with less time to reach the maintenance dose when treated with warfarin as compared with patients with CYP2C9*2, *3, or *13.[60]

Andersson and colleagues[61] reveal that the CYP2C9*3 polymorphism predisposes toward pharmacologic interaction between warfarin and simvastatin. This influence on the magnitude of simvastatin–warfarin drug–drug interaction was seen only in patients with the CYP2C9*3 allele. CYP2C9*3 requires reducing the dose of warfarin when treated with simvastatin to avoid the risk of bleeding.

CYP2B6

CYP2B6 polymorphism is linked to the interindividual variability in the management of opioid dependence[62] as well as smoking cessation.[63,64]

Opioid dependence and CYP2B6
Patients with the AA genotype of CYP2B6 may require a higher methadone dose as compared with patients with the GG genotype for opioid dependence management.[65]

CYP2B6*6 homozygotes had significantly higher trough (R)- and (S)-enantiomer methadone plasma levels than noncarriers.[62] However, CYP2B6*6 homozygotes did not differ from noncarriers in therapeutic response to daily doses of methadone.[62]

Ketamine has shown an opioid-sparing effect when used as an analgesic adjuvant in perioperative multimodal analgesia after THA[66] and TKA[67] with a significant impact on early mobilization. CYP2B6 *6 is associated with decreased clearance of ketamine as compared with CYP2B6 *1. Median plasma clearance in the *6/*6 and *1/*1 genotypes were 21.6 L/h and 68.1 L/h, respectively.[68]

Anesthesia and CYP2B6
A cohort study of 51 patients with average age of 65 years shows that patients with the AA genotype undergoing anesthesia with propofol may have decreased clearance of the drug as compared with patients with the GG genotype.[69] However, a different study found no association for the CYP2B6*4, *6 and *7 haplotypes.[70]

Smoking cessation and CYP2B6
Smoking has a complex impact on pain perception[71] and it is also associated with increased risk of opioid requirements and dependence after TJA.[72] Elaine and colleagues discussed the correlation between CYP2A6 enzymatic activity and cigarette smoking behavior. Individuals who had the G allele had an average 25% higher metabolite ratio (trans-3′-hydroxycotinine to cotinine ratio) when compared with the AA genotype allele. Allele G is associated with increased metabolism of nicotine in people with tobacco use disorder.[73]

The antismoking effect of bupropion does not seem to be related to its antidepressant effect as bupropion is equally effective as a smoking cessation therapy in smokers with and without depression.[63] Smoking cessation success requires patients to complete 6 months of smoking abstinence plus some adjuvants such as bupropion.[63] Individuals with tobacco use disorders and GG genotype may have a decreased response to bupropion as compared with individuals with the AA genotype. Forty-eight percent of patients with CYP2B6 rs2279343 AA genotype in the bupropion-only group succeeded in smoking cessation as compared with 35.5% of patients carrying the AG or GG genotypes (CYP2B6*4).[64]

CYP3A4

CYP3A4 is one of the most essential cytochrome P450 enzymes. It is responsible for the clearance of approximately 45%-60% of currently prescribed medications.[74,75] With regard to opioids, CYP3A4 regulates the excretion of fentanyl, buprenorphine, and methadone.[11] Moreover, it processes some of the cardiovascular medications such as antihypertensive medications (felodipine,[76] amlodipine,[77] nifedipine,[78] statins[79]) and lipid-lowering medications (atorvastatin and simvastatin). CYP3A4 is also responsible for the clearance of some immune suppressant drugs such as cyclosporine,[80] tacrolimus,[81] antibiotics (Erythromycin[82]), and sedatives (Midazolam[83]).

Opioids and CYP3A4
CYP3A4 mediated hepatic-biotransformation is the main metabolic pathway for Fentanyl.[84] Yuan and colleagues[85] investigated the impact of CYP3A4*1G polymorphism on the plasma fentanyl concentration and fentanyl consumption for postoperative pain control. The results showed that patients with CYP3A4 *1 G/*1G variant consumed significantly less fentanyl than those with either the 1/*1 group or the *1/*1G group (P < .05) to achieve a similar degree of pain control.

CYP3A4 and CYP2B6 are the main metabolic enzymes for methadone.[86] Chen and colleagues performed a large cohort study for opioid-dependent patients undergoing methadone maintenance treatment. This study showed that Allele G of CYP3A4 (rs2246709) is associated with increased severity of withdrawal symptoms for methadone treatment as compared with allele A.[87]

Cardiovascular medications and CYP3A4
Calcium channel blockers (CCBs) are among the most often prescribed drugs for the treatment of

hypertension.[88] CYP3A4*1G carriers are more likely to reach the target mean arterial pressure of less than 92 mm Hg when treated with amlodipine compared with AA homozygotes.[77] Wang and colleagues[89] investigate the effect of CYP3A4*1 polymorphism on the nifedipine pharmacokinetics in healthy volunteers. They conclude that there is no significant association between CYP3A4*1G polymorphism and pharmacokinetics of nifedipine.

The association between statins and CYP3A4 polymorphism has been investigated. Gao and colleagues[90] reveal that CYP3A4*1G increases the lipid-lowering efficacy of atorvastatin and may have no significant effect on simvastatin treatment. It has a gene-dose-dependent effect on atorvastatin with a reduction in serum TC ($P < .01$). However, the investigation shows that CYP3A4*1G might not be a significant contributor to the variability in pharmacokinetic and pharmacodynamic response to clopidogrel therapy.[91]

DISCUSSION

In addition to highlighting the role of CYP enzymes in this current article, as well as other genetic polymorphisms involved in drug–gene responses in our previous literature, we provide insight into how pharmacogenomic testing can be used in improving opioid dosing and efficacy in postoperative pain control. The genetic variability present on an individual-to-individual basis in drug metabolization can present an extremely challenging task when prescribing opioid medications for proper pain control. This article, in addition to our preceding literature, highlights the genetic interplay and how physicians can use genetic testing to their advantage. Future articles may aim to investigate genetic polymorphisms in the mu-opioid receptor (OPRM1) and kappa-opioid receptor (OPRK1), uridine glucuronosyltransferase (UGT), or catecholamine-O-methyltransferase (COMT) genes. For more integration and widespread adoption of pharmacogenomic testing in clinical practice, further clinical studies are required to develop clear dosing and treatment algorithms to facilitate the use of information obtained from pharmacogenomic testing. However, the continuous development of US Food and Drug Administration (FDA)-approved genetic pain modulation panels is required to gather and analyze more evidence-based information with regard to pharmacogenomic testing (7).

Additional cost–benefit analysis studies and process methods for the legalization of pharmacogenomic testing are needed for the appropriate incorporation of knowledge surrounding pharmacogenomic testing into standard total joint arthroplasty practice. Meanwhile, orthopedic surgeons should become familiar with the genetic aspect of opioid use and abuse, as well as how these interplay into how patients respond differently postoperatively on an individual basis (7). Advancements in pharmacogenomic testing as a part of clinical medicine may provide insights into more effectively optimizing postoperative pain, specifically following total joint arthroplasty; improving patient procedural satisfaction; reducing patient nonadherence; diminishing tendency toward opioids dependency and/or adverse reactions; cutting current expenditures at not only the medical but also legal and bureaucratic levels; as well as potentially targeting and contesting the opioid epidemic as a whole.

The Current and Future Health Care Policies for Pharmacogenomic Testing

Pharmacogenomics testing is expected to reduce the amount of trial and error that currently exists in prescribing and while leading to more efficient and safer drug therapies. The benefits of pharmacogenomic testing are the ability in predicting the optimal drug dosage; identify patients at risk of drug-induced toxicity or adverse side effects, and indicating whether a drug will be efficacious.[92] One in 4 primary care patients in North America is prescribed at least one medication that commonly causes adverse drug reactions due to genetic variability in drug metabolism, it is understandable that pharmacogenomics is expected to play a large role in personalized medicine.[93] Acceptance of Pharmacogenomic testing is lacking due to the global health care economy. The cost and coverage of Pharmacogenomic testing are debatable with insurance companies. Currently, the health care economy faces escalating drug budgets, aging populations, expanding population size, and limited health care resources.[93] These specific challenges have contributed to difficulties in the level of resources and acceptance of personalized medicine.

Current health care policies and coverage are determined by specific insurance providers. In many cases, the health insurance plan will cover the costs of genetic testing when it is recommended by patients' providers. There are different policies based on which Genetic test is covered. For insurers to cover specific genetic testing and personalized medicine they all follow protocols that are based on the strength of evidence for testing, availability of clinical guidelines, and health technology assessments by independent organizations.[3] Usually, the lack of evidence is the contributing factor for noncoverage.[4] While FDA plays a minor role in the insurance policy decision to cover genetic testing, the FDA inclusion of PGx (pharmacogenomic) information in drug package inserts plays an important factor.[3] Drugs without revisions to the packages inserts are usually not covered by insurers.[4]

Many countries seem to recognize the potential of personalized medicine, whether it is pharmacogenomics or molecular diagnostics. Currently, insurance coverage for disease-related genomic and PGx testing is low and variable.[4] Pharmacogenomic testing in clinical practice will help to improve patient outcomes. The implementation of genetic tests is a necessity, to improve patient safety, quality of health care, and allocation of resources for all settings. Implementation will help to create successful changes in clinical practice as well as increase the development of other pharmacogenetic tests.

The Insurance Coverage of Pharmacogenomic Testing

Insurance coverage policies are a major determinant of patient access to genomic tests. Approximately $5 billion was spent on genomic testing in 2010 and as of 2018, there are over 54,538 tests for 11,169 conditions, 16,415 genes, and 506 laboratories according to the National Institutes of Health's Genetic Testing Registry.[3] The cost of pharmacogenomic testing is an important barrier because of limited reimbursement. Insurance companies have suggested that there are many low-cost generic drugs that are available to patients before the use of a new drug that would require genotyping.[94] Pharmacogenomic testing coverage by insurance companies is dependent on medications with major guidelines for clinical implementation based on evidence. Currently, single-gene tests have limited coverage, especially if they lack clinical evidence and clinical guidelines. Medicare contractors and private payers often do not have policies for specific genomic tests.[4] Approved genetic testing by insurers includes medication with specific genotypes with a black box warning by the FDA and the disease-related test Oncotype Dx. Coverage for testing varies based on insurers, cost-effectiveness, and differences in insurers' coverage pools.[4]

How This Data Can Be Used to Develop a Predictive Model for Postop Pain Optimization?

The management of pain is challenging, drug intervention is usually the first-line therapy for resolving pain. Personalizing analgesia during the perioperative period to maximize pain relief while minimizing adverse events can help in postoperative pain optimization. Genetic factors can be major influences on how patients respond to a specific treatment. Genetic factors such as modulatory proteins that are involved in pain perceptions, analgesic metabolism, and receptor signaling.[95] Focusing on genetic evaluation can help to long-term investigate patients' compatibility with specific medication.

Future direction and industry effort to develop more accurate and precise kits

Genetic testing of drug response represents an important goal for targeted therapy.[96] Pharmacogenomic (PGx) information provides clarifying appropriate treatments. Patients receiving postoperative care with the use of pain medication, genetic testing can improve outcomes and reduce total health care costs. Optimizing the choice and dosage of specific pain medication can limit the adverse events prescribers see in their patients. The implementation of pharmacogenomic testing for pain management can help to advance and provide more clinical evidence for genetic testing. The more genetic testing is conducted in this subspecialty, the more it creates testable outcomes and modification of pain precise kits in the pharmaceutical industry.

SUMMARY

Orthopedic surgeons should become familiar with the genetic aspect of opioid use and abuse, as well as the influence of the patient genetic makeup in opioid selection and response, and polymorphic variants in pain modulation. Furthermore, special attention should be paid to DGIs and DDGIs in the orthopedic community because using pharmacogenomic approaches may lead to powerful and personalized pain management systems.

CLINICS CARE POINTS

- CYP2D6 poor metabolizers experience suboptimal pain relief, require higher doses of codeine and be at a significant risk of adverse events of other coadministered medications primarily metabolized by CYP2D6 such as beta-blockers (metoprolol), SSRIs (citalopram, escitalopram, fluoxetine, fluvoxamine, paroxetine or sertraline), and amitriptyline.

- Patients with CYP3A4 *1 G/*1G variant consumed significantly less fentanyl than those with either the 1/*1 group or the *1/*1G group ($P < .05$) to achieve a similar degree of pain control.

- Patients with the AA genotype of CYP2B6 undergoing anesthesia with propofol may have decreased clearance of the drug as compared with patients with the GG genotype.
- CYP2B6 *6 is associated with decreased clearance of ketamine as compared with CYP2B6 *1
- CYP2C9*3 requires reducing the dose of warfarin when prescribed with simvastatin to avoid the risk of bleeding.

THE AUTHORS' CONTRIBUTIONS

Author	Position, Affiliation	Contribution
Brendan Farley, BS	• Resident- Department of Orthopedic Surgery, West Virginia University, Morgantown, WV, USA 26506	Study design, data acquisition, analysis, interpretation of data, and writing the article.
Mohamed Awad, MD, MBA	• Senior Research Fellow- Michigan State University, East Lansing, MI, USA • Chief research Officer- FAJR Scientific, Resident Research Partnership, Northville, MI, USA	Data extraction, data acquisition, and participating in article writing
Paige Anderson, BS	• Research Assistant- FAJR Scientific, Resident Research Partnership, Northville, MI, USA	Data extraction, data acquisition, and participating in article writing
Ali Esseili	• Research Assistant- FAJR Scientific, Resident Research Partnership, Northville, MI, USA • College Student, University of Michigan, Dearborn, MI, USA	Data extraction and editing the article
Justin Hruska, MD	• Anesthesiology Attending- NorthStar Anesthesia, Detroit Medical Center, Detroit, MI, USA.	Critical analysis, interpretation of data, and editing the article
Mostafa Gamal. MD	• Professor of Surgery, Wayne State University, Detroit, MI, USA	Critical analysis, interpretation of data, and editing the article.
Khaled J. Saleh, MD, MSc, FRCS(C), MHCM	• Clinical Professor, Michigan State University Department of Surgery • Attending Surgeon and Section Chief J Dingell Veteran Affairs Medical Center Department of Surgery • CEO & Founder of FAJR Scientific, Resident Research Partnership, Northville, MI, USA	Study design, data acquisition, analysis, and editing the article.

DISCLOSURE

The authors have no source of funding and no conflict of interest to disclose.

REFERENCES

1. Morris BJ, Mir HR. The opioid epidemic: impact on orthopaedic surgery. J Am Acad Orthop Surg 2015; 23(5):267–71.
2. Manchikanti L, Helm S 2nd, Fellows B, et al. Opioid epidemic in the United States. Pain Physician 2012; 15(3 Suppl):Es9–38.
3. Hansen RN, Oster G, Edelsberg J, et al. Economic costs of nonmedical use of prescription opioids. Clin J Pain 2011;27(3):194–202.
4. CDC Grand Rounds: Prescription Drug Overdoses—a U.S. Epidemic. JAMA 2012;307(8):774–6.
5. Awad ME, Padela MT, Sayeed Z, et al. Pharmacogenomics Testing for Postoperative Pain Optimization Before Total Knee and Total Hip Arthroplasty. JBJS Rev 2018;6(10):e3.
6. Okafor L, Chen AF. Patient satisfaction and total hip arthroplasty: a review. Arthroplasty 2019;1(1):6.
7. Neuprez A, Delcour JP, Fatemi F, et al. Patients' Expectations Impact Their Satisfaction following Total Hip or Knee Arthroplasty. PLoS ONE 2016;11(12): e0167911.
8. Baker PN, van der Meulen JH, Lewsey J, et al. The role of pain and function in determining patient satisfaction after total knee replacement. The Journal of Bone and Joint Surgery. British volume 2007; 89-B(7):893–900.
9. Awad ME, Padela MT, Sayeed Z, et al. Pharmacogenomic Testing for Postoperative Pain Optimization Before Total Joint Arthroplasty: A Focus on Drug-Drug-Gene Interaction with Commonly Prescribed Drugs and Prior Opioid Use. JBJS Rev 2019;7(5):e2.
10. Smith HS. Opioid metabolism. Mayo Clin Proc 2009;84(7):613–24.
11. Agarwal D, Udoji MA, Trescot A. Genetic testing for opioid pain management: a primer. Pain Ther 2017;6(1):93–105.
12. Al-Omari A, Murry D. Pharmacogenetics of the Cytochrome P450 Enzyme System: Review of Current Knowledge and Clinical Significance. J Pharm Pract 2007;20:206–18.
13. Weckselblatt B, Rudd MK. Human Structural Variation: Mechanisms of Chromosome Rearrangements. Trends Genet 2015;31(10):587–99.
14. Robert F, Pelletier J. Exploring the Impact of Single-Nucleotide Polymorphisms on Translation. Front Genet 2018;9(507).
15. Ventola CL. Pharmacogenomics in clinical practice: reality and expectations. P t 2011;36(7):412–50.
16. Zanger UM, Schwab M. Cytochrome P450 enzymes in drug metabolism: Regulation of gene expression, enzyme activities, and impact of genetic variation. Pharmacol Ther 2013;138(1):103–41.
17. Database, C.D. Free U.S. Outpatient Drug Usage Statistics. 2021 [cited 2021 January 14]. Available at: https://clincalc.com/DrugStats/.
18. Whirl-Carrillo M, McDonagh EM, Hebert JM, et al. Pharmacogenomics knowledge for personalized medicine. Clin Pharmacol Ther 2012;92(4):414–7.
19. Sangar MC, Anandatheerthavarada HK, Martin MV, et al. Identification of genetic variants of human cytochrome P450 2D6 with impaired mitochondrial targeting. Mol Genet Metab 2010;99(1):90–7.
20. Andreassen TN, Eftedal I, Klepstad P, et al. Do CYP2D6 genotypes reflect oxycodone requirements for cancer patients treated for cancer pain? A cross-sectional multicentre study. Eur J Clin Pharmacol 2012;68(1):55–64.
21. VanderVaart S, Berger H, Sistonen J, et al. CYP2D6 polymorphisms and codeine analgesia in postpartum pain management: a pilot study. Ther Drug Monit 2011;33(4):425–32.
22. Susce MT, Murray-Carmichael E, de Leon J. Response to hydrocodone, codeine and oxycodone in a CYP2D6 poor metabolizer. Prog Neuropsychopharmacol Biol Psychiatry 2006;30(7):1356–8.
23. Zineh I, Beitelshees AL, Gaedigk A, et al. Pharmacokinetics and CYP2D6 genotypes do not predict metoprolol adverse events or efficacy in hypertension. Clin Pharmacol Ther 2004;76(6):536–44.
24. de Leon J, Dinsmore L, Wedlund P. Adverse drug reactions to oxycodone and hydrocodone in CYP2D6 ultrarapid metabolizers. J Clin Psychopharmacol 2003;23(4):420–1.
25. Elkalioubie A, Allorge D, Robriquet L, et al. Near-fatal tramadol cardiotoxicity in a CYP2D6 ultrarapid metabolizer. Eur J Clin Pharmacol 2011;67(8):855–8.
26. Stamer UM, Stüber F, Muders T, et al. Respiratory depression with tramadol in a patient with renal impairment and CYP2D6 gene duplication. Anesth Analg 2008;107(3):926–9.
27. Vevelstad M, Pettersen S, Tallaksen C, et al. O-demethylation of codeine to morphine inhibited by low-dose levomepromazine. Eur J Clin Pharmacol 2009;65(8):795–801.
28. Kirksey M, Chiu YL, Ma Y, et al. Trends in in-hospital major morbidity and mortality after total joint arthroplasty: United States 1998-2008. Anesth Analg 2012;115(2):321–7.
29. Pulido L, Parvizi J, Macgibeny M, et al. In hospital complications after total joint arthroplasty. J Arthroplasty 2008;23(6 Suppl 1):139–45.
30. Belmont PJ Jr, Goodman GP, Kusnezov NA, et al. Postoperative myocardial infarction and cardiac arrest following primary total knee and hip

arthroplasty: rates, risk factors, and time of occurrence. J Bone Joint Surg Am 2014;96(24):2025–31.

31. Fleischmann KE, Goldman L, Young B, et al. Association between cardiac and noncardiac complications in patients undergoing noncardiac surgery: outcomes and effects on length of stay. Am J Med 2003;115(7):515–20.

32. Edelstein AI, Kwasny MJ, Suleiman LI, et al. Can the American College of Surgeons Risk Calculator Predict 30-Day Complications After Knee and Hip Arthroplasty? J Arthroplasty 2015;30(9 Suppl):5–10.

33. Fleisher LA, Beckman JA, Brown KA, et al. ACC/AHA 2007 guidelines on perioperative cardiovascular evaluation and care for noncardiac surgery: a report of the American College of Cardiology/American Heart Association Task Force on Practice Guidelines (Writing Committee to Revise the 2002 Guidelines on Perioperative Cardiovascular Evaluation for Noncardiac Surgery): developed in collaboration with the American Society of Echocardiography, American Society of Nuclear Cardiology, Heart Rhythm Society, Society of Cardiovascular Anesthesiologists, Society for Cardiovascular Angiography and Interventions, Society for Vascular Medicine and Biology, and Society for Vascular Surgery. Circulation 2007;116(17):e418–99.

34. van Klei WA, Bryson GL, Yang H, et al. Effect of beta-blocker prescription on the incidence of postoperative myocardial infarction after hip and knee arthroplasty. Anesthesiology 2009;111(4):717–24.

35. Bijl MJ, Visser LE, van Schaik RH, et al. Genetic variation in the CYP2D6 gene is associated with a lower heart rate and blood pressure in beta-blocker users. Clin Pharmacol Ther 2009;85(1):45–50.

36. Ciszkowski C, Madadi P, Phillips MS, et al. Codeine, ultrarapid-metabolism genotype, and postoperative death. N Engl J Med 2009;361(8):827–8.

37. Batty JA, Hall AS, White HL, et al. An investigation of CYP2D6 genotype and response to metoprolol CR/XL during dose titration in patients with heart failure: a MERIT-HF substudy. Clin Pharmacol Ther 2014;95(3):321–30.

38. Hamadeh IS, Langaee TY, Dwivedi R, et al. Impact of CYP2D6 polymorphisms on clinical efficacy and tolerability of metoprolol tartrate. Clin Pharmacol Ther 2014;96(2):175–81.

39. Shord SS, Cavallari LH, Gao W, et al. The pharmacokinetics of codeine and its metabolites in Blacks with sickle cell disease. Eur J Clin Pharmacol 2009;65(7):651–8.

40. Lotsch J, Rohrbacher M, Schmidt H, et al. Can extremely low or high morphine formation from codeine be predicted prior to therapy initiation? Pain 2009;144(1–2):119–24.

41. Takekuma Y, Takenaka T, Kiyokawa M, et al. Evaluation of effects of polymorphism for metabolic enzymes on pharmacokinetics of carvedilol by population pharmacokinetic analysis. Biol Pharm Bull 2007;30(3):537–42.

42. Bijl MJ, Visser LE, Hofman A, et al. Influence of the CYP2D6*4 polymorphism on dose, switching and discontinuation of antidepressants. Br J Clin Pharmacol 2008;65(4):558–64.

43. Van Nieuwerburgh FC, Denys DA, Westenberg HG, et al. Response to serotonin reuptake inhibitors in OCD is not influenced by common CYP2D6 polymorphisms. Int J Psychiatry Clin Pract 2009;13(1):345–8.

44. Wijnen PA, Limantoro I, Drent M, et al. Depressive effect of an antidepressant: therapeutic failure of venlafaxine in a case lacking CYP2D6 activity. Ann Clin Biochem 2009;46(Pt 6):527–30.

45. Nickinson RS, Board TN, Kay PR. Post-operative anxiety and depression levels in orthopaedic surgery: a study of 56 patients undergoing hip or knee arthroplasty. J Eval Clin Pract 2009;15(2):307–10.

46. Scott JE, Mathias JL, Kneebone AC. Depression and anxiety after total joint replacement among older adults: a meta-analysis. Aging Ment Health 2016;20(12):1243–54.

47. Dharmshaktu P, Tayal V, Kalra BS. Efficacy of antidepressants as analgesics: a review. J Clin Pharmacol 2012;52(1):6–17.

48. de Vos A, van der Weide J, Loovers HM. Association between CYP2C19*17 and metabolism of amitriptyline, citalopram and clomipramine in Dutch hospitalized patients. Pharmacogenomics J 2011;11(5):359–67.

49. Smith JC, Curry SC. Prolonged toxicity after amitriptyline overdose in a patient deficient in CYP2D6 activity. J Med Toxicol 2011;7(3):220–3.

50. Mazaleuskaya LL, Theken KN, Gong L, et al. PharmGKB summary: ibuprofen pathways. Pharmacogenet Genomics 2015;25(2):96–106.

51. Parvizi J, Miller AG, Gandhi K. Multimodal pain management after total joint arthroplasty. J Bone Joint Surg Am 2011;93(11):1075–84.

52. Lin J, Zhang L, Yang H. Perioperative administration of selective cyclooxygenase-2 inhibitors for postoperative pain management in patients after total knee arthroplasty. J Arthroplasty 2013;28(2):207–13.e2.

53. Llerena A, Alvarez M, Dorado P, et al. Interethnic differences in the relevance of CYP2C9 genotype and environmental factors for diclofenac metabolism in Hispanics from Cuba and Spain. Pharmacogenomics J 2014;14(3):229–34.

54. Pilotto A, Seripa D, Franceschi M, et al. Genetic susceptibility to nonsteroidal anti-inflammatory drug-related gastroduodenal bleeding: role of cytochrome P450 2C9 polymorphisms. Gastroenterology 2007;133(2):465–71.

55. Prieto-Perez R, Ochoa D, Cabaleiro T, et al. Evaluation of the relationship between polymorphisms in CYP2C8 and CYP2C9 and the pharmacokinetics of celecoxib. J Clin Pharmacol 2013;53(12):1261–7.

56. Bae JW, Forslund-Bergengren C, Tybring G, et al. Effects of CYP2C9*1/*3 and *1/*13 on the pharmacokinetics of losartan and its active metabolite E-3174. Int J Clin Pharmacol Ther 2012;50(9):683–9.

57. Liang R, Li L, Li C, et al. Impact of CYP2C9*3, VKORC1-1639, CYP4F2rs2108622 genetic polymorphism and clinical factors on warfarin maintenance dose in Han-Chinese patients. J Thromb Thrombolysis 2012;34(1):120–5.

58. Mega JL, Walker JR, Ruff CT, et al. Genetics and the clinical response to warfarin and edoxaban: findings from the randomised, double-blind ENGAGE AF-TIMI 48 trial. Lancet 2015;385(9984):2280–7.

59. Lee JE, Ryu DH, Jeong HJ, et al. Extremely elevated international normalized ratio of warfarin in a patient with CYP2C9*1/*3 and thyrotoxicosis. J Korean Med Sci 2014;29(9):1317–9.

60. Kim HS, Lee SS, Oh M, et al. Effect of CYP2C9 and VKORC1 genotypes on early-phase and steady-state warfarin dosing in Korean patients with mechanical heart valve replacement. Pharmacogenet Genomics 2009;19(2):103–12.

61. Andersson ML, Eliasson E, Lindh JD. A clinically significant interaction between warfarin and simvastatin is unique to carriers of the CYP2C9*3 allele. Pharmacogenomics 2012;13(7):757–62.

62. Dennis BB. Impact of ABCB1 and CYP2B6 genetic polymorphisms on methadone metabolism, dose and treatment response in patients with opioid addiction: a systematic review and meta-analysis 2014;9(1).

63. Roddy E. Bupropion and other non-nicotine pharmacotherapies. Bmj 2004;328(7438):509–11.

64. Tomaz PR, Santos JR, Issa JS, et al. CYP2B6 rs2279343 polymorphism is associated with smoking cessation success in bupropion therapy. Eur J Clin Pharmacol 2015;71(9):1067–73.

65. Levran O, Peles E, Hamon S, et al. CYP2B6 SNPs are associated with methadone dose required for effective treatment of opioid addiction. Addict Biol 2013;18(4):709–16.

66. Remerand F, Le Tendre C, Baud A, et al. The early and delayed analgesic effects of ketamine after total hip arthroplasty: a prospective, randomized, controlled, double-blind study. Anesth Analg 2009;109(6):1963–71.

67. Adam F, Chauvin M, Du Manoir B, et al. Small dose ketamine improves postoperative analgesia and rehabilitation after total knee arthroplasty. Anesth Analg 2005;100(2):475–80.

68. Li Y, Jackson KA, Slon B, et al. CYP2B6*6 allele and age substantially reduce steady-state ketamine clearance in chronic pain patients: impact on adverse effects. Br J Clin Pharmacol 2015;80(2):276–84.

69. Eugene AR. CYP2B6 genotype guided dosing of propofol anesthesia in the elderly based on nonparametric population pharmacokinetic modeling and simulations. Int J Clin Pharmacol Toxicol 2017;6(1):242–9.

70. Loryan I, Lindqvist M, Johansson I, et al. Influence of sex on propofol metabolism, a pilot study: implications for propofol anesthesia. Eur J Clin Pharmacol 2012;68(4):397–406.

71. Warner DO. Perioperative abstinence from cigarettes: physiologic and clinical consequences. Anesthesiology 2006;104(2):356–67.

72. Bedard NA, DeMik DE, Dowdle SB, et al. Trends and risk factors for prolonged opioid use after unicompartmental knee arthroplasty. Bone Joint J 2018;100-b(1 Supple A):62–7.

73. Johnstone E, Benowitz N, Cargill A, et al. Determinants of the rate of nicotine metabolism and effects on smoking behavior. Clin Pharmacol Ther 2006;80(4):319–30.

74. Guengerich FP, Hosea NA, Parikh A, et al. Twenty years of biochemistry of human P450s: purification, expression, mechanism, and relevance to drugs. Drug Metab Dispos 1998;26(12):1175–8.

75. Li AP, Kaminski DL, Rasmussen A. Substrates of human hepatic cytochrome P450 3A4. Toxicology 1995;104(1–3):1–8.

76. Lown KS, Bailey DG, Fontana RJ, et al. Grapefruit juice increases felodipine oral availability in humans by decreasing intestinal CYP3A protein expression. J Clin Invest 1997;99(10):2545–53.

77. Bhatnagar V, Garcia EP, O'Connor DT, et al. CYP3A4 and CYP3A5 polymorphisms and blood pressure response to amlodipine among African-American men and women with early hypertensive renal disease. Am J Nephrol 2010;31(2):95–103.

78. Werk AN, Cascorbi I. Functional gene variants of CYP3A4. Clin Pharmacol Ther 2014;96(3):340–8.

79. Kitzmiller JP, Luzum JA, Baldassarre D, et al. CYP3A4*22 and CYP3A5*3 are associated with increased levels of plasma simvastatin concentrations in the cholesterol and pharmacogenetics study cohort. Pharmacogenet Genomics 2014;24(10):486–91.

80. Min DI, Ku YM, Perry PJ, et al. Effect of grapefruit juice on cyclosporine pharmacokinetics in renal transplant patients. Transplantation 1996;62(1):123–5.

81. Shi WL, Tang HL, Zhai SD. Effects of the CYP3A4*1B Genetic Polymorphism on the Pharmacokinetics of Tacrolimus in Adult Renal Transplant Recipients: A Meta-Analysis. PLoS One 2015;10(6):e0127995.

82. Ishikawa Y, Akiyoshi T, Imaoka A, et al. Inactivation kinetics and residual activity of CYP3A4 after treatment with erythromycin. Biopharm Drug Dispos 2017;38(7):420–5.

83. Foti RS, Rock DA, Wienkers LC, et al. Selection of alternative CYP3A4 probe substrates for clinical drug interaction studies using in vitro data and in vivo simulation. Drug Metab Dispos 2010;38(6):981–7.

84. Tateishi T, Krivoruk Y, Ueng YF, et al. Identification of human liver cytochrome P-450 3A4 as the enzyme responsible for fentanyl and sufentanil N-dealkylation. Anesth Analg 1996;82(1):167–72.

85. Yuan R, Zhang X, Deng Q, et al. Impact of CYP3A4*1G polymorphism on metabolism of fentanyl in Chinese patients undergoing lower abdominal surgery. Clinica Chim Acta 2011;412(9):755–60.

86. Kapur BM, Hutson JR, Chibber T, et al. Methadone: a review of drug-drug and pathophysiological interactions. Crit Rev Clin Lab Sci 2011;48(4):171–95.

87. Chen CH, Wang SC, Tsou HH, et al. Genetic polymorphisms in CYP3A4 are associated with withdrawal symptoms and adverse reactions in methadone maintenance patients. Pharmacogenomics 2011;12(10):1397–406.

88. Muntwyler J, Follath F. Calcium channel blockers in treatment of hypertension. Prog Cardiovasc Dis 2001;44(3):207–16.

89. Wang XF, Yan L, Cao HM, et al. Effect of CYP3A4*1G, CYP3A5*3, POR*28, and ABCB1 C3435T on the pharmacokinetics of nifedipine in healthy Chinese volunteers. Int J Clin Pharmacol Ther 2015;53(9):737–45.

90. Gao Y, Zhang LR, Fu Q. CYP3A4*1G polymorphism is associated with lipid-lowering efficacy of atorvastatin but not of simvastatin. Eur J Clin Pharmacol 2008;64(9):877–82.

91. Danielak D, Karaźniewicz-Łada M, Wiśniewska K, et al. Impact of CYP3A4*1G Allele on Clinical Pharmacokinetics and Pharmacodynamics of Clopidogrel. Eur J Drug Metab Pharmacokinet 2017;42(1): 99–107.

92. Kapoor R, Tan-Koi WC, Teo YY. Role of pharmacogenetics in public health and clinical health care: a SWOT analysis. Eur J Hum Genet 2016;24(12): 1651–7.

93. Bartlett G, Zgheib N, Manamperi A, et al. Pharmacogenomics in Primary Care: A Crucial Entry Point for Global Personalized Medicine? Curr Pharmacogenomics Person Med 2012;10(2):101–5.

94. Volkow ND, McLellan AT. Opioid abuse in chronic pain–misconceptions and mitigation strategies. N Engl J Med 2016;374(13):1253–63.

95. Cregg R, Russo G, Gubbay A, et al. Pharmacogenetics of analgesic drugs. Br J Pain 2013;7(4): 189–208.

96. Di Francia R, Berretta M, Catapano O, et al. Molecular diagnostics for pharmacogenomic testing of fluoropyrimidine based-therapy: costs, methods and applications. Clin Chem Lab Med 2011;49(7): 1105–11.

Osteonecrosis of the Knee
Not all Bone Edema is the Same

Matthew C. Pearl, MD[a,b,*], Michael A. Mont, MD[a,c], Giles R. Scuderi, MD[a,d]

KEYWORDS

• Bone marrow edema • Knee pain • Osteonecrosis • MRI

KEY POINTS

- Knee MRIs are becoming more common in workup of knee pain, and bony edema is common.
- Thorough evaluation of edema patterns combined with history and physical examination can aid in diagnosis.
- Osteonecrotic causes to consider include spontaneous, secondary, and postarthroscopic osteonecrosis.
- Traumatic causes to consider include bone bruises and subchondral fractures, as well as meniscal root tears.
- Nontraumatic causes include bone marrow edema syndrome and transient osteoporosis, as well as osteochondritis dissecans.

INTRODUCTION

In the evaluation of knee pain, often patients are seen by their general practitioners or other specialists before orthopedic referral Figs. 1–6. During a workup, MRI is often obtained, and rates of knee MRIs being performed continue to increase both in the United States and internationally.[1,2] One common finding on MRI of the knee is bony edema represented by high signal intensity on fluid-sensitive sequences (ie, T2, short tau inversion) and a relatively low signal intensity on T1 sequences.

Although MRI is a powerful diagnostic tool, these findings can present diagnostic challenges to those attempting to diagnose the underlying cause of knee complaints. Although the differential diagnosis of bony edema is broad, attention to history, physical examination, and MRI findings can aid in determining causes of knee complaints.

The aim of this article was to review the literature to aid in the workup and potential treatment of these bony lesions with a particular focus on radiologic appearances.

OSTEONECROSIS SYNDROMES

One important group of diseases that can lead to knee pain and bony edema is osteonecrosis. The knee is the second most common location to be affected by osteonecrosis, at about 10% of the incidence in the hip.[3] Osteonecrosis of the knee can be divided into 3 distinct entities: spontaneous osteonecrosis of the knee (SPONK), secondary osteonecrosis of the knee (SONK), and postarthroscopic osteonecrosis of the knee (PAONK). Although there are differences in these processes, similarities also exist, particularly in later stages as collapse occurs resulting in the loss of articular contour and joint degeneration. This delineation of precollapse and postcollapse disease is critical because it is used to guide treatment.

[a] Department of Orthopaedic Surgery, Lenox Hill Hospital, New York, NY, USA; [b] Northwell Orthopedic Institute, 130 East 77th Street, 11th Floor, Black Hall, New York, NY 10075, USA; [c] Rubin Institute for Advanced Orthopedics, Sinai Hospital of Baltimore, 2401 W. Belvedere Avenue, Baltimore, MD, USA; [d] Northwell Orthopedic Institute, 210 East 64th Street, New York, NY 10065, USA
* Corresponding author. Northwell Orthopedic Institute, 130 East 77th Street, 11th Floor, Black Hall, New York, NY 10075.
E-mail address: matthewcpearl@gmail.com

Orthop Clin N Am 53 (2022) 377–392
https://doi.org/10.1016/j.ocl.2022.06.002
0030-5898/22/© 2022 Elsevier Inc. All rights reserved.

Spontaneous Osteonecrosis of the Knee

The first description of osteonecrosis of the knee was that of SPONK by Ahlback and colleagues,[4] in 1968, before the advent of MRI. Their diagnosis and description were based on history and physical examination, radiographs, Strontium-85 scintimetry, and biopsy. They observed radiolucent lesions in 39 patients aged older than 60 years, without any trauma, which were consistent with osteonecrosis. Because no underlying cause was determined at the time, it was deemed to be spontaneous. Although still recognized as a distinct entity, technologic advances and further study have suggested that SPONK may be a misnomer as an underlying cause is likely. Both vascular and traumatic theories of origin have been proposed.[5] Pathogenesis secondary to subchondral insufficiency fracture (SIF) was first described by Yamamoto and colleagues,[6] in 2000, and has been supported by publications since.[5,7–9] Further correlation with decreased bone mineral density[10] as well as meniscal pathologic condition, particularly meniscal root tears,[8,11,12] is supportive of this traumatic theory of altered biomechanics being the likely mechanism of pathogenesis. Others have described this as a prearthritic condition of unknown origin. Mears and colleagues described radiographic and pathologic characteristics in 21 patients (22 knees), with SPONK. They found that 14 of 22 specimens (64%) showed significant osteopenia and 15 of 22 specimens (68%) showed evidence of osteoarthritis, with no evidence of true osteonecrosis and only one potentially consistent with a fracture.[13]

Ahlback's initial description of the patient population remains consistent with contemporary understanding. Patients are predominantly women (3:1) aged older than 65 years,[10] with unilateral disease. One evaluation of 176 knees by MRI reported a prevalence of 3.4% and 9.4% in those aged older than 50 and 65 years, respectively.[14] Typically, there is no reported trauma but pain may have a sudden onset. The most common complaint is that of unilateral medial sided knee pain as the medial femoral condyle is typically affected.[8,9,13,15] Pain tends to be worse with weight-bearing as well as at night, resulting in varying levels of functional impairment. Patients may have a history of osteoporosis, corticosteroid use, metabolic or endocrine abnormalities, resulting in decreased bone mineral density. On examination, point tenderness to the medial femoral condyle may be present.[9]

Radiographs of SPONK lesions are typically normal early and may remain normal throughout the disease process.[16] If progression is noted, flattening of the condyle is the first sign. This is followed by the presence of a radiolucent lesion surrounded by an area of sclerosis. This may

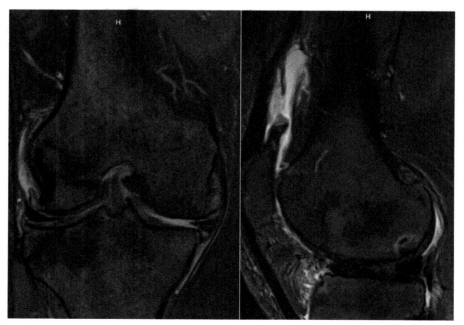

Fig. 1. Coronal proton density and sagittal short tau inversion MRI showing multifocal SONK and associated degenerative changes.

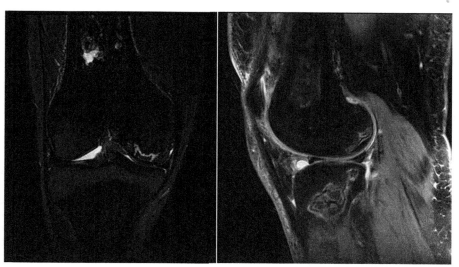

Fig. 2. Coronal and sagittal fluid-sensitive imaging of secondary osteonecrosis with "double-line" sign at margin of necrotic lesions.

progress to collapse of the subchondral bone. Ultimately, degenerative changes of the tibio-femoral joint may be observed. Lesions are typically wedge-shaped and located in the epiphysis. It is important to note that although there are areas of radiolucency and sclerosis, the serpentine pattern classically attributed to secondary osteonecrosis is never seen in radio-graphs of SPONK.[16]

MRI has allowed for better understanding of SPONK. The typical appearance is an ill-defined region of bone marrow edema in the subchondral, epiphyseal bone of the central weight-bearing portion of the medial femoral condyle. On T1 imaging, hypointensity is seen replacing the normal signal of yellow marrow. On fluid-sensitive sequences, the area can have a variable appearance but are most commonly hyperintense representing fluid. Due to the ischemic nature, if contrast is used, decreased uptake will be noted. As mentioned previously, SPONK and SIF are often observed concomi-tantly and may represent a spectrum of the same process. As a result, deformation or frac-ture line in the subchondral bone is often observed. In later disease, collapse of the sub-chondral bone may be seen followed by degen-erative changes in the articular cartilage.[16–19] The large, poorly defined area of edema can be seen in other causes as well, such as bone bruising and transient bone marrow edema syn-drome (BMES) but may be differentiated based on history and specific location as well as the possible presence of the subchondral fracture line. Additionally, because these causes are not

ischemic in nature, an MRI obtained with intrave-nous contrast should show evidence of hypervascularity.[19]

The natural progression of SPONK is variable ranging from a self-limited course to degenera-tive changes.[9,10,16] Size of the subchondral lesion and staging of lesion, as well as the pres-ence or absence of associate meniscal patho-logic condition, have been shown to be prognostic to progression.[9,11] Extent of the edema has been suggested to be of little or no prognostic value.[17]

Multiple staging systems have been proposed based on radiographs starting with Koshino in 1979. The most widely used is Aglietti's system, whose adaptation of the Koshino classification was described in 1983[20] with 5 stages represent-ing radiographic progression of the disease pro-cess as outlined in Table 1. In addition to this staging system, Aglietti and colleagues also described 2 additional methods of describing le-sions based on radiographs. The first is calcu-lating total lesion area by measuring maximum diameter in anteroposterior and transverse di-mensions. They found lesions greater than 5 cm^2 had a worse prognosis. The second method was looking at anteroposterior projec-tions and calculating the percentage of condylar width occupied by the lesion. They found that le-sions exceeding 40% of the affected condylar width had a worse prognosis. Lotke and col-leagues[21] similarly found poorer prognosis with lesions more than 50% of condylar width.

For small lesions (<3.5 cm^2), diagnosed early, nonoperative measures are often appropriate and have shown excellent results in multiple studies. Modalities include protected weight-bearing, analgesics, and nonsteroidal anti-inflammatory medications (NSAIDs).[22] Lateral wedge insoles have been suggested as an adjunct.[23] Bisphosphonates have been suggested to prevent collapse in some studies,[24] whereas other studies have found no improvement over NSAIDs, calcium carbonate, and vitamin D.[25]

Patients who have large (>5 cm²), or advanced lesions, or progressive symptoms despite nonoperative management should be considered for surgical intervention, and multiple surgical options have been proposed.

In precollapse, joint preserving procedures have shown good results in preventing or delaying collapse and degeneration. One such procedure is core decompression (CD), which is theorized to decrease local tissue pressures and promote vascular flow and healing. It has been shown to increase Knee Society Scores[26] and has a low failure rate with some studies suggesting the addition of autogenous and osteochondral grafts may further decrease the need for additional surgery.[27,28] Cartilage transfer procedures including osteochondral autologous transplant (OAT),[29] and osteochondral allograft (OCA)[30] have also been shown to postpone further surgical intervention.

Due to the unicompartmental nature of SPONK, high tibial osteotomies have been used historically and may still be appropriate in select patients. However, they have shown inferior results to arthroplasty as early as 1983.[20]

If the disease is advanced at the time of presentation or fails joint preservation, arthroplasty may be indicated. If the pathologic condition is contained within a single compartment, unicompartmental knee arthroplasty (UKA) can be considered with studies showing good functional results[31] and similar survivorship to total knee arthroplasty (TKA).[32] However, if there is multicompartmental degenerative changes TKA should be performed.

Secondary Osteonecrosis of the Knee

Secondary osteonecrosis occurs in the hip in 90% of cases but may occur about the knee 10% of the time.[3,9,10] Due to this discrepancy, descriptions and data from the hip are often extrapolated to SONK. Secondary osteonecrosis is an ischemic entity influenced by both local and systemic factors. Patients tend to be younger than those afflicted by SPONK, typically in their 20s to 50s. The femur is still most commonly affected but specific anatomic location is less predictable than in SPONK. Multiple lesions, bilateral involvement, as well as distant involvement is the rule, in contrast to SPONK. Risk factors include alcohol, tobacco, corticosteroid use, obesity, coagulopathies such as sickle cell disease, systemic lupus erythematosus, Caisson disease, Gaucher disease, and myeloproliferative disorders with corticosteroid and/or alcohol abuse accounting for approximately 90% of cases. In the pediatric population, it can be seen in the setting of leukemia.

Because of the multifocal nature, complaints can vary and include deep-seated bony, vague pain especially in early stages. A careful history is paramount to identify any associated risk factors or history of distant osteonecrosis and should be correlated with examination and appropriate imaging. Physical examination can note point tenderness on direct palpation of the affected bony areas. Additionally, the evaluation of distant sites may also be appropriate based on careful screening of additional clinical complaints.

Plain radiographs may be normal in preliminary stages and are thus not sensitive for the detection of early disease.[33] As the disease progresses, hallmark serpiginous lines of sclerosis can be seen surrounding more radiolucent geographic areas representing areas of necrosis and a local healing response in the diaphysis, metaphysis, and epiphysis. Later in the disease process, collapse of these lesions can be seen ultimately leading to degeneration changes of the tibio-femoral articulation.[17] The most common staging system for SONK is the Ficat and Arlet classification, as modified for the knee[3,9,10] seen in Table 2.

Use of MRI has greatly improved the detection of SONK with sensitivities and specificities reported to be greater than 97%.[33] In early, uncomplicated secondary osteonecrosis, normal bone marrow signal will be maintained. Edema appears early surrounding the lesion but spares the infarcted segment. A serpentine rim can be observed that is hypointense on T1. A "double-line" sign may also be seen on fluid-sensitive sequences representing an inner area of granulation tissue abutting sclerotic new bone formation, which is pathognomonic for secondary osteonecrosis.[7,17,19] Collapse begins at the coronal border of lesions and propagates along the subchondral region. It is critical to scrutinize this area between the lesion and the articular surface because edema in this location is suggestive of impending articular collapse.[17] Evidence of collapse includes the loss of subchondral contour or synovial fluid in continuity with fluid deep to the articular cartilage. Late in the disease process, there is loss of T1 intensity because the lesion begins to fragment.

Due to high rates of progression, as high at 80% by 2 years,[10] as well as poor patient satisfaction with nonoperative measures,[9] this management should be restricted to asymptomatic patients. Due to its relative rarity, many pharmacologic therapies that have shown efficacy in the hip have not been adequately studied in the knee to properly evaluate their efficacy[10] but may be considered. This leaves surgical intervention as the mainstay of treatment. In precollapse stages, joint preservation has been successful. CD has been shown to have high success rates of 79%[3] to 92%.[34] Other joint preserving surgeries include bone grafting. Although not been studied as extensively as in the hip, small studies suggest that it may delay the need for arthroplasty.[35,36] OCA has also been studied and contemporary studies support it as a joint salvage option.[30]

Despite early diagnosis and treatment, many patients will eventually require arthroplasty. Given the diffuse, often bicondylar nature of SONK, UKA is typically not recommended.[9,10] Outcomes of TKA performed for the treatment of SONK have historically been less optimal than when performed for osteoarthritis. However, modern implant designs, cementation techniques, and appropriate utilization of stems and augments now provide more reliable outcomes.[3,9,10,37,38]

Postarthroscopic Osteonecrosis of the Knee

The third, and least common, type of osteonecrosis seen about the knee is PAONK. First described by Brahme and colleagues[39] in 1991, PAONK is osteonecrosis that occurs following arthroscopic surgery. Santori and colleagues,[40] evaluated more than 2,000 arthroscopies and found only 2 cases of subsequent osteonecrosis. Prues-Latour and colleagues[41] also examined rates of osteonecrosis after arthroscopy during 50 years, finding a slightly higher rate of 1.5% (9 out of 585). This typically occurs in older patients[9,41,42] with a mean age of 58 years.[43] Although PAONK was classically described following Yttrium aluminium garnet (YAG) laser-associated surgeries, meniscectomy and chondroplasty,[39,44–46] it has also been observed following anterior cruciate ligament (ACL) reconstruction.[46]

The most common anatomic location is the medial femoral condyle[10,43,44,46] followed by the lateral femoral condyle,[10,43,46] the tibial plateau,[43–45] and rarely the patella.[46,47] Pape

and colleagues, in their systematic review, reported occurrence rates of 82% in the medial femoral condyle, 8.5% in the lateral femoral condyle, 2.1% in the lateral tibial plateau, and 2.1% in the medial tibial plateau. They also found that osteonecrosis always occurred in the same compartment as the preoperative pathologic condition and site of the procedure.[43]

The pathophysiology of PAONK remains ambiguous but shares many characteristics with SPONK including clinical symptoms, location, and imaging findings, suggesting that they may be similar processes.[43] The histology shares similarities as well. One investigation, by MacDessi and colleagues, of TKAs performed within 2 years of arthroscopy, found 8 cases in which osteonecrosis was not present on prearthroscopic imaging but was present on postarthroscopic imaging. Histology of the bone resected at the time of arthroplasty was consistent with SIF and SPONK.[10,44] Potential modes of pathogenesis exist from surgery-induced or pathologic condition-induced alterations in biomechanics, fluid or tourniquet pressure at the time of surgery, direct trauma from passing instruments, and thermal injury from radiofrequency ablation without any compelling evidence for any particular hypothesis.

Although the name suggests a rigid definition of the disease, diagnosis can be challenging. Suspicion should be high for any patient with prolonged recovery following arthroscopy,[42,43,46] particularly with the onset of symptoms 6 to 8 weeks following surgery. More common complications such as infection, arthrofibrosis, and so forth should be ruled out before investigation of osteonecrosis.[46] Physical examination is similar to that of spontaneous osteonecrosis in that tenderness to palpation may or may not be present and when present, the medial femoral condyle is the most common location.

Similar to other types of osteonecrosis, radiographs are unlikely to demonstrate specific changes early in the disease. Later, they may show evidence of collapse and eventually degenerative changes.

MRI is the diagnostic modality of choice and timing is just as important as the findings. As described earlier, PAONK knee shares MRI findings with SPONK. Fluid-sensitive images show a subchondral area of low intensity surrounded by an area of high intensity representing edema. There may be lines of low signal intensity deeper within the affected condyle and loss of articular contour.[42,43] However, these findings are only consistent with the diagnosis of postarthroscopic osteonecrosis in the correct clinical and temporal setting. First, these findings must have been absent from preoperative studies. Their appearance preoperatively would lead to a diagnosis of SPONK and one must delineate them from other forms of bony edema when present. Additionally, to be consistent with a diagnosis of PAONK, these findings must be present on postoperative imaging. This presents an additional diagnostic challenge because it takes time for MRI findings to develop. The most common timing window is 4 to 6 weeks postprocedure.[42,43] This is based largely on data from a canine femoral head model[48] as well as Kubo and colleagues[49] who performed preoperative and serial postoperative hip MRIs following renal transplant.

Management of PAONK is similar to that of other forms of osteonecrosis and is largely based on lesion size, progression, and collapse. A similar nonoperative approach should be considered at first with protected weight-bearing and analgesia. Bisphosphonates have been explored as a treatment option with some encouraging results[50] but more research is needed regarding specific pharmacologic treatments. Similar joint preserving surgeries can be considered in small, precollapse lesions, particularly in younger patients. For lesions that have already undergone collapse, arthroplasty is likely the best surgical option. One study by Bonutti and colleagues[51] of 19 patients with

PAONK who underwent 4 UKA and 15 TKA, showed excellent results.

TRAUMATIC CAUSES

The second important subset of pathologic condition to consider when evaluating a patient with bony edema is those who have undergone trauma. Understanding the mechanism as well as the diagnostic imaging can help determine the underlying diagnosis. The following section will describe the traumatic entities of bone bruises, subchondral fractures, and meniscal root tears.

Bone Bruise and Subchondral Fractures

Among the most common traumatic causes are bone bruises and subchondral fractures. These can be seen as a continuum of disease with bone bruises resulting in injury only of the trabecular portion of the bone rather than subchondral or peripheral cortical bone. Bone bruises, or occult intraosseous fractures, were first described in 1988 by Yao and Lee who observed epiphyseal bony edema in 8 patients with normal radiographs following trauma. All were managed nonoperatively. At 3 months, 6 patients reported marked improvement in symptoms.[52]

Because these lesions are the result of trauma, several classic mechanisms exist for producing them regardless of their anatomic location: direct blow, compressive force of adjacent

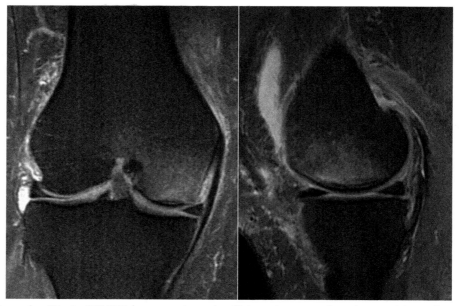

Fig. 3. Coronal and Sagittal T2 MRI demonstrating an insufficiency fracture in the right medial femoral condyle with associated edema.

bones, and traction forces resulting from ligamentous injury. With regards to the knee, several mechanisms of injury have been elucidated each resulting in a specific pattern of bony edema as described by Sanders and colleagues[53] in 2000. They classified injuries as falling into 5 categories: pivot shift injuries, dashboard injuries, hyperextension, clip injuries, and lateral patella dislocations. In addition to mechanism, bone bruise patterns also provide insight to potential-associated soft tissue injuries. A pivot shift injury classically results in an ACL injury. This occurs as the femur externally rotates relative to the tibia causing the lateral femoral condyle, typically at the sulcus terminalis, to affect the posterior lateral tibial plateau. This impact produces bony edema in these regions[53–57] in up to 80% of complete ACL ruptures.[54,55] The second mechanism is a dashboard injury. This is described as impaction to the anterior proximal tibia with the knee in flexion and is commonly associated with injury to the posterior cruciate ligament (PCL). Edema seen in this injury from the direct blow is seen in the anterior tibia and compressive force of adjacent bones in the posterior patella[53,56] because it affects the trochlea. Traction forces from the stressed PCL can produce bony edema in the central posterior tibia as well as the centro-lateral and postero-lateral femur.[56] The third mechanism is hyperextension, which can also result in PCL injury and a similar bony edema pattern. The dominant edema pattern seen in hyperextension injuries is so called "kissing lesion" because the anterior distal femur impacts the anterior proximal tibia.[53,56,58] Additional soft tissue injuries that should be investigated in these injuries are posterior capsule and ACL injuries.[58] The fourth mechanism of injury is that of a clip injury, described as a lateral impact on a knee in midflexion resulting in valgus force. Direct blow in this mechanism is seen as bony edema in the lateral femoral condyle. Additional bony edema is likely to be seen in the medial femoral condyle resulting from tensile forces from the stressed medial collateral ligament (MCL). MCL injuries should be carefully ruled out in this pattern of bony edema as lateral femoral condyle edema is seen in 45% of MCL injuries and is reported more often than edema in the medial femoral condyle.[55] The final mechanism is lateral patella dislocation. This injury is often seen in twisting injuries with the knee in flexion. As the patella dislocates, contact is between the antero-lateral femoral condyle and the medial or odd facet of the patella,[53,54,56] and focal edema is

seen in these 2 sites. Care should be taken to examine the patella for osteochondral or chondral fracture and resultant loose bodies. Additionally, the medial patello-femoral ligament is placed under stress in this injury and may cause bony edema in the medial femoral condyle[53] between the medial epicondyle and adductor tubercle.

Since their initial description, these lesions have been reported as having negative radiographs in initial evaluation. In the case of subchondral fractures, subchondral areas of sclerosis may be noted late in the process as the fracture goes on to have a healing response. Bone bruising on MRI is demonstrated as geographic, nonlinear areas of low intensity on T1 and high intensity on fluid-sensitive sequences[53–55,57,59] due to the replacement of normal marrow with inflammatory fluid. There is a hypervascular response to these bony injuries resulting in increased contract enhancement.[54] As described by Vellet and colleagues,[59] patterns of T1 abnormalities consistent with fracture include reticular, geographic, linear, impaction, and osteochondral. Additionally, the presence of hemarthrosis in the absence of intra-articular ligament injury should raise suspicion for intra-articular fracture because they are identified in up to 72% of patients with posttraumatic hemarthroses.[59] Duration of MRI findings resulting from these injuries is variable. The abnormalities seen on fluid-sensitive sequences typically resolve more quickly than that of T1 imaging, typically in 12 to 24 weeks. However, overall resolution time has been reported from 3 weeks to 2 years.[55]

Ligamentous injuries should be managed as deemed appropriate by the treating physician, and their management is beyond the scope of this review. Most simple bone bruises and subchondral fractures, those not associated with ligamentous injury or loose bodies, can be managed nonoperatively. Treatment typically consists of protected or nonweight-bearing, bracing or immobilization, and analgesics. Wright and colleagues[60] reported the mean time of return to preinjury level of activity level was 3.2 (0.5–12) months with 91% of patients returning by 6 months. Although short-to mid-term recovery is promising, it should be noted that these injuries may be indicative of more serious metabolic and mechanical cartilage injury and may have negative long-term sequelae.[55] Histologic sampling of cartilage overlying bone bruises and subchondral fractures has demonstrated chondrocyte degeneration and necrosis, and loss of proteoglycans.[57]

Meniscal Root Tears

The meniscus is critical for reducing the forces on the articular cartilage and subchondral bone within the tibio-femoral joint by converting compressive forces into hoop stresses. Significant injury to the meniscus results in altered biomechanics and tibio-femoral joint stresses[61–64] seen on MRI as bone marrow edema. Meniscal root injuries account for 10% to 21% of meniscal tears[65] are defined as injuries occurring within 9 to 10 millimeters of the meniscal root attachment, and result in complete delinking of the meniscus from its tibial attachment and extrusion of the meniscus from its native footprint. This has demonstrated equivalent biomechanics to complete meniscectomy as first described by Allaire and colleagues in 2008.[66]

Meniscal root tears tend to occur in 2 distinct populations. The first is in older patients, mostly aged older than 50 years. These tend to be degenerative in nature and occur more frequently in the medial compartment. Risk factors for these tears mirror those of osteoarthritis of the knee including female sex, increased body mass index, varus mechanical axis, and lower activity level. These tears are often reported after minor twisting in deep knee flexion activities. Conversely, lateral meniscus tears tend to be associated with more major trauma. They are seen in younger, more active patients and are frequently diagnosed in combination with ligamentous injuries.[63,65,67]

Mechanical symptoms such as locking, catching, and buckling are less commonly reported than in meniscal body injuries, and when they do occur, they are more frequent in activities of deep flexion but recurrent effusions can occur.[65,67] Physical examination can be particularly challenging. Joint line tenderness may or may not be present given the deep location of the meniscal root. Provocative maneuvers such as the McMurray test (in which the knee is flexed, rotated, and brought into extension) are less likely to be positive than in meniscal body tears.[65,67] Pain with deep flexion is the most commonly positive physical examination finding, reported in 14 of 21 patients (67%) in one study[68] and 41 of 45 patients (91%) in another.[69]

On plain radiographs, avulsion injuries of the meniscal root ligaments may be seen but are uncommon. In young patients, associated injuries seen with ligamentous injury may be apparent. Care should be taken to evaluate for degenerative changes because these can guide treatment. Full-length films should be considered to evaluate limb malalignment.

Similar to other meniscal injuries, MRI is the gold standard for diagnosis with sensitivity and specificity greater than 90%.[64,70] Due to the resultant overloading of compartments, subchondral bone marrow edema is found in most patients.[71] The pattern of bone marrow edema is similar to that of other overload syndromes such as bone bruising, and SPONK as an increase in signal intensity on fluid-sensitive imaging. Decreased signal intensity on T1 imaging with an ill-defined margin and subchondral fractures has also been reported.[61,63,64,70–73] Edema tends to occur more commonly within a central position in the compartment than in other meniscal tears.[61] Additional patterns of bone marrow edema that may be seen are insertional edema of the posterior medial meniscus root ligament attachment site and submeniscal cysts.[64,70,71] For diagnosis of the meniscal lesion itself, the T2-weighted sequence typically provides the best assessment. Classically, 4 MRI findings are described indicating a meniscal root tear: 1) a radial tear in the root on axial imaging, 2) a vertical linear defect in the root on coronal imaging (truncation sign), 3) sudden absence of normal low signal root on sagittal imaging (ghost sign), and 4) meniscal extrusion beyond the tibial plateau on coronal imaging.[63,65,67,70]

Management of meniscal root tears depends on 3 major factors: age and activity level of the patient and the degree of degenerative changes in the knee. Nonoperative management should be reserved for elderly, low-demand patients with advanced degenerative changes to the articular cartilage,[65] with a goal of symptomatic control. Analgesics, cortisone injections, activity modification, and unloader braces can be considered. Krych and colleagues, looked at

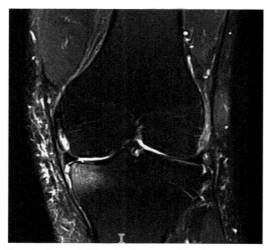

Fig. 4. Coronal T2 MRI demonstrating bony edema and meniscal extrusion secondary to meniscal root tear.

nonoperative management of these injuries and found an 87% failure rate of conservative management. At midterm follow-up, no patient had normal or near normal International Knee Documentation Committee scores, and average Kellgren-Lawrence grade increased from 1.5 to 2.4 on plain radiographs, with 31% of patients undergoing TKA.[71] As a result of poor outcomes with nonoperative management, surgery is typically recommended. In older patients or those with degenerative changes, partial meniscectomy is typically performed. In younger, more active patients, where restoration of meniscal integrity is desired, both trans-tibial and suture anchor meniscal repair techniques have been described. Unlike meniscal body injuries, the meniscal root is relatively vascular and has greater healing potential. If there is major limb malalignment, this should be addressed before or at the time of meniscal repair because varus alignment of greater than 5° was found to be an independent predictor of inferior outcomes in those undergoing meniscal root repair.[74]

ATRAUMATIC CAUSES

Additional causes to consider include those that are developmental, degenerative, or idiopathic in nature and include osteochondritis dissecans (OCD), and the spectrum of conditions of BMES and transient osteoporosis (TO). These occur with no history of trauma or inciting event, which can complicate the diagnostic process.

Osteochondritis Dissecans

OCD affects the articular cartilage and subchondral bone in patients in the first 3 decades of life. It involves separation and detachment of an osteochondral fragment from the surrounding articular surface. It was first described by König in 1887 in a patient who had mechanical symptoms related to a detached fragment.[75] OCD can occur in multiple joints in the body but most commonly the knee[76] at a rate of 9.5/100,000.[77] Both pediatric or juvenile and adult forms of the disease have been described, which are delineated by the presence or absence of open physes but there is debate of whether adult lesions represent unresolved pediatric OCD.[78] According to a recent, large, multicenter epidemiological study of 1004 knees in 903 patients, the majority of OCDs in the knee are the pediatric form with 75.3% occurring in patients who have open physes, 15% in patients who have closing physes, and 9.7% in patients who have fully closed physes. This same study found that men are affected

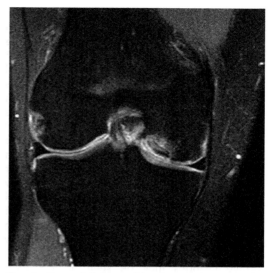

Fig. 5. Coronal fluid-sensitive image demonstrating unstable adult OCD in classic location on medial femoral condyle.

at a nearly 2 to 1 rate. Additionally, 91.4% of patients in this study self-identified as athletes with the majority playing multiple sports,[79] and although an association with increased activity level is possible,[78] it remains controversial. The precise cause remains unclear, and there is no universally accepted pathogenetic mechanism.[79] Vascular, local ossification, biomechanical, and genetic factors have all been suggested to play some role.[78] The most common location of the OCD in the knee is the medial femoral condyle representing 63.6% to 85% of lesions.[77,80] More specifically, the posterior central aspect of the medial femoral condyle is the classic anatomic description. OCD also occurs in the lateral femoral condyle, trochlea, patella, and lateral tibial plateau 18.1%, 9.5%, 6%, and 0.2% of the time, respectively, in that study of 1004 OCD lesions.[79] Bilateral lesions occur with a rate from 7.3 to 12.6%[77,79,81] and should always be considered.[78] Lesions are classified either as stable if overlying articular cartilage is intact or as unstable if there is an articular cartilage defect in which synovial fluid can track between the lesion and underlying bone. This is an important distinction as unstable lesions are typically more symptomatic and problematic.

Patients with OCD of the knee are unlikely to report an inciting injury.[78,79] In a patient who has a stable lesion, they may have mild, vague, or intermittent pain in the affected knee. Unstable lesions, as first described by König, can result in loose bodies and mechanical symptoms.[78] Recurrent, unexplained effusions are a common presenting symptom. There may or may not be tenderness to palpation due to the location of the lesions. For lesions of the medial femoral condyle, the Wilson test has been described as reproducible pain with tibial internal rotation during knee extension from 90° to 30° that is relieved with tibial external rotation.

Plain radiographs of early lesions may be normal or show contour abnormalities with an ill-defined area of radiolucency at the articular surface.[17,19,78] More advanced lesions will show sharper demarcation of a semicircle or semioval area of lucency potentially with fragmentation of the ossified fragment from the underlying bone.[19,78] If a lesion heals, this area may show evidence of ossification and sclerosis.[78] Degenerative changes may be seen as long-term sequelae. Bilateral films are recommended due to the frequency at which bilateral lesions may occur.

MRI is standard of care for care in the workup of OCD. T1 imaging is useful in determining lesion size,[78] with the lesion having lower signal intensity to the surrounding, unaffected bone. Fluid-sensitive imaging is variable but should be carefully reviewed for evidence of high-signal rim, fluid-filled cysts, or high intensity lines that are in continuity with the synovial fluid because these may represent instability.[7,17,19,78,82] These characteristics of instability were described by Kijowski and colleagues, in 2008, for both pediatric and adult lesions. They found that any high T2-signal-intensity rim or cysts surrounding an adult OCD is an unequivocal sign of instability. However, in juvenile lesions, a high T2-signal-intensity rim surrounding an OCD lesion indicates instability only if it has the same signal intensity as adjacent joint fluid, is surrounded by a second outer rim of low T2 signal intensity, or is accompanied by multiple breaks in the subchondral bone plate. Cysts only indicate instability if they are multiple in number or larger than 5 mm in size.[82] High fluid-sensitive signal intensity around the lesion can represent fluid but may also indicate a healing response in the form of granulation tissue; postcontrast sequences may be helpful in delineating the two.[17,78]

Treatment of OCD lesions depend on the patient's skeletal maturity as well as the size and stability of the lesion. In small, stable lesions in patients who have open physes, nonoperative management is often appropriate.[78,79] This consists of activity restriction, bracing, protected weight-bearing, physical therapy, and casting in decreasing frequencies[79] and has shown

variable success rate of 49% to 100%.[78] For most lesions, surgery is recommended.[79] This is supported by Sanders and colleagues[83] who demonstrated that in pediatric patients managed nonoperatively for OCD lesions followed for 35 years, there was a 30% incidence of an osteoarthritis diagnosis and an 8% incidence of undergoing arthroplasty. Surgical options are also guided by lesion characteristics. For stable lesions, transarticular or retrograde drilling is recommended with similar patient-oriented and radiographic outcomes seen in both methods.[84] In unstable, but reducible lesions, fragment fixation with or without bone marrow stimulation or grafting is recommended with various fixation constructs available including various designs of metal screws and bioabsorbable implants with no significant difference seen in fixation methods.[85] If the lesion is unstable and irreducible or fragmented, then the recommended treatment is excision. For lesions smaller than 1.5 cm^2 debridement and microfracture can be considered. Due to the relatively poor biomechanical properties of fibrocartilage, excised OCD lesions larger than 1.5 cm^2 should undergo additional cartilage procedures. Autologous chondrocyte implantation (ACI), matrix-associated ACI, OAT, and OCA have been studied and have shown success in improving function and reducing need for arthroplasty.[78,86,87]

Bone Marrow Edema Syndrome and Transient Osteoporosis

Another set of conditions that one may encounter presenting as knee pain and bone

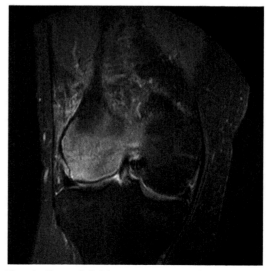

Fig. 6. Coronal fluid-sensitive image demonstrating transient BMES.

Table 1
Description of Aglietti staging system of spontaneous osteonecrosis of the knee as described in 1983

Stage	Description
I	Normal radiographs
II	Some flattening in weight-bearing portion of femoral condyle
III	Radiolucent subchondral lesion surrounded by sclerosis without sequestration
IV	Subchondral collapse with additional sclerosis and sequestration
V	Degenerative changes such as subchondral sclerosis and osteophytes on both tibia and femur

marrow about the knee is BMES and TO (or transient osteopenia). These conditions are the result of acute, spontaneous demineralization and are delineated only by the absence or presence of osteopenia on radiographic examination or bone mineral density testing which is seen in TO but not in BMES.[7,16,19] Similar to other causes previously discussed, these occur elsewhere in the body, most commonly in the proximal femur and have mostly been described in case reports and case series. Curtiss and Kincaid were first to describe transient demineralization of the hip during pregnancy in 1959.[88] It has since been described to occur in other joints including the knee, ankle, and within the foot.[89] Migratory forms have been reported and bilateral disease has reported as occurring up to 20% of the time.[90] As supported by its initial description, transient BMES can occur in pregnancy, typically in the

Table 2
Description of the modified Ficat and Arlet staging system of secondary osteonecrosis of the knee

Stage	Description
I	Normal radiographic appearance
II	Cystic or sclerotic lesion but normal bony contour
III	Crescent sign or subchondral collapse
IV	Narrowing of joint space with secondary degenerative changes

third trimester or immediately postpartum but is more commonly seen in healthy, middle-aged men[5,89,90] with two-thirds of cases occurring in the fourth to seventh decades of life.[91] In a case series of 10 patients with transient BMES of the knee, the medial femoral condyle was affected in 8 patients, whereas the lateral femoral condyle was affected in 4 patients.[91] The pathogenesis is unclear but neurogenic and vascular mechanisms have been proposed.[89] Some suggest the synovium may play a role as joint effusions are common and synovial biopsies in the disease commonly show mild inflammation.[89,90] Biopsy of the affected bone shows irregularly woven bone with osteoid seams and lining cells.[89]

Patients with transient BMES of the knee complain of acute, spontaneous onset of knee pain, which may be localized to the affected condyle(s) and is exacerbated by weight-bearing.[89–91] Physical examination may show an antalgic gait and reluctance to squat. There may be pain to palpation of the joint line and affected condyle(s) and effusions are common. Typically, passive range of motion is preserved with pain only at extremes. Provocative maneuvers for the meniscus may be positive, which can make diagnosis more difficult.[89,91]

Radiographs are, by definition, normal in BMES but show local decreased bone mineralization in TO typically within 3 to 6 weeks after the onset of symptoms. The subchondral and cortical bone is spared.[16,89,91] In TO, normal mineralization may not normalize for up to 2 years.[89]

Bone marrow edema is a hallmark of these disease processes. The pattern is ill-defined and diffuse extending beyond weight-bearing surfaces. Fluid-sensitive sequences will frequently show an associated joint effusion. In comparison to osteonecrotic causes, there is marked enhancement on postcontrast imaging owing to the preserved vascularity.[16,89,90]

Symptoms are self-limiting and typically resolve within 3 to 12 months. Therefore, management is typically symptomatic with analgesics, NSAIDs, and protected weight-bearing. Nonweight-bearing is not recommended because disuse osteopenia may worsen demineralization. Use of bisphosphonates has been proposed, and there are limited studies suggesting that they provide improvement or shorten the disease cycle.[16,89,90,92]

DISCUSSION

With the increasing utilization of MRI, orthopedic surgeons will likely be seeing many more patients present with a diagnosis of some form of bone marrow edema about the knee. This nonexhaustive list should provide some framework for the evaluation of these patients and their MRIs to aid in the diagnosis and management.

For osteonecrotic causes, a careful history including surgical history can help delineate PAONK from other causes. This is particularly important with SPONK because they have similar physical examination and radiographic findings of wedge-shaped epiphysial edema and may be associated with subchondral fractures. For SPONK, a high level of clinical suspicion should exist in patients aged older than 60 years presenting with atraumatic medial knee pain. For SONK, a history of coagulopathy, steroid or alcohol use may be elicited. These lesions are often multifocal, and may affect other parts of the skeletal system, particularly the femoral head. The classic appearance is that of serpiginous lines on MRI. In early stages or low-demand patients, nonoperative management may be appropriate. For all osteonecrotic causes, it is critical to evaluate for collapse because this will determine the efficacy for joint salvage versus arthroplasty.

Traumatic causes such as bone bruises, subchondral fractures, and meniscal root tears will most often present with a history of trauma, although in older patients, meniscal root tears may be degenerative in nature. The pattern of bone bruises may suggest associated injuries and thorough evaluation of imaging as well as a detailed physical examination are of utmost importance. Often bone bruises and small subchondral fractures can be treated with restricted weight-bearing with or without a period of immobilization. Given the meniscal root's role in meniscal function, these injuries are often best managed surgically. It is important to consider the patient's age, functional level, and degenerative changes in the knee to determine if nonoperative treatment, meniscectomy, meniscal repair, or arthroplasty is most appropriate.

Nontraumatic causes of OCD and BMES or TO may also be encountered in clinical practice. OCD is most common in pediatric or juvenile patients, particularly young men. On imaging, the lesion will be discrete from the remainder of the epiphysis. The evaluation for articular integrity is critical because it determines the stability of the lesion. The treatment of stable lesions is more controversial, and nonoperative management can be considered. However, unstable lesions are typically best managed with surgery and a variety of procedures and techniques have been shown to be efficacious. Conversely BMES and TO are largely self-limiting and can be treated with protected weight-bearing and symptomatic management, although bisphosphonates have been suggested as pharmacotherapeutic agents.

CLINICS CARE POINTS

- Rates of knee MRIs are increasing, and bone marrow edema is a common finding. Coupled with history and physical examination, patterns of bone marrow edema aid in diagnosis.

- Spontaneous osteonecrosis occurs in mostly elderly patients without trauma, appears as edema within the medial femoral condylar epiphysis and may be related to SIFs.

- Although less common than in the hip, SONK has similar associated risk factors and radiographic serpiginous appearance with additional local and distant lesions being common.

- Although rare, postarthroscopic osteonecrosis can occur after arthroscopy and has many clinical and radiographic similarities with spontaneous osteonecrosis.

- In precollapse osteonecrosis, joint preservation can be considered, whereas in postcollapse osteonecrosis, arthroplasty is the operative treatment of choice.

- Bone bruises and subchondral fractures are traumatic injuries to the trabecular and subchondral bone and the majority can be managed nonoperatively.

- Meniscal root tears demonstrate edema related to compartmental overload because of loss of mechanical properties of the meniscus, and the majority should be addressed with surgery.

- OCD occurs mostly in young men. Stable pediatric lesions can be managed nonoperatively but surgery should be considered for all unstable lesions. Stability is determined based on the articular integrity surrounding the lesion.

- BMES and TO appear on MRI as diffuse edema extending through the epiphysis and metaphysis, and the majority are self-limiting with nonoperative management being appropriate.

ACKNOWLEDGMENTS

Thank you to Daniel M. Walz, MD, Chief, Division of Musculoskeletal Imaging, Associate Professor of Radiology, Hofstra–Northwell School of Medicine for assisting in image acquisition.

DISCLOSURE

M.C. Pearl: None. M.A. Mont: Royalty and Consultant: Stryker. Consultant: Stryker, 3M, Centrexion, CERAS Health, Johnson & Johnson, Kolon Tissuegene, Mirror-AR, NXSCI, Pacira, Peerwell, Pfizer-Lily, Skye Biologics, SOLVED Health, Smith & Nephew. Stock or Stock options: CERAS Health, MirrorAR, Peerwell, USMI. Leadership/Editorial: The Knee Society, The Hip Society, Journal of Arthroplasty, Journal of Knee Surgery, Surgical Technology, International Orthopedics. G.R. Scuderi: Royalty and Consultant: Zimmer Biomet. Consultant: 3M, ROM Tech, EMN. Stock or Stock options: ROM Tech, EMN, Force Therapeutics. Royalties: Springer, Elsevier, Theime Editorial Board: Journal Knee Surgery.

REFERENCES

1. Smith L, Barratt A, Buchbinder R, et al. Trends in knee magnetic resonance imaging, arthroscopies and joint replacements in older Australians: still too much low-value care? ANZ J Surg 2020;90(5): 833–9.
2. Solomon D, Katz J, Carrino J, et al. Trends in knee magnetic resonance imaging. Med Care 2003; 41(5):687–92.
3. Mont MA, Baumgarten KM, Rifai A, et al. Atraumatic osteonecrosis of the knee. J Bone Joint Surg Am 2000;82(9):1279–90.
4. Ahlbäck S, Bauer GCH, Bohne WH. Spontaneous osteonecrosis of the knee. Arthritis Rheum 1968; 11(6):705–33.
5. Ochi J, Nozaki T, Nimura A, et al. Subchondral insufficiency fracture of the knee: review of current concepts and radiological differential diagnoses. JPN J Radiol 2022;40(5):443–57.
6. Yamamoto T, Bullough PG. Spontaneous osteonecrosis of the knee: the result of subchondral insufficiency fracture. J Bone Jt Surg Am 2000;82:858–66.
7. Rajmane KC, Schweitzer ME. MR imaging of bone marrow about the knee. Semin Musculoskelet Radiol 2009;13(4):371–83.
8. Pareek A, Parkes CW, Bernard C, et al. Spontaneous osteonecrosis/subchondral insufficiency fractures of the knee: high rates of conversion to surgical treatment and arthroplasty. J Bone Joint Surg Am 2020;102(9):821–9.
9. Karim AR, Cherian JJ, Jauregui JJ, et al. Osteonecrosis of the knee: review. Ann Transl Med 2015;3(1):6.
10. Mont MA, Marker DR, Zywiel MG, et al. Osteonecrosis of the knee and related conditions. J Am Acad Orthop Surg 2011;19(8):482–94.
11. Oda S, Fujita A, Moriuchi H, et al. Medial meniscal extrusion and spontaneous osteonecrosis of the knee. J Orthop Sci 2019;24(5):867–72.
12. Hussain ZB, Chahla J, Mandelbaum BR, et al. The role of meniscal tears in spontaneous osteonecrosis of the knee: a systematic review of suspected etiology and a call to revisit nomenclature. Am J Sports Med 2019;47(2):501–7.
13. Mears SC, McCarthy EF, Jones LC, et al. Characterization and pathological characteristics of spontaneous osteonecrosis of the knee. Iowa Orthop J 2009;29:38–42.
14. Pape D, Seil R, Fritsch E, et al. Prevalence of spontaneous osteonecrosis of the medial femoral condyle in elderly patients. Knee Surg Sports Traumatol Arthrosc 2002;10(4):233–40.
15. al-Rowaih A, Bjorkengren A, Egund N, et al. Size of osteonecrosis of the knee. Clin Orthop Relat Res 1993;(287):68–75.
16. Fotiadou A, Karantanas A. Acute nontraumatic adult knee pain: the role of MR imaging. Radiol Med 2009;114(3):437–47.
17. Gorbachova T, Melenevsky Y, Cohen M, et al. Osteochondral lesions of the knee: differentiating the most common entities at mri. Radiographics 2018;38(5):1478–95.
18. Ramnath RR, Kattapuram SV. MR appearance of SONK-like subchondral abnormalities in the adult knee: SONK redefined. Skeletal Radiol 2004; 33(10):575–81.
19. Roemer FW, Frobell R, Hunter DJ, et al. MRI-detected subchondral bone marrow signal alterations of the knee joint: terminology, imaging appearance, relevance and radiological differential diagnosis. Osteoarthr Cartil 2009;17(9):1115–31.
20. Aglietti P, Insall JN, Buzzi R, et al. Idiopathic osteonecrosis of the knee. Aetiology, prognosis and treatment. J Bone Joint Surg Br 1983;65(5):588–97.
21. Lotke PA, Abend JA, Ecker ML. The treatment of osteonecrosis of the medial femoral condyle. Clin Orthop Relat Res 1982;171:109–16.
22. Yates PJ, Calder JD, Stranks GJ, et al. Early MRI diagnosis and non-surgical management of spontaneous osteonecrosis of the knee. Knee 2007; 14(2):112–6.
23. Uchio Y, Ochi M, Adachi N, et al. Effectiveness of an insole with a lateral wedge for idiopathic osteonecrosis of the knee. J Bone Joint Surg Br 2000; 82(5):724–7.
24. Jureus J, Lindstrand A, Geijer M, et al. Treatment of spontaneous osteonecrosis of the knee (SPONK) by a bisphosphonate. Acta Orthop 2012;83:511–4.
25. Meier C, Kraenzlin C, Friederich NF, et al. Effect of ibandronate on spontaneous osteonecrosis of the

knee: a randomized, double-blind, placebo-controlled trial. Osteoporos Int 2014;25:359–66.

26. Forst J, Forst R, Heller KD, et al. Spontaneous osteonecrosis of the femoral condyle: causal treatment by early core decompression. Arch Orthop Trauma Surg 1998;117(1–2):18–22.

27. Lieberman JR, Varthi AG, Polkowski GG. Osteonecrosis of the knee - which joint preservation procedures work? J Arthroplasty 2014;29(1):52–6.

28. Deie M, Ochi M, Adachi N, et al. Artificial bone grafting [calcium hydroxyapatite ceramic with an interconnected porous structure (Ip-cha)] and core decompression for spontaneous osteonecrosis of the femoral condyle in the knee. Knee Surg Sports Traumatol Arthrosc 2008;16(8):753–8.

29. Duany NG, Zywiel MG, McGrath MS, et al. Joint-preserving surgical treatment of spontaneous osteonecrosis of the knee. Arch Orthop Trauma Surg 2010;130(1):11–6.

30. Tírico LEP, Early SA, McCauley JC, et al. Fresh osteochondral allograft transplantation for spontaneous osteonecrosis of the knee: a case series. Orthop J Sports Med 2017;5(10). 2325967117730540.

31. Fukuoka S, Fukunaga K, Taniura K, et al. Medium-term clinical results of unicompartmental knee arthroplasty for the treatment for spontaneous osteonecrosis of the knee with four to 15 years of follow-up. Knee 2019;26(5):1111–6.

32. Bruni D, Iacono F, Raspugli G, et al. Is unicompartmental arthroplasty an acceptable option for spontaneous osteonecrosis of the knee? Clin Orthop Relat Res 2012;470(5):1442–51.

33. Yong KL, El-Haddad C, Pillay S. Progression of knee osteonecrosis on MRI. Radiol Case Rep 2021;16(3):678–83.

34. Marulanda G, Seyler TM, Sheikh NH, et al. Percutaneous drilling for the treatment of secondary osteonecrosis of the knee. J Bone Joint Surg Br 2006;88(6):740–6.

35. Rijnen WH, Luttjeboer JS, Schreurs BW, et al. Bone impaction grafting for corticosteroid-associated osteonecrosis of the knee. J Bone Joint Surg Am 2006;88(suppl 3):62–8.

36. Lee K, Goodman SB. Cell therapy for secondary osteonecrosis of the femoral condyles using the Cellect DBM System: a preliminary report. J Arthroplasty 2009;24(1):43–8.

37. Mont MA, Rifai A, Baumgarten KM, et al. Total knee arthroplasty for osteonecrosis. J Bone Joint Surg Am 2002;84-A:599–603.

38. Myers TG, Cui Q, Kuskowski M, et al. Outcomes of total and unicompartmental knee arthroplasty for secondary and spontaneous osteonecrosis of the knee. J Bone Joint Surg 2006;88(suppl_3):76–82.

39. Brahme SK, Fox JM, Ferkel RD, et al. Osteonecrosis of the knee after arthroscopic surgery: diagnosis with MR imaging. Radiology 1991;178(03):851–3.

40. Santori N, Condello V, Adriani E, et al. Osteonecrosis after arthroscopic medial meniscectomy. Arthroscopy 1995;11:220–4.

41. Prues-Latour V, Bonvin JC, Fritschy D. Nine cases of osteonecrosis in elderly patients following arthroscopic meniscectomy. Knee Surg Sports Traumatol Arthrosc 1998;6:142–7.

42. Zhuang Z, Chhantyal K, Shi Y, et al. Post-arthroscopic osteonecrosis of the knee: a case report and literature review. Exp Ther Med 2020;20(4):3009–16.

43. Pape D, Seil R, Anagnostakos K, et al. Postarthroscopic osteonecrosis of the knee. Arthroscopy 2007;23(4):428–38.

44. MacDessi SJ, Brophy RH, Bullough PG, et al. Subchondral fracture following arthroscopic knee surgery: a series of eight cases. The J Bone Joint Surgery-American Volume 2008;90(5):1007–12.

45. Marx A, Beier A, Taheri P, et al. Post-arthroscopic osteonecrosis of the medial tibial plateau: a case series. J Med Case Rep 2016;10(1):291.

46. Lansdown DA, Shaw J, Allen CR, et al. Osteonecrosis of the knee after anterior cruciate ligament reconstruction: a report of 5 cases. Orthopaedic J Sports Med 2015;3(3). 232596711557612.

47. Carstensen SE, Domson GF. Patellar osteonecrosis following knee arthroscopy. Orthopedics 2019;42(6):e552–4.

48. Nakamura T, Matsumoto T, Nishino M, et al. Early magnetic resonance imaging and histologic findings in a model of femoral head necrosis. Clin Orthop Relat Res 1997;(334):68–72.

49. Kubo T, Yamazoe S, Sugano N, et al. Initial MRI findings of non-traumatic osteonecrosis of the femoral head in renal allograft recipients. Magn Reson Imaging 1997;15(9):1017–23.

50. Kraenzlin ME, Graf C, Meier C, et al. Possible beneficial effect of bisphosphonates in osteonecrosis of the knee. Knee Surg Sports Traumatol Arthrosc 2010;18(12):1638–44.

51. Bonutti PM, Seyler TM, Delanois RE, et al. Osteonecrosis of the knee after laser or radiofrequency-assisted arthroscopy: Treatment minimallt invasive knee arthroplasty. J Bone Joint Surg Am 2006;88(Suppl3):S69–75.

52. Yao L, Lee JK. Occult intraosseous fracture: detection with MR imaging. Radiology 1988;167:749–51.

53. Sanders TG, Medynski MA, Feller JF, et al. Bone contusion patterns of the knee at MR imaging: footprint of the mechanism of injury. Radiographics 2000;20:S135–51.

54. Deangelis JP, Spindler KP. Traumatic bone bruises in the athlete's knee. Sports Health 2010;2(5):398–402.

55. Mandalia V, Henson JHL. Traumatic bone bruising– a review article. Eur J Radiol 2008;67(1):54–61.

56. Berger N, Andreisek G, Karer AT, et al. Association between traumatic bone marrow abnormalities of the knee, the trauma mechanism and associated soft-tissue knee injuries. Eur Radiol 2017;27(1): 393–403.

57. Mandalia V, Fogg AJB, Chari R, et al. Bone bruising of the knee. Clin Radiol 2005;60(6):627–36.

58. Ali AM, Pillai JK, Gulati V, et al. Hyperextension injuries of the knee: do patterns of bone bruising predict soft tissue injury? Skeletal Radiol 2018;47(2): 173–9.

59. Vellet AD, Marks PH, Fowler PJ, et al. Occult post-traumatic osteochondral lesions of the knee: prevalence, classification, and short-term sequelae evaluated with MR imaging. Radiology 1991; 178(1):271–6.

60. Wright RW, Phaneuf MA, Limbird TJ, et al. Clinical outcome of isolated subcortical trabecular fractures (Bone bruise) detected on magnetic resonance imaging in knees. Am J Sports Med 2000;28(5):663–7.

61. Krych AJ, Wu IT, Desai VS, et al. Osteomeniscal impact edema (Omie): description of a distinct mri finding in displaced flap tears of the medial meniscus, with comparison to posterior root tears. J Knee Surg 2020;33(7):659–65.

62. Koenig JH, Ranawat AS, Umans HR, et al. Meniscal root tears: diagnosis and treatment. Arthroscopy 2009;25(9):1025–32.

63. Kennedy MI, Strauss M, LaPrade RF. Injury of the meniscus root. Clin Sports Med 2020;39(1):57–68.

64. Choi JY, Chang EY, Cunha GM, et al. Posterior medial meniscus root ligament lesions: mri classification and associated findings. Am J Roentgenol 2014;203(6):1286–92.

65. Pache S, Aman ZS, Kennedy M, et al. Meniscal root tears: current concepts review. Arch Bone Jt Surg 2018;6(4):250–9.

66. Allaire R, Muriuki M, Gilbertson L, et al. Biomechanical consequences of a tear of the posterior root of the medial meniscus. Similar to total meniscectomy. J Bone Joint Surg Am 2008;90(9):1922–31.

67. Zhou ML, Haley CC. Meniscal ramp lesions and root tears: a review of the current literature. Sports Med Arthrosc Rev 2021;29(3):158–67.

68. Lee JH, Lim YJ, Kim KB, et al. Arthroscopic pullout suture repair of posterior root tear of the medial meniscus: radiographic and clinical results with a 2-year follow-up. Arthroscopy 2009;25(9):951–8.

69. Kim JH, Chung JH, Lee DH, et al. Arthroscopic suture anchor repair versus pullout suture repair in posterior root tear of the medial meniscus: a prospective comparison study. Arthroscopy 2011; 27(12):1644–53.

70. Palisch AR, Winters RR, Willis MH, et al. Posterior root meniscal tears: preoperative, intraoperative, and postoperative imaging for transtibial pullout repair. Radiographics 2016;36(6):1792–806.

71. Krych AJ, Reardon PJ, Johnson NR, et al. Non-operative management of medial meniscus posterior horn root tears is associated with worsening arthritis and poor clinical outcome at 5-year follow-up. Knee Surg Sports Traumatol Arthrosc 2017;25(2):383–9.

72. Krych AJ, Johnson NR, Mohan R, et al. Arthritis progression on serial mris following diagnosis of medial meniscal posterior horn root tear. J Knee Surg 2018;31(7):698–704.

73. Yao L, Stanczak J, Boutin RD. Presumptive subarticular stress reactions of the knee: MRI detection and association with meniscal tear patterns. Skeletal Radiol 2004;33(5):260–4.

74. Moon HK, Koh YG, Kim YC, et al. Prognostic factors of arthroscopic pull-out repair for a posterior root tear of the medial meniscus. Am J Sports Med 2012;40(5):1138–43.

75. König F. The classic: on loose bodies in the joint. Clin Orthopaedics Relat Res 2013;471(4):1107–15.

76. Heyworth BE, Kocher MS. Osteochondritis dissecans of the knee. JBJS Rev 2015;3(7):1–12.

77. Kessler JI, Nikizad H, Shea KG, et al. The demographics and epidemiology of osteochondritis dissecans of the knee in children and adolescents. Am J Sports Med 2014;42(2):320–6.

78. Chau MM, Klimstra MA, Wise KL, et al. Osteochondritis dissecans: current understanding of epidemiology, etiology, management, and outcomes. J Bone Joint Surg Am 2021;103(12): 1132–51.

79. Nissen CW, Albright JC, Anderson CN, et al. Descriptive epidemiology from the research in osteochondritis dissecans of the knee (ROCK) prospective cohort. Am J Sports Med 2022;50(1): 118–27.

80. Aichroth P. Osteochondritis dissecans of the knee. A clinical survey. J Bone Joint Surg Br 1971;53(3): 440–7.

81. Hefti F, Beguiristain J, Krauspe R, et al. Osteochondritis dissecans: a multicenter study of the European Pediatric Orthopedic Society. J Pediatr Orthop B 1999;8(4):231–45.

82. Kijowski R, Blankenbaker DG, Shinki K, et al. Juvenile versus adult osteochondritis dissecans of the knee: appropriate MR imaging criteria for instability. Radiology 2008;248(2):571–8.

83. Sanders TL, Pareek A, Johnson NR, et al. Nonoperative management of osteochondritis dissecans of the knee: progression to osteoarthritis and arthroplasty at mean 13-year follow-up. Orthopaedic J Sports Med 2017;5(7). 232596711770464.

84. Gunton MJ, Carey JL, Shaw CR, et al. Drilling juvenile osteochondritis dissecans: retro- or trans-articular? Clin Orthop Relat Res 2013;471(4): 1144–51.

85. Kocher MS, Czarnecki JJ, Andersen JS, et al. Internal fixation of juvenile osteochondritis dissecans lesions of the knee. Am J Sports Med 2007;35(5): 712–8.

86. Gudas R, Simonaitytė R, Čekanauskas E, et al. A prospective, randomized clinical study of osteochondral autologous transplantation versus microfracture for the treatment of osteochondritis dissecans in the knee joint in children. J Pediatr Orthop 2009;29(7):741–8.

87. Lyon R, Nissen C, Liu XC, et al. Can fresh osteochondral allografts restore function in juveniles with osteochondritis dissecans of the knee? Clin Orthopaedics Relat Res 2013;471(4):1166–73.

88. Curtiss PH, Kincaid WE. Transitory demineralization of the hip in pregnancy. A report of three cases. J Bone Joint Surg Am 1959;41-A:1327–33.

89. Korompilias AV, Karantanas AH, Lykissas MG, et al. Transient Osteoporos J Am Acad Orthopaedic Surgeons 2008;16(8):480–9.

90. Berman N, Brent H, Chang G, et al. Transient osteoporosis: Not just the hip to worry about. Bone Rep 2016;5:308–11.

91. Vardi G, Turner PJ. Transient osteoporosis of the knee. Knee 2004;11(3):219–23.

92. Varenna M, Zucchi F, Binelli L, et al. Intravenous pamidronate in the treatment of transient osteoporosis of the hip. Bone 2002;31(1):96–101.

Tendinopathies and Allied Disorders of the Hip

Gerard A. Sheridan, MD, FRCSI*, Michael E. Neufeld, MD, FRCSC, Rotem Moshkovitz, Donald S. Garbuz, MD, FRCSC, Bassam A. Masri, MD, FRCSC

KEYWORDS

- Greater trochanteric pain syndrome • Piriformis syndrome • Iliopsoas tendinopathy
- Rectus femoris tendinopathy

KEY POINTS

- Greater trochanteric pain syndrome is common both prior to and after total hip replacement surgery.
- Endoscopic abdutor tendon repair has a lower complication rate when compared to open repair.
- Iliopsoas tendon infiltration is effective in almost half of patients with iliopsoas tendonitis.

INTRODUCTION

There are many soft tissue structures around the hip joint that may serve as a source of pain in both the native and prosthetic hip. In this review, the role of the gluteal, piriformis, iliopsoas, and rectus femoris musculotendinous units in the etiology of pathology around the hip joint will be discussed. Management options ranging from tailored physical therapy regimens to local steroid infiltration along with more invasive open and arthroscopic surgical techniques will be reviewed for each pathological entity. While not all conditions are well understood, advancements have been made in the management of each of these often challenging cases in both the native and prosthetic hip settings. This review explores these advancing treatment methods which will supplement the practice of any hip surgeon who is presented with problematic tendinopathy around both the native and prosthetic hip joint.

GREATER TROCHANTERIC PAIN SYNDROME

Introduction

Greater trochanteric pain syndrome (GTPS) is a common but rarely debilitating clinical condition characterized by localized lateral hip pain that may radiate to the knee, often exacerbated by walking, stairs, or lying directly on the affected hip.[1,2] Although previously thought to be caused by "trochanteric bursitis," tendinopathy of the gluteus medius or minimus is now recognized as the primary cause of GTPS.[1,2] The anatomy of the major hip abductors are very well known. The gluteus medius and minimus originate from different portions of the ilium, are innervated by the superior gluteal nerve, and insert onto the posterolateral and anterior aspects of the greater trochanter, respectively.[3] Gluteus medius tears are usually caused by a degenerative process but can also be caused by acute trauma. The degenerative progression in gluteal tendinopathy is common and tendinopathy can progress to partial-thickness tears, or even more advanced full-thickness tears with varying levels of retraction and atrophic changes in the muscle substance.[4]

Etiology, Diagnosis, and Clinical Characteristics

The reported prevalence of GTPS and symptomatic gluteal tendon tears in the general population ranges between 10 and 25% and most commonly occurs in women patients between the age of 40–60.[1,2,5] Up to two-thirds of people with GTPS have coexisting lower back pain or hip joint osteoarthritis and these patients are often excluded from trials evaluating treatment

---

Department of Orthopaedics, University of British Columbia, Vancouver, BC, Canada
* Corresponding author.
E-mail address: sheridga@tcd.ie

Orthop Clin N Am 53 (2022) 393–401
https://doi.org/10.1016/j.ocl.2022.06.003

options for GT and gluteal tendon pathology.[5–7] Although the exact cause remains unknown, female sex, advancing age, and anatomic factors are known risk factors for symptomatic gluteal tendinopathy.[1,2,5,7]

There are no defined clinical or imaging criteria for GTPS. However, patients often complain about lateral hip pain made worse with activity or lying directly on the hip. Patients with gluteus medius tears will often complain about a painful limp and illicit a Trendelenburg gait secondary to hip abductor weakness on examination.[1,7] A variety of clinical tests such as gait analysis, various resisted abduction maneuvers, and palpation has been described for the diagnosis of gluteal tendinopathy but have limited validity in terms of diagnostic value.[7,8] In a study of 65 participants, Grimaldi and colleagues[8] demonstrated that patients with lateral pain to palpation of the greater trochanter and pain with 30 seconds of single-leg stance have a 98% probability (100% specificity, Positive Likelihood Ratio of 12.2) of having MRI confirmed gluteal tendinopathy. Patients with no pain to palpation of the greater trochanter were very unlikely to have MRI detected gluteal tendinopathy.[8]

MRI remains the gold standard for the diagnosis of GTPS and gluteal tendon tears with a reported specificity of 95% and sensitivity of 73%.[4,9] Ultrasound has been reported to have a higher sensitivity and positive predictive value when compared to MRI; however, this modality is dependent on the technical skill of the ultrasonographer.[10] Babari and colleagues[11] developed an MRI and histopathological grading system for tendinopathy (bursitis, tendinopathy, partial-thickness tear, full-thickness tear) that was used in a recent systematic review on stage-adjusted treatment recommendations for gluteal tendinopathy. Other gluteal tendinopathy classifications such as the Melbourne Hip MRI score have shown excellent intra and inter-observer reliability and may allow standardized comparisons between results in future studies.[12]

Management Options
Nonoperative management
Conservative (nonoperative) measures are first-line treatment of GTPS/gluteal tendinopathy with success rates of approximately 80-90%, however, authors are now reporting a higher proportion of patients with gluteus medius tears that are refractory to conservative management.[2,5–7] Many nonoperative interventions have been described for the treatment of GTPS/gluteal tendinopathy including systemic

analgesics, physical therapy and exercise programs, injections (corticosteroids (CSI), platelet-rich plasma (PRP), autologous tenocyte injection (ATI)), and ultrasound/shock-wave therapy (SWT). A detailed description of levels of evidence and individual studies are out of the scope of this review, but can be found in a recent systematic review with stage-adjusted treatment recommendations for gluteal tendinopathy by Ladurner and colleagues[6]

Physical Therapy
A small randomized controlled trial showed that an exercise program by a physical therapist resulted in better pain scores at 8 weeks (but no other time point) and better patient satisfaction out to 1 year when compared to a single cortisone steroid injection (CSI) with a wait and see approach.[13] The optimal exercise program or the additional benefit of physical therapy beyond that of education is not clear and requires further study.[14]

Injections
Randomized controlled trials have demonstrated that CSI provide good short-term (4–8 week) pain relief and improved functional outcomes in patients with GTPS and grade 1-3 gluteal tendinopathy.[6] However, the therapeutic benefit does not last more than 3-6 months in most studies and structural abnormalities in the gluteal tendons have a poorer treatment effect.[6] Level 1 b evidence supports that PRP injections provide better short-term pain relief versus CSI and have a longer lasting effect with good improvements in pain and function out to 2 years.[6] The addition of percutaneous needle tenotomy did not have any benefit over PRP injection alone, and evidence for needle tenotomy as a stand-alone treatment is limited.[6] In a small series of 12 patients, Bucher and colleagues[6,15] showed that ATI resulted in improved pain and functional outcomes scores at 1 and 2 years, but more data is needed on ATI.

Shock Wave Therapy
A randomized controlled trial and a small number of studies have demonstrated SWT to provide good long-term results in patients with grades 1–2 tendinopathy; however, overall patient satisfaction was not high, the benefit was questionable for those with grade 3 tendinopathy, and the optimal protocol remains unknown.[6,16]

Operative management
Operative management may be indicated after failure of a minimum of 3 months of conservative

treatment (recalcitrant cases) or in younger patients with acute partial or full-thickness tears of the gluteus medius.[2,5,7] Detail on individual study results, levels of evidence, and gluteal tendon pathology grade-based recommendations can be found in a recent systematic review by Ladurner and colleagues including 16 studies.[6]

In the absence of partial or full-thickness gluteal tendon tears, both open or arthroscopic bursectomy ± ITB release have demonstrated good results for patients with GTPS providing improved patient functional outcome scores, satisfaction, pain scores, abduction power, and gait parameters, even out to long-term follow-up.[6]

For higher grade partial or full-thickness gluteus medius tears, multiple series have demonstrated that open or endoscopic tendon repairs provide good clinical and functional outcomes, as well as patient satisfaction in the short, medium, and long-term (5 years).[6] The effect of muscle retraction and fatty infiltration of the gluteus medius on outcomes is controversial.[6] In cases of full-thickness tears with retraction, Ebert and colleagues[17] showed promising clinical outcomes at two years postsurgery using synthetic augmentation of the hip abductors.

A recent systematic review by Longstaffe and colleagues[18] revealed that both open and endoscopic tendon repairs have similar patient-reported outcomes, clinical outcomes, and retear rates (3.4% open vs. 4.1% endoscopic); however, endoscopic repair demonstrated a decreased complication rate (0.7% vs. 7.8%). The overall complication and retear rates were 5.2% and 3.8%, respectively.[18] It should be noted that despite these promising outcomes, patients are seldom symptom-free and a proportion can experience chronic pain and dysfunction.[6] This needs to be clearly discussed with patients prior to surgery to avoid disappointment.

Greater Trochanteric Pain Syndrome After a Total Hip Replacement

Up to 25% of patients report having GTPS and/or gluteal tears prior to total hip arthroplasty (THA) and approximately 4–17% report this post-THA.[2,19,20] The evaluation of patients with THA reporting GTPS must rule out component loosening, infection, adverse reaction to metal debris due to trunnion corrosion, referred pain from spinal conditions, and other conditions not related to GTPS and symptomatic gluteal tendon tears. Gluteal tendinopathy is an important source of pain post-THA to consider when these other conditions have been ruled out.[20]

In addition to the risk factors outlined above, surgical approach (direct lateral/anterolateral) and excessive leg length and offset have been associated with GTPS post-THA.[20,21] Additionally, in a propensity score-matched study Rosinksy and colleagues[22] showed that asymptomatic gluteal tendinopathies impact outcomes after total hip replacement.

The conservative and operative treatment post-THA is the same as above. There are fewer studies evaluating operative treatment of GT and gluteal tendon tears after THA and they are limited to series with small sample sizes.[20] However, these small series do show improvements in patient reported and clinical outcomes after bursectomy with or without ITB release and gluteal tendon repairs or reconstruction.[20] The complication rate is acceptable but can be catastrophic in the setting of a THA (ie, prosthetic joint infection) and patients with gluteus medius tears should be counseled that they may not be symptom-free even after surgery. Additionally, in patients with GTPS and low-grade gluteal tendinopathy, bursectomy and IT band release have been shown to have inferior outcomes when compared to patients without a THA.[19] Higher quality of evidence is needed for surgical management of GTPS and gluteal tendinopathy after THA.

PIRIFORMIS SYNDROME
Anatomy and Etiology

The term "Piriformis syndrome" (later Piriformis syndrome) was first coined by Robinson in 1947.[23] Recent attempts at categorizing this condition have resulted in a simple classification system described by Foster and colleagues where the piriformis syndrome can be divided into either a primary or secondary category.[24] Examples of primary piriformis syndrome would include intrinsic muscular conditions such as trauma, pyomyositis or myositis ossificans.[25,26] Secondary piriformis syndrome arises in the context of an external source of irritation on the muscle from the sacroiliac joint, structures around the sciatic notch or a mass effect originating from the posterior region of the hip joint.[27,28]

Shah and colleagues recently investigated the epidemiology and etiology of secondary piriformis syndrome.[28] In that study, 143 patients were diagnosed with sciatica pain of nonspinal origin. All patients underwent pelvic MRI and of these, 17% (n = 24) demonstrated objective piriformis muscle and sciatic nerve findings. Seven patients (5%) presented with tumor, 7 (5%) had chronic inflammatory changes and one patient had adhesions between the obturator internus muscle and the sciatic nerve. Three female patients (2%) had aberrant anatomy of the piriformis muscle. The remaining patients had findings in keeping with nerve atrophy or muscular hypertrophy without an identifiable cause.

Regarding sciatic nerve anatomy, it has previously been postulated that anatomical variants of the sciatic nerve may contribute to the clinical symptomatology of piriformis syndrome. A recent radiological study analyzing 783 noncontrast hip MRIs for varying indications, concluded that sciatic nerve variants were present in 19.2% of the cohort.[29] Piriformis syndrome was found to be present in 11.3% of the variant hips compared to 9.0% of normal hips. This difference was not statistically significant (p = 0.39). With buttock pain and sciatica as secondary endpoints, the authors concluded that sciatic nerve anatomical variants are not associated with piriformis syndrome, sciatica, or buttock pain–contrary to popular opinion.

Management options
Management options vary from conservative measures including physical therapy to injections including steroid and botox which have been described as effective in certain settings. Dry needling is another example of minimally invasive intervention. When nonoperative management options have failed, surgical options available include endoscopic sciatic nerve decompression with or without piriformis muscle release. Open surgical approaches have also been described for the management of this condition, but suitable surgical candidates are very rare.

Nonoperative management
First-line treatment includes physical therapy. Massage and stretching have long held an important role in the conservative management of the condition. However, more tailored patient physical strengthening and exercise regimes may be more appropriate. Abductor strengthening and movement reeducation has been shown to be effective in certain cases.[30] Other techniques including myofascial stretching have been compared to postfacilitation stretching techniques in a recent RCT reported by Shahzad and colleagues.[31] This RCT included 40 patients and found that the postfacilitation stretching technique shows more improvement in pain, muscle length, straight leg raise, and lower extremity functional scale.

Injections
Peri-sciatic injections of steroid have been shown to provide symptomatic relief in patients that have not responded well to physical therapy.[32] Surface landmarks should be used to avoid injuring the sciatic nerve when injecting in this region. Ultrasound guidance provides a useful means of accurately identifying the piriformis muscle prior to injection in an effort to avoid injury to surrounding structures.[33]

Given the likely role of spasticity in the pain process of piriformis syndrome, many authors have investigated the effect of locally injecting botulinum neurotoxin type B. Clinical efficacy as high as 90% has been demonstrated in some studies.[34] Dosages vary between studies and Fishman and colleagues found that a dose of 12,500 units of botox was safe and effective.[35] This dose was superior for pain relief at 2 weeks. The most severe side effects were dry mouth and dysphagia at 2-4 weeks after injection. Effects of the injection were seen for up to 3 months in some patients.

More novel injection treatments include substances such as platelet-rich plasma (PRP). Ozturk and colleagues compared the effect of PRP to saline injections in the management of piriformis syndrome.[36] Pain scores and disability indices were improved 1 week after surgery in the PRP group when compared to the saline group but the difference in effect had resided at 1 month after the injection. Given the expense incurred with PRP, there is insufficient evidence to support its current use in mainstream piriformis syndrome management.

Dry needling has also been shown to be effective in certain patients.[37] A recent comparative study analyzing 32 patients with piriformis syndrome demonstrated that pain intensity using the visual analog scale was significantly less in the dry needling group when compared to controls that did not undergo an intervention (p = 0.007).

Operative management
Open resection of the piriformis tendon may be supplemented by trochanteric bursectomy and sciatic nerve neurolysis depending on the specific pathology noted. Han and colleagues[38] report a series of 12 open tendon releases. Ten of the 12 cases were considered a success. Morbidity for the open release includes increased incision length (often greater than 10 cm), longer length of hospital stay, and higher intraoperative blood loss. For this reason, endoscopic treatment methods have been developed. Ilizaliturri and colleagues described a 15 patient cohort undergoing endoscopic release of the piriformis tendon with sciatic nerve exploration. The Benson outcome ratings

in that study were noted to be excellent for 11 patients, good for 3, and fair for 1.[39]

To assess whether endoscopic surgery is effective and safe, a cadaveric study analyzing the outcome of endoscopic release demonstrated that in 10 cadaveric hips, complete tendon release was reported in 9 patients.[40] The sciatic nerve was on average 5.2 cm from the tenotomy site. The inferior gluteal artery was noted to be 7.1 cm from the tenotomy site. Neither structure was injured in the study reported by Coulomb and colleagues

A recent review by Vij and colleagues[41] states that surgical management options for piriformis syndrome remain the gold standard provided nonoperative options have been exhausted without success. Both endoscopic and open approach options exist for the surgical management of this condition. It would appear that endoscopic options are preferable to open surgery due to both an improved functional outcome and lower complication rates, provided that surgeon is skilled in arthroscopic techniques.

ILIOPSOAS TENDINOPATHY
Etiology
The iliopsoas tendon may be irritated in a number of clinical settings. One of the main causes follows total hip arthroplasty and includes decreased anteversion or inadequate abduction or both of the acetabular component, leading to irritation of the tendon on the anterior rim of the acetabular component.

A more obscure cause of postoperative iliopsoas tendonitis includes femoral component head–neck corrosion at the modular interface.[42] In a series of 120 revision total hip arthroplasties, 8 were deemed to have iliopsoas sign (groin pain on resisted hip flexion) secondary to iliopsoas irritation due to femoral component corrosion at the modular interface.

Another source of possible irritation is the large head of a dual mobility articulation.[43]

Although uncommon after total hip arthroplasty, in this setting the specific cause of iliopsoas tendinopathy must be identified prior to instigating a management plan. For example, if prominent screws are penetrating the iliopsoas muscle, these may need to be exchanged for shorter screws.[44] If the acetabular component is excessively retroverted, which may lead to tendon irritation, the acetabular component may need to be revised to a more optimal version.[44] Positioning the acetabular component parallel to the transverse acetabular ligament (TAL) may reduce tendon irritation due to excess acetabular retroversion.[45] The TAL has proven to be a very useful anatomical landmark for avoiding complications associated with acetabular component malpositioning after total hip arthroplasty.

Femoroacetabular impingement may lead to iliopsoas tendonitis also.[46] Femoral neck CAM lesions may lead to overgrowth of bone in the anterior region of the hip joint. These in turn may impinge on the tendon leading to iliopsoas tendonitis.

Management
Injection
Infiltration of the iliopsoas bursa under image guidance is a good option with reasonable rates of success. Some series report success rates (defined as a clinically relevant improvement in patient pain scores) in up to 49% of patients undergoing this intervention.[47] There are a considerable number of patients who will not experience any benefit from fluoroscopically guided injection. For this cohort, surgical options are available.

Surgical intervention
A number of management options exist for this condition, namely open and arthroscopic tendon release. A recent systematic review by Longstaffe and colleagues[48] compared the results of open and arthroscopic iliopsoas tendon release for the indications of internal snapping hip, iliopsoas impingement, and iliopsoas tendinopathy after total hip arthroplasty. The results supported arthroscopic techniques as being superior to open techniques regarding the reoccurrence of snapping (5.1% vs 21.7%) and groin pain relief (89.1% vs 85.6%) with fewer complications (4.2% vs 21.1%) overall.[48]

Focusing specifically on the issue of iliopsoas tendonitis after total hip arthroplasty, O'Connell and colleagues[49] systematically reviewed 7 articles and compared outcomes for the treatment of iliopsoas tendon release both under arthroscopic (n = 88) and open (n = 27) approaches. In the arthroscopy group, 91.8% experienced successful outcomes, whereas only 77.8% experienced successful outcomes in the open tenotomy group.

The advantages of endoscopic techniques are significant. Minimal incision length, reduced operative time, and reduced intraoperative bleeding are some of the advantages of using endoscopic as opposed to open techniques. Endoscopic release has also been shown to provide good functional improvement even when acetabular overhang and anteversion are not optimal and are not corrected surgically.[50] This is helpful for the arthroplasty surgeon in the setting of suboptimal acetabular component position, with iliopsoas tendonitis, as it may be possible to control symptoms through arthroscopic release alone without the need to remove a well-fixed acetabular implant.[50] This may be preferable as implant removal always carries the potential complication of bone loss or fracture during the removal stage of the procedure.

The clinical implications that iliopsoas release has on hip flexion strength are not well described. To prevent this specific complication, alternative surgical techniques have been explored to both relieve symptoms and also retain hip flexion strength.[51] Benad and colleagues describe a novel technique involving ambulatory iliopsoas bursectomy through the Hueter approach. This is followed by the placement of a polyglactin 910 (vicryl) mesh in the anterior hip capsule which then induces thickening of the anterior hip capsule. From a modest sample of 5 patients, all experienced symptom relief with an improvement in functional scores. One patient did develop a deep infection which required surgical drainage. The introduction of nonbiological foreign material into the hip region after total hip arthroplasty will likely remain an unfavorable option for most surgeons due to the risk of inducing a prosthetic joint infection.

RECTUS FEMORIS TENDINOPATHY
Background
The rectus femoris muscle is the most common site of acute injury in athletes' quadricep muscle group.[52] Specifically, it is at risk from sporting activities that involve sprinting, jumping, or kicking, as they subject the lower limb to strong, repeated, eccentric loading.[52,53] Injuries of the rectus femoris origin can result in groin pain, functional limitation and they may also progress to a chronic tendinopathy.[54] The most common site of injury is at the distal myotendinous junction, and in soccer players specifically, at the deep myotendinous junction of the reflected head.[54] Grade I tears describe a myotendinous junction with integrity maintained, grade II tears describe partial myotendinous junction disruption and grade III tears describe complete disruption of the junction.[55]

More rarely, acute calcific tendinitis can present in the rectus femoris and presents with severe localized pain, swelling, edema, erythema, and loss of function or range of motion.[56,57] The etiology is not entirely known, but traumatic, genetic, and local metabolic factors have been thought to potentially contribute.[57]

The rectus femoris is generally an atypical location for calcific tendinitis, and so it is often misdiagnosed and mistreated when it presents in this region.[56] While acute calcific tendinitis resolves spontaneously, generally within two weeks of symptom onset, chronic cases impairing function may require intervention.[57]

Management options
Management options depend on the mechanism of injury to the tendon, so appropriate management relies on imaging to confirm an accurate diagnosis. For example, partial tears are managed effectively with physiotherapy, whereas complete tears may require surgical intervention such as a suture anchor repair for a proximal head avulsion.[52,58]

Symptomatic calcific tendonitis of the rectus femoris also has conservative and surgical treatment options. Nonsurgical treatment options include nonsteroidal antiinflammatory drugs, physical therapy, rest, injection of CSI, and injection of local anesthetics.[57,59] Surgical removal of the calcification by open or arthroscopic techniques, is indicated for unresolved pain following conservative treatment.[57]

SUMMARY

While not all tendinopathies and related conditions around the hip are well understood, significant advances have been made in the management of each of these often challenging cases in both the native and prosthetic hip settings. This review presents the best available evidence relating to these advancing treatment methods which should prove useful in supplementing the practice of any hip surgeon who is faced with problematic tendinopathy around both the native and prosthetic hip joint.

CLINICS CARE POINTS

- Although previously thought to be caused by "trochanteric bursitis," tendinopathy of the gluteus medius or minimus is now recognized as the primary cause of greater trochanteric pain syndrome (GTPS)

- For the treatment of greater trochanteric pain syndrome (GTPS), open and endoscopic tendon repairs have similar patient-reported outcomes, clinical outcomes, and retear rates; however, endoscopic repair demonstrates a decreased complication rate (0.7% vs. 7.8%)

- Up to 25% of patients report having GTPS and/or gluteal tears prior to total hip arthroplasty (THA) and approximately 4–17% report this post-THA
- Piriformis syndrome can be divided into either a primary or secondary category
- Contrary to popular opinion, sciatic nerve anatomical variants are not associated with piriformis syndrome, sciatica, or buttock pain
- Infiltration of the iliopsoas bursa under image guidance leads to success is up to 49% of patients
- In both the native and prosthetic hip, results support the use of arthroscopic techniques as being superior to open techniques in treating iliopsoas tendonitis regarding the reoccurrence of snapping and groin pain relief with fewer complications in the arthroscopic cohort overall
- In rectus femoris tendinopathy, the most common site of injury is at the distal myotendinous junction and in soccer players specifically, at the deep myotendinous junction of the reflected head.

REFERENCES

1. Fearon AM, Scarvell JM, Neeman T, et al. Greater trochanteric pain syndrome: defining the clinical syndrome. Br J Sports Med 2013; 47(10):649–53.
2. Pierce TP, Issa K, Kurowicki J, et al. Abductor tendon tears of the hip. JBJS Rev 2018;6(3):1–7.
3. Robertson WJ, Gardner MJ, Barker JU, et al. Anatomy and dimensions of the gluteus medius tendon insertion. Arthroscopy 2008;24(2):130–6.
4. Kong A, Vliet A, Zadow S. MRI and US of gluteal tendinopathy in greater trochanteric pain syndrome. Eur Radiol 2007;17(7):1772–83.
5. Reid D. The management of greater trochanteric pain syndrome: a systematic literature review. J Orthop 2016;13(1):15–28.
6. Ladurner A, Fitzpatrick J, O'Donnell JM. Treatment of gluteal tendinopathy: a systematic review and stage-adjusted treatment recommendation. Orthop J Sport Med 2021;9(7):1–12.
7. LaPorte C, Vasaris M, Gossett L, et al. Gluteus medius tears of the hip: a comprehensive approach. Phys Sportsmed 2019;47(1):15–20.
8. Grimaldi A, Mellor R, Nicolson P, et al. Utility of clinical tests to diagnose MRI-confirmed gluteal tendinopathy in patients presenting with lateral hip pain. Br J Sports Med 2017;51(6):519–24.
9. Cvitanic O, Henzie G, Skezas N, et al. MRI diagnosis of tears of the hip abductor tendons (gluteus medius and gluteus minimus). AJR Am J Roentgenol 2004;182(1):137–43.
10. Westacott DJ, Minns JI, Foguet P. The diagnostic accuracy of magnetic resonance imaging and ultrasonography in gluteal tendon tears–a systematic review. Hip Int 2011;21(6):637–45.
11. Bhabra G, Wang A, Ebert JR, et al. Lateral elbow tendinopathy: development of a pathophysiology-based treatment algorithm. Orthop J Sport Med 2016;4(11). https://doi.org/10.1177/2325967116670635.
12. Tso CKN, O'Sullivan R, Khan H, et al. Reliability of a novel scoring system for mri assessment of severity in gluteal tendinopathy: the melbourne hip MRI score. Orthop J Sport Med 2021;9(4). https://doi.org/10.1177/2325967121998389.
13. Mellor R, Bennell K, Grimaldi A, et al. Education plus exercise versus corticosteroid injection use versus a wait and see approach on global outcome and pain from gluteal tendinopathy: prospective, single blinded, randomised clinical trial. BMJ 2018;361. https://doi.org/10.1136/BMJ.K1662.
14. Ganderton C, Semciw A, Cook J, et al. Gluteal loading versus sham exercises to improve pain and dysfunction in postmenopausal women with greater trochanteric pain syndrome: a randomized controlled trial. J Womens Health (Larchmt) 2018; 27(6):815–29.
15. Bucher TA, Ebert JR, Smith A, et al. Autologous tenocyte injection for the treatment of chronic recalcitrant gluteal tendinopathy: a prospective pilot study. Orthop J Sport Med 2017;5(2). https://doi.org/10.1177/2325967116688866.
16. Carlisi E, Cecini M, Di Natali G, et al. Focused extracorporeal shock wave therapy for greater trochanteric pain syndrome with gluteal tendinopathy: a randomized controlled trial. Clin Rehabil 2019;33(4):670–80.
17. Ebert JR, Bucher TA, Mullan CJ, et al. Clinical and functional outcomes after augmented hip abductor tendon repair. Hip Int 2018;28(1):74–83.
18. Longstaffe R, Dickerson P, Thigpen CA, et al. Both open and endoscopic gluteal tendon repairs lead to functional improvement with similar failure rates: a systematic review. J ISAKOS 2021;6(1):28–34.
19. Robertson-Waters E, Berstock JR, Whitehouse MR, et al. Surgery for greater trochanteric pain syndrome after total hip replacement confers a poor outcome. Int Orthop 2018;42(1):77–85.
20. Capogna BM, Shenoy K, Youm T, et al. Tendon disorders after total hip arthroplasty: evaluation and management. J Arthroplasty 2017;32(10):3249–55.
21. Worlicek M, Messmer B, Grifka J, et al. Restoration of leg length and offset correlates with trochanteric pain syndrome in total hip arthroplasty. Sci Rep 2020;10:7107.
22. Rosinsky PJ, Bheem R, Meghpara MB, et al. Asymptomatic gluteal tendinopathies negatively impact

outcomes of total hip arthroplasty: a propensity score-matched study. J Arthroplasty 2021;36(1):242–9.

23. Robinson DR. Pyriformis syndrome in relation to sciatic pain. Am J Surg 1947;73(3):355–8.

24. Foster MR. Piriformis syndrome. Orthopedics 2002;25(8):821–5.

25. Wun-Schen C. Bipartite piriformis muscle: an unusual cause of sciatic nerve entrapment. Pain 1994;58(2):269–72.

26. Beauchesne RP, Schutzer SF. Myositis ossificans of the piriformis muscle: an unusual cause of piriformis syndrome. A case report. J Bone Joint Surg Am 1997;79(6):906–10.

27. Pace JB, Nagle D. Piriform syndrome. West J Med 1976;124(6):435–9.

28. Shah SS, Consuegra JM, Subhawong TK, et al. Epidemiology and etiology of secondary piriformis syndrome: A single-institution retrospective study. J Clin Neurosci 2019;59:209–12.

29. Bartret AL, Beaulieu CF, Lutz AM. Is it painful to be different? Sciatic nerve anatomical variants on MRI and their relationship to piriformis syndrome. Eur Radiol 2018;28(11):4681–6.

30. Tonley JC, Yun SM, Kochevar RJ, et al. Treatment of an individual with piriformis syndrome focusing on hip muscle strengthening and movement reeducation: a case report. J Orthop Sports Phys Ther 2010;40(2):103–11.

31. Shahzad M, Rafique N, Shakil-Ur-Rehman S, et al. Effects of ELDOA and post-facilitation stretching technique on pain and functional performance in patients with piriformis syndrome: A randomized controlled trial. J Back Musculoskelet Rehabil 2020;33(6):983–8.

32. Hanania M, Kitain E. Perisciatic injection of steroid for the treatment of sciatica due to piriformis syndrome. Reg Anesth Pain Med 1998;23(2):223–8.

33. Bardowski EA, Byrd JWT. Piriformis Injection: An Ultrasound-Guided Technique. Arthrosc Tech 2019;8(12):e1457–e61.

34. Lang AM. Botulinum toxin type B in piriformis syndrome. Am J Phys Med Rehabil 2004;83(3):198–202.

35. Fishman LM, Konnoth C, Rozner B. Botulinum neurotoxin type B and physical therapy in the treatment of piriformis syndrome: a dose-finding study. Am J Phys Med Rehabil 2004;83(1):42-50; quiz 1–3.

36. Öztürk GT, Erden E, Ulaşlı AM. Effects of ultrasound-guided platelet rich plasma injection in patients with piriformis syndrome. J Back Musculoskelet Rehabil 2021.

37. Fusco P, Di Carlo S, Scimia P, et al. Ultrasound-guided Dry Needling Treatment of Myofascial Trigger Points for Piriformis Syndrome Management: A Case Series. J Chiropr Med. 2018;17(3):198–200.

38. Han SK, Kim YS, Kim TH, et al. Surgical treatment of piriformis syndrome. Clin Orthop Surg 2017;9(2):136–44.

39. Ilizaliturri VM Jr, Arriaga R, Villalobos FE, et al. Endoscopic release of the piriformis tendon and sciatic nerve exploration. J Hip Preserv Surg 2018;5(3):301–6.

40. Coulomb R, Khelifi A, Bertrand M, et al. Does endoscopic piriformis tenotomy provide safe and complete tendon release? A cadaver study. Orthop Traumatol Surg Res 2018;104(8):1193–7.

41. Vij N, Kiernan H, Bisht R, et al. Surgical and non-surgical treatment options for piriformis syndrome: a literature review. Anesth Pain Med 2021;11(1):e112825.

42. Matsen Ko L, Coleman JJ, Stas V, et al. Iliopsoas irritation as presentation of head-neck corrosion after total hip arthroplasty: a case series. Orthop Clin North Am 2015;46(4):461–8.

43. Fessy MH, Riglet L, Gras LL, et al. Ilio-psoas impingement with a dual-mobility liner: an original case report and review of literature. SICOT J 2020;6:27.

44. Hessmann MH, Hübschle L, Tannast M, et al. Irritation der Iliopsoassehne nach totalendoprothetischem Hüftgelenkersatz [Irritation of the iliopsoas tendon after total hip arthroplasty]. Orthopade 2007;36(8):746–51.

45. Archbold HA, Mockford B, Molloy D, et al. The transverse acetabular ligament: an aid to orientation of the acetabular component during primary total hip replacement: a preliminary study of 1000 cases investigating postoperative stability. J Bone Joint Surg Br 2006;88(7):883–6.

46. Mardones R, Via AG, Tomic A, et al. Arthroscopic release of iliopsoas tendon in patients with femoro-acetabular impingement: clinical results at mid-term follow-up. Muscles Ligaments Tendons J 2016;6(3):378–83.

47. Agten CA, Rosskopf AB, Zingg PO, et al. Outcomes after fluoroscopy-guided iliopsoas bursa injection for suspected iliopsoas tendinopathy. Eur Radiol 2015;25(3):865–71.

48. Longstaffe R, Hendrikx S, Naudie D, et al. Iliopsoas release: a systematic review of clinical efficacy and associated complications. Clin J Sport Med 2021;31(6):522–9.

49. O'Connell RS, Constantinescu DS, Liechti DJ, et al. A systematic review of arthroscopic versus open tenotomy of iliopsoas tendonitis after total hip replacement. Arthroscopy 2018;34(4):1332–9.

50. Viamont-Guerra MR, Ramos-Pascual S, Saffarini M, et al. Endoscopic tenotomy for iliopsoas tendinopathy following total hip arthroplasty can relieve pain regardless of acetabular cup overhang or anteversion. Arthroscopy 2021;37(9):2820–9.

51. Benad K, Delay C, Putman S, et al. Technique to treat iliopsoas irritation after total hip replacement: Thickening of articular hip capsule through an abridged direct anterior approach. Orthop Traumatol Surg Res 2015;101(8):973–6.

52. Pesquer L, Poussange N, Sonnery-Cottet B, et al. Imaging of rectus femoris proximal tendinopathies. Skeletal Radiol 2016;45(7):889–97.

53. Dragoni S, Bernetti A. Rectus femoris tendinopathy. In: Bisciotti G, Volpi P, editors. The lower limb tendinopathies. Cham, Switzerland: Springer; 2016. p. 67–84.

54. Zini R, Panasci M. Post-traumatic ossifications of the rectus femoris: arthroscopic treatment and clinical outcome after 2 years. Injury 2018;49(Suppl 3): S100–4.

55. Mendiguchia J, Alentorn-Geli E, Idoate F, et al. Rectus femoris muscle injuries in football: a clinically relevant review of mechanisms of injury, risk factors and preventive strategies. Br J Sports Med 2013;47(6):359–66.

56. Kim YS, Lee HM, Kim JP. Acute calcific tendinitis of the rectus femoris associated with intraosseous involvement: a case report with serial CT and MRI findings. Eur J Orthop Surg Traumatol 2013; 23(Suppl 2):S233–9.

57. Comba F, Piuzzi NS, Zanotti G, et al. Endoscopic Surgical Removal of Calcific Tendinitis of the Rectus Femoris: Surgical Technique. Arthrosc Tech 2015; 4(4):e365–9.

58. Ueblacker P, Müller-Wohlfahrt HW, Hinterwimmer S, et al. Suture anchor repair of proximal rectus femoris avulsions in elite football players. Knee Surg Sports Traumatol Arthrosc 2015;23(9):2590–4.

59. Jethwa T, Abadin A, Pujalte G. Rare case of symptomatic calcific tendinopathy of the origin of rectus femoris tendon. BMJ Case Rep 2020; 13(12):e236809.

Acetabular Retroversion

Dysplasia in Disguise that Leads to Early Arthritis of the Hip

Mohammad S. Abdelaal, MD, Ryan M. Sutton, MD,
Steven Yacovelli, MD, Joshua D. Pezzulo, BS,
Dominic M. Farronato, BS, Javad Parvizi, MD, FRCS*

KEYWORDS

- Acetabulum retroversion • Acetabular morphology • Hip dysplasia • Hip osteoarthritis
- Total hip replacement

KEY POINTS

- One in three patients undergoing total hip replacement (THA) younger than 40 years of age had acetabular retroversion.
- Acetabular retroversion is predictive of premature osteoarthritis even in absence of acetabular dysplasia.
- The findings of this study suggest that the prevalence of acetabular retroversion in younger patients is underrecognized and should be taken into account when managing cases of hip pain that may require THA.

INTRODUCTION

Structural abnormalities of the hip are assumed to play a substantial role in the development of osteoarthritis (OA).[1,2] Acetabular retroversion (AR) is an abnormal morphologic variation that involves posterolateral orientation of the acetabulum with subsequent posterior wall deficiency and anterior over-coverage of the femoral head.[1,3] As the acetabular walls progress more caudally from the roof, the edges evolve gradually in a spiral fashion into anteversion like normal hips. However, the anterior wall of the acetabulum remains in a more lateral position than normal and the posterior wall remains more medial, leading to alteration in the orientation of the whole socket, not just its cranial aspect.[4,5] Although most of the dysplastic hips are associated with excessive acetabular anteversion, it has been reported that one in six cases of congenital acetabular dysplasia have concomitant AR.[6]

The pathologic orientation of the acetabulum in AR has been implicated as a cause of hip pain in young adults.[4,7] The posterior under coverage of the femoral head with concomitant increased anterior contact stresses of the hip can lead to an accelerated rate of articular cartilage degeneration.[2,5,8] Consequently, earlier progression to end-stage hip OA for younger patients makes treatment options more challenging, especially with the potential for higher activity levels and longer life expectancy in this population.[9]

In clinical practice, acetabular orientation is most often judged based on the projection of the acetabular walls on standardized anteroposterior (AP) pelvic radiographs.[10] Cross-over sign (COS) is the main hallmark used to establish the presence of AR,[3,11,12] with other radiographic features including posterior wall sign (PWS),[13] prominence of ischial spine sign (ISS),[14] and elephant's ear sign.[15]

Previous studies have suggested some relationship between subtle deformities of the hip such as AR or femoroacetabular impingent and subsequent development of OA of the hip.[16,17] Concomitant hip malformations were detected

Rothman Orthopaedic Institute at Thomas Jefferson University, Philadelphia, PA, USA
* Corresponding author. Rothman Orthopaedic Institute, 125 South 9th Street Suite 1000, Philadelphia, PA 19107.
E-mail address: javadparvizi@gmail.com

0030-5898/22/© 2022 Elsevier Inc. All rights reserved.

in 36.6% of women and 71.0% of men with hip OA.[18] Nevertheless, the structural abnormality that predisposes certain hips to eventual degenerative change and subsequent THA remains ambiguous. There is a current deficit in our knowledge of whether a certain radiographic parameter can suggest worse outcomes regarding the predisposition of end-stage hip disease. In addition, the prevalence of these conditions in those undergoing THA needs to be identified.

It is hypothesized that AR is an underrecognized problem that can be predictive of premature development of hip OA in younger patients that require THA. Also, with growing number of young patients requiring THA, there is a potential risk of suboptimal cup placement in those with anatomic malformation of the acetabulum. Therefore, we sought to assess the prevalence of AR in a cohort of patients undergoing THA before 40 years of age compared with older population. We also aimed to evaluate the association between AR and acetabular dysplasia in both groups.

METHODS

In accordance with institutional review board approval, preoperative AP pelvic radiographs of 645 consecutive patients who underwent THA before 40 years of age at a single institution from January 2012 to June 2020 were retrospectively examined. Of this group, 70 radiographs were excluded because of excessive pelvic tilt or asymmetry, making them unsuitable for evaluation of acetabular orientation. Furthermore, radiographs in which exposure of the film did not clearly show the outline of the acetabulum, particularly the anterior and posterior walls, the ischial spine, the acetabular sourcil, and the lateral edge of the acetabulum were also excluded (n = 64). The resulting cohort consisted of 511 radiographs in 431 patients. The control group, THA patients who were 40 years and older and operated during the same time period, was obtained from our institutional joint arthroplasty database via propensity matching based on gender and body mass index (BMI) (n = 1800). Radiographs of the matched group were similarly evaluated for excessive pelvic tilt or asymmetry, resulting in 650 radiographs (624 patients).

Radiographic Evaluation
AP radiographs of the pelvis were taken with the patient in the supine position. Our institution uses standardized protocol for AP pelvis radiographs. The tube is placed at a distance of 120 cm from the x-ray film and at a right angle to the table. The x-ray central beam is centralized on a point halfway between the upper border of symphysis pubis and the transverse line connecting both anterior superior iliac spines.

In order to ensure normal images were not misdiagnosed as AR, radiographic evaluation of proper pelvic inclination and rotation was evaluated for each patient. Extent of pelvic inclination was evaluated using the method described by Siebenrock and colleagues.[19] The distance between the pubic symphysis and the sacrococcygeal joint was measured on each standard AP radiograph for comparison with the reported control values of average 47 mm in women and 32 mm in men. Any pelvic x-ray that did not lie within the range of the control values was considered to have excessive pelvic inclination and was therefore excluded. The rotational alignment of the pelvis was evaluated through the positions of the sacral midpoint and the pubic symphysis and by the symmetric radiographic appearance of bilateral obturator foramen.

Radiographs were evaluated to identify AR using the following radiographic criteria: (1) COS,[11] which occurs when the anterior and posterior walls of the acetabulum meet caudal to the acetabular roof, so that the superior part of the anterior acetabular wall is lateral to (intersect) the superior part of posterior wall; (2) PWS,[12] which exists when the center of the femoral head is located lateral to the posterior wall of the acetabulum; (3) ISS[14] that is defined as the exaggerated projection of the triangular shaped ischial spine medially from the pelvic brim toward the pelvic inlet; (4) elephant's ear sign, which is the outward flaring of iliac wings appearing as an elephant's ears (Fig. 1).

Classically, acetabular dysplasia has been defined as upsloping of the acetabular sourcil and under-coverage of the femoral head by the weight-bearing acetabular cartilage. Radiographic evaluation of acetabular dysplasia was based on the lateral center edge angle (LCEA) of Wiberg and the Tönnis angle. The LCEA measures lateral coverage of the femoral head, with values less than 20° considered dysplastic.[20] LCEA was measured as the angle between a line from the center of the femoral head parallel to the longitudinal axis and a line from the center of the femoral head to the most lateral edge of the acetabulum. The Tonnis angle measures the inclination of the acetabular sourcil and is considered abnormal if greater than 13°.[21] The

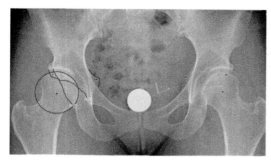

Fig. 1. An AP pelvis radiograph showing bilateral *COS (single blue star),**ISS (double blue stars), and PWS (the blue dot in the center of the femoral head is located lateral to the posterior wall). A best-fit circle was used to determine the center of the femoral head. AW: anterior wall, PW: posterior wall.

Table 1 Baseline characteristics			
Variable	**THA ≥40 y N = 650**	**THA <40 y N = 511**	**P-Value**
Age, years (SD)	62.9 (9.63)	33.1 (5.60)	<.001[a]
Gender:			<.001[a]
Women	360 (55.4%)	210 (41.1%)	
Men	290 (44.6%)	301 (58.9%)	
BMI, kg/m²(SD)	28.0 (5.32)	28.1 (5.20)	.521
Laterality			.199
Left	291 (44.8%)	249 (48.7%)	
Right	359 (55.2%)	262 (51.3%)	

[a] Significant P value.
[b] Unless otherwise indicated, the values are expressed as the mean plus the standard deviation for continuous variables and the number of patients (and the percentage of the group) for categorical variables.

center of the femoral head was estimated from a circle fit to the medial and inferior contour of the femoral head. The longitudinal axis of the body was defined perpendicular to a line connecting the inferior ischial tuberosities or inferior margins of the acetabular tear drops.

Cohorts were stratified according to the presence of dysplasia to assess the frequency of AR signs in those with versus those without dysplasia. Logistic regression analysis was performed to determine the association between having positive COS and confounding variables (dysplasia, gender, and BMI). Continuous data were presented as mean (standard deviation), and categorical data are presented as cell count (percentage). Normality was assessed via Shapiro-Wilk test. Mann–Whitney U tests were used to calculate P values for continuous data and chi-square tests were used for categorical data. A difference was considered statistically significant when the P value is < 0.05. All statistical analyses were performed using R Studio (Version 3.6.1, Vienna, Austria).

RESULTS

There were more men in the younger age group (58.9% vs 41.1%), and more women in the older age group (55.4% vs 44.6%). The mean age for the younger age group was 33.1 ± 5.60 years and for the older age group was 62.9 ± 9.63 years. No difference in BMI or laterality was found between groups (Table 1).

Regarding radiographic findings mean LCEA was smaller in the younger group (27.9○±○12.60 vs 36.0○ ± 12.10, P < .001). The average mean Tönnis angle was larger in the younger group (11.5○± 99.9) compared with the older group (7.32○ ±7.80, P < .001). When

dysplasia was identified according to the presence of either LCEA less than 20○ or Tönnis angle greater than 13○, the younger group had a higher prevalence of dysplastic cases (40.7% vs 21.4%, P < .001) (Table 2).

Prevalence of Radiographic Signs of Acetabular Retroversion

Positive COS was observed in 29.5% of the younger cohort that was significantly higher than the older cohort (16.2%, P < .001). Elephant's ear sign was detected more frequently in the younger group compared with the older group (20.1% vs 14.7%, P = .020). Similar prevalence of positive ISS (20.2% vs 16.2%, P = .091) and positive PWS (21.7% vs 21.2%, P = .913) was observed between younger and older groups, respectively. When the coexistence of the AR radiological signs was assessed, there was higher prevalence of coexisting positive COS plus either positive ISS or positive PWS in the younger cohort compared with older cohort (22.9% vs 10.9%, P < .001). Pelvic x-rays free of any signs of retroversion were noted in 62.6% of the younger cohort compared with 65.5% of the older cohort (P = .329) (see Table 2).

Groups Stratified According to Associated Acetabular Dysplasia

In the group with developmental dysplasia of the acetabulum (LCEA < 20○ and/or Tonnis angle >13○), no difference in gender, BMI, or laterality was observed between the younger

Table 2
Radiographic parameters of hips in both groups

Variable	THA ≥40 y N = 650	THA < 40 y N = 511	P-Value
LCEA, mean(SD)	36.0 (12.11)	27.9 (12.60)	<.001[a]
Tönnis angle, mean(SD)	7.32 (7.80)	11.5 (9.99)	<.001[a]
Dysplasia (LCEA<20 or Tönnis >13)	139 (21.4%)	208 (40.7%)	<.001[a]
COS	105 (16.2%)	151 (29.5%)	<.001[a]
ISS	105 (16.2%)	103 (20.2%)	.091
PWS	138 (21.2%)	103 (21.7%)	.913
Elephant's ear sign	95 (14.7%)	100 (20.1%)	.020[a]
Combined positive COS + ISS or PWS	71 (10.9%)	115 (22.9%)	<.001[a]
Negative for any signs of retroversion	426 (65.5%)	311 (62.6%)	.329

[a] Significant P value.
[b] Unless otherwise indicated, the values are expressed as the mean plus the standard deviation for continuous variables and the number of patients (and the percentage of the group) for categorical variables.

and older cohorts, respectively. The younger cohort had lower mean LCEA (18.5° ±11.0 vs 26.9°± 10.6, P < .001) and higher mean Tönnis angle (20.7° ±7.31 vs 16.7° ±8.50, P < .001) compared with the older cohort. Similar prevalence of COS, ISS, and elephant's ear sign was noted between groups. Positive PWS was higher in the older cohort (43.2% vs 26.0%, P = .002) (Fig. 2, Table 3).

In the group without evidence of acetabular dysplasia, the younger cohort was found to have smaller mean LCEA (34.4° ±8.91 vs 38.3°±11.4, P < .001) and higher average Tönnis angle (5.22° ±5.83 vs 4.41°±4.66, P < .001), although all measurements were within the normal ranges for the respective angles. Regarding the AR signs, a significantly higher prevalence of COS (31.4% vs 14.7%, P < .001), elephant's ear sign (19.8% vs 13.2%, P = .017), and coexistence of AR signs (23.3% vs 9.39%, P < .001) were seen in the younger cohort compared with the older cohort. The prevalence of positive ISS and PWS was similar between cohorts. (Fig. 3; see Table 3).

When accounting for acetabular dysplasia, BMI, and gender, there was no association with a positive COS. THA at a younger age was associated with higher prevalence of COS (odds ratio 2.15, CI: 1.61–2.88, P < .001) (Table 4).

DISCUSSION

AR represents a structural anomaly that alters the orientation of the acetabulum and has

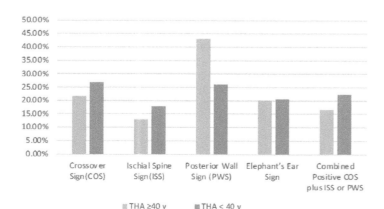

Fig. 2. Prevalence of AR signs in patients with dysplasia.

Table 3
Data stratified according to the presence of dysplasia

Variable	Dysplasia THA ≥40 y N = 139	THA < 40 y N = 208	P Value	No Dysplasia THA ≥40 y N = 511	THA < 40 y N = 303	P-Value
Age, mean(SD)	59.6 (10.00)	33.3 (5.62)	<.001[a]	63.8 (9.34)	32.9 (5.59)	<.001[a]
Gender:			1.000			<.001[a]
Women	74 (53.2%)	110 (52.9%)		286 (56.0%)	100 (33.0%)	
Men	65 (46.8%)	98 (47.1%)		225 (44.0%)	203 (67.0%)	
BMI, mean(SD)	27.6 (4.93)	28.1 (5.46)	0.376	28.1 (5.42)	28.1 (5.03)	0.965
Laterality:			0.827			0.171
Left	63 (45.3%)	98 (47.1%)		228 (44.6%)	151 (49.8%)	
Right	76 (54.7%)	110 (52.9%)		283 (55.4%)	152 (50.2%)	
LCEA, mean(SD)	26.9 (10.6)	18.5 (11.0)	<0.001[a]	38.3 (11.4)	34.4 (8.91)	<0.001[a]
Tönnis Angle, mean(SD)	16.7 (8.50)	20.7 (7.31)	<0.001[a]	4.41 (4.66)	5.22 (5.83)	<0.001[a]
COS	30 (21.6%)	56 (26.9%)	0.316	75 (14.7%)	95 (31.4%)	<0.001[a]
ISS	18 (12.9%)	37 (17.8%)	0.289	87 (17.0%)	66 (21.8%)	0.113
PWS	60 (43.2%)	46 (26.0%)	0.002[a]	78 (15.3%)	57 (19.1%)	0.186
Elephant's ear sign	28 (20.1%)	41 (20.5%)	1.000	67 (13.2%)	59 (19.8%)	0.017[a]
Combined positive COS + ISS or PWS	23 (16.5%)	45 (22.3%)	0.245	48 (9.39%)	70 (23.3%)	<0.001[a]
Negative for any signs of retroversion	70 (50.4%)	116 (59.8%)	0.110	356 (69.7%)	195 (64.4%)	0.137

[a] Significant P value.
[b] Unless otherwise indicated, the values are expressed as the mean plus the standard deviation for continuous variables and the number of patients (and the percentage of the group) for categorical variables.

been identified as a predictive factor for early cartilage degeneration and premature development of OA.[8] The diagnosis of AR has mainly been based on the evaluation of COS on plain AP pelvic radiographs. Other supportive signs include ISS, elephant's ear sign, and PWS. The results of this study demonstrated an association between AR and the early development of OA

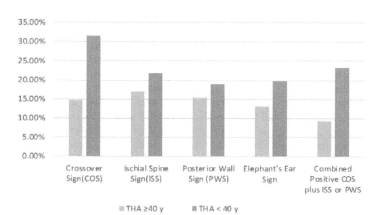

Fig. 3. Prevalence of AR signs in patients without dysplasia.

Table 4
Logistic regression using cross-over sign as the dependent outcome

Variable	Estimate	P-Value	Odds Ratio	Lower 95	Upper 95
Case (THA<40)	0.77	<.001*	2.15	1.61	2.88
Dysplasia	0.05	.737	1.05	0.77	1.43
BMI	−0.01	.469	0.99	0.96	1.02
Gender	0.03	.847	1.03	0.77	1.38

and subsequent THA. Younger patients undergoing THA have a significantly higher prevalence of AR even when controlling for gender, BMI, and acetabular dysplasia. This study is unique in identifying these specific findings in an age-dependent comparative cohort.

Previous studies have analyzed the acetabular joint reaction forces and concluded that these forces are directed posteriorly and superiorly.[22,23] The acetabular contact pressures are hence highest in the posterior aspect of the acetabulum especially when performing an action such as rising from a chair.[24] Deficiency of the posterior acetabular wall, as in AR, would therefore result in increased contact stresses during the activities of daily living, with theoretically higher unit loads imposed on the available posterior cartilage. In addition, the excessive anterior overcoverage secondary to AR can be provocative of impingement especially with mid-range of hip flexion. The repetitive abutment of the acetabular rim against the femoral head–neck junction can lead to degeneration of the labrum with fragmentation and ossification of the superior rim of the acetabulum.[25] The pathomechanics provoked by both posterior wall insufficiency and anterior overcoverage are believed to carry substantial weight in the development of premature OA of the hip.[26]

The results of this study are in agreement with the findings obtained by previous reports, which suggested an association between AR and OA of the hip.[5,25,26] Kim and colleagues[25] found a positive correlation between AR and joint space narrowing in 117 hips of patients undergoing CT virtual colonoscopy, and they suggested an early treatment of the underlying structural abnormality to prevent progressive degeneration. Ezoe and colleagues[26] described retroversion in 20% of patients with OA, 18% with developmental dysplasia, and 42% with Legg–Calve–Perthes disease compared with 6% in healthy subjects. Although these studies used pelvic radiographs to associate AR with radiological evidence of OA that may not correlate with the actual severity of symptoms, our study used THA as a

hard endpoint of the correlation between AR and end-stage hip disease.

This study demonstrated that the prevalence of AR in patients with dysplastic hips was 26.9% in patients younger than 40 years of age and 21.6% in patients older than 40 years of age. This observation falls within the spectrum of values reported in the literature with frequencies ranging from one out of three to one out of six patients with hip dysplasia having associated AR.[6,27,28] Although the details of the methodology and findings may vary between studies, the overall prevalence of AR in our dysplastic group was slightly higher than that determined by Ezoe and colleagues[26] and Li and Ganz[6] (18% and 17.2%, respectively). In contrast, Mast and colleagues[28] reported AR prevalence of up to 37% in dysplastic hips, however they used very strict criteria to exclude excessive pelvic tilt, instead of the criteria of Siebenrock and colleagues that is commonly used in the literature.[19] The complexity of acetabular dysplasia warrants careful evaluation of the spatial orientation of the acetabulum, especially when planning for periacetabular osteotomy to achieve appropriate reorientation of the socket and halt the progression to OA.[2]

In the group without dysplasia, we identified a significantly higher frequency of patients with AR in the younger cohort (31.4%) compared with the older cohort (14.7%). These values were in concordance with previous studies. Recently, Wassilew and colleagues[29] analyzed data from three-dimensional (3D) computed tomography scans of 200 asymptomatic hips with average of 26.7% ± 3.7 undertaken for conditions unrelated to disorders of the hip. They reported a 28.5% prevalence of AR with COS in 24.5% of cases and PWS in 5.5% of cases. Also, Fujii and colleagues[30] found that after adjusting for indices of acetabular dysplasia, hip symptoms (pain) started at a significantly younger age (average 27.4 years), in patients with AR compared with an average age of 40.5 years in those without AR. Further, Nehme and colleagues[27] compared the AR prevalence in non-operated hips of patients with unilateral osteotomy using similar criteria to identify dysplasia (LCEA < 20° and/or Tonnis angle >13°). In the non-operated group, they found 19% prevalence of AR in dysplastic hips and 22% prevalence of AR in hips without dysplasia, concluding that the presence of AR is independent of the presence of acetabular dysplasia. Our study confirmed that AR can be associated with premature OA even in absence of acetabular dysplasia. A possible explanation for this is that the determinants of the orientation of the acetabular socket during development are independent of those that determine other features of acetabulum dysplasia, such as coverage of the femoral head or the inclination of the roof. Although factors determining the acetabular orientation might be unclear, they seem to be related to the embryologic development of the pelvic ring. Conditions such as bladder exstrophy and pubic diastasis can lead to AR.[31] On the other hand, features of dysplasia such as degree of roof slope and the coverage of the femoral head are more related to the concentric positioning of the head into the acetabulum during development.[32]

Traditionally, a hip with LCEA of less than 20° is considered dysplastic, but recent literature suggests that the risk of developing OA extends into higher values of LCEA, ranging from 25° to 30°.[33] In this study, the younger population had significantly lower LCEA and higher Tönnis angle compared with the older population. Wyles and colleagues[2] investigated the contralateral hips of patients who underwent THA before 55 years of age. They found that LCEA less than 25° and a Tönnis angle greater than 10° were associated with the development of contralateral hip OA and the eventual need for THA. Thomas and colleagues[17] reported that for each degree reduction of the LCEA below 28°, there was 13% increase in the risk of hip OA and 18% increase in the risk of THA over a 20-year period. Only women were included in the study by Thomas and colleagues, but the mechanism by which morphologic abnormalities lead to increased contact stress and cartilage degeneration are likely to be similar in both men and women.[34]

When THA is performed in patients with AR, specific attention should be taken to the native contours of the anterior and posterior walls of the acetabulum. In hips with AR, the altered anatomic landmarks may prompt surgeons to reduce the anteversion of the acetabular component or over-medialize the cup to achieve proper coverage. This can result in overhanging of the anterior wall of the acetabulum, abnormal loading of the bearing surface, and increase wear. Consequently, inadequate cup position can lead to osteolysis, aseptic loosening, or dislocation.[35,36] Careful evaluation of a good quality preoperative radiograph, especially in young patients, allows the surgeon to prevent theses adverse outcomes.

A major limitation to this study was the number of radiographs that was excluded because of lack of standardization. Interpretation of the AP pelvic radiograph, especially for COS, is very sensitive to the position of the pelvis at the time of exposure, thus even small movements could exclude a radiograph for evaluation.[19] Most of the excluded radiographs were not well centered, laterally rotated, or were of poor quality that limited visibility of the anterior and posterior acetabular walls. Cohorts such as this have traditionally been very difficult to obtain, which was especially true for this study, with stringent eligibility criteria of the radiographs involved. Furthermore, all measurements and categorization were based off-plain pelvis radiographs. Unfortunately, this was the only imaging modality available for every patient in the study. It is well recognized that alternative radiologic modalities, such as 3D imaging or MRI, are often used to provide more complete information about morphologic features of the hip. In addition, this study did not assess the effect of femoral version in patients with AR that may have a compensatory effect on the acetabular morphology and may in part explain why some patients with AR do not develop early OA of the hip. The possibility of cam impingement or abnormalities of the head–neck junction of the femur were not analyzed because of the presence of osteophytes at the head–neck junction, which made the assessment of alpha angle difficult and unreliable, especially in older patients. Finally, it should be emphasized that this study results describe associations and do not present evidence of a true causal relationship between AR and premature OA of the hip.

SUMMARY

In conclusion, this study evaluated the prevalence of AR in subjects undergoing THA before 40 years of age. One in three patients in this population had AR compared with the historical one-in-six ratio of the OA patients stated by previous studies. AR seems to be a common, yet underrecognized, anomaly that may increase the risk of developing hip OA over time. Understanding and searching for this pathoanatomical and pathomechanical variant is important when evaluating young patients with hip pain. Furthermore, these findings have important applicability during preoperative planning for THA in younger populations to achieve adequate soft tissue tension and avoid impingement. Prospective studies with longitudinal data that can provide evidence of the causal relationship between AR and OA development are warranted.

REFERENCES

1. Tönnis D, Heinecke A. Acetabular and femoral anteversion: relationship with osteoarthritis of the hip. J Bone Joint Surg Am 1999;81(12):1747–70.
2. Wyles CC, Heidenreich MJ, Jeng J, et al. The John Charnley Award: Redefining the Natural History of Osteoarthritis in Patients With Hip Dysplasia and Impingement. Clin Orthop Relat Res 2017;475(2): 336–50.
3. Peters CL, Anderson LA, Erickson JA, et al. An algorithmic approach to surgical decision making in acetabular retroversion. Orthopedics 2011;34(1): 10.
4. Reynolds D, Lucas J, Klaue K. Retroversion of the acetabulum. A cause of hip pain. J Bone Joint Surg Br 1999;81(2):281–8.
5. Giori NJ, Trousdale RT. Acetabular retroversion is associated with osteoarthritis of the hip. Clin Orthop Relat Res 2003;417:263–9.
6. Li PLS, Ganz R. Morphologic features of congenital acetabular dysplasia: one in six is retroverted. Clin Orthop Relat Res 2003;416:245–53.
7. Vahedi H, Aalirezaie A, Schlitt PK, et al. Acetabular Retroversion Is a Risk Factor for Less Optimal Outcome After Femoroacetabular Impingement Surgery. J Arthroplasty 2019;34(7):1342–6.
8. Beck M, Kalhor M, Leunig M, et al. Hip morphology influences the pattern of damage to the acetabular cartilage: femoroacetabular impingement as a cause of early osteoarthritis of the hip. J Bone Joint Surg Br 2005;87(7):1012–8.
9. Clohisy JC, Dobson MA, Robison JF, et al. Radiographic structural abnormalities associated with premature, natural hip-joint failure. J Bone Joint Surg Am 2011;93(Suppl 2):3–9.
10. Tannast M, Siebenrock KA, Anderson SE. Femoroacetabular Impingement: Radiographic Diagnosis— What the Radiologist Should Know. Am J Roentgenol 2007;188(6):1540–52.
11. Jamali AA, Mladenov K, Meyer DC, et al. Anteroposterior pelvic radiographs to assess acetabular retroversion: high validity of the "cross-over-sign. J Orthop Res 2007;25(6):758–65.
12. Werner CML, Copeland CE, Ruckstuhl T, et al. Radiographic markers of acetabular retroversion: correlation of the cross-over sign, ischial spine sign and posterior wall sign. Acta Orthop Belg 2010;76(2):166–73.
13. Ina J, Raji Y, Strony JT, et al. The Role of Imaging in Femoroacetabular Impingement: History, Current Practices, and Future Applications. JBJS Rev 2021; 9(8):e21, 00007.
14. Kalberer F, Sierra RJ, Madan SS, et al. Ischial spine projection into the pelvis : a new sign for acetabular retroversion. Clin Orthop Relat Res 2008;466(3): 677–83.
15. Sutton R, Azboy I, Restrepo C, et al. Ptosis of the hip: a new radiographic finding in patients undergoing femoroacetabular osteoplasty. J Hip Preserv Surg 2018;5(4):425–34.
16. Murphy SB, Ganz R, Müller ME. The prognosis in untreated dysplasia of the hip. A study of radiographic factors that predict the outcome. J Bone Joint Surg Am 1995;77(7):985–9.
17. Thomas GER, Palmer AJR, Batra RN, et al. Subclinical deformities of the hip are significant predictors of radiographic osteoarthritis and joint replacement in women. A 20 year longitudinal cohort study. Osteoarthritis Cartilage 2014;22(10):1504–10.
18. Gosvig KK, Jacobsen S, Sonne-Holm S, et al. Prevalence of Malformations of the Hip Joint and Their Relationship to Sex, Groin Pain, and Risk of Osteoarthritis: A Population-Based Survey. JBJS 2010; 92(5):1162–9.
19. Siebenrock KA, Schoeniger R, Ganz R. Anterior femoro-acetabular impingement due to acetabular retroversion. Treatment with periacetabular osteotomy. J Bone Joint Surg Am 2003;85(2):278–86.
20. Wiberg G. The anatomy and roentgenographic appearance of a normal hip joint. Acta Chir Scand 1939;83(Suppl 58):7–38.
21. Clohisy JC, Carlisle JC, Beaulé PE, et al. A systematic approach to the plain radiographic evaluation of the young adult hip. J Bone Joint Surg Am 2008;90(Suppl 4):47–66.
22. Wtte H, Eckstein F, Recknagel S. A Calculation of the Forces Acting on the Human Acetabulum during Walking. CTO 1997;160(4):269–80.
23. Pedersen DR, Brand RA, Davy DT. Pelvic muscle and acetabular contact forces during gait. J Biomech 1997;30(9):959–65.
24. Hodge WA, Carlson KL, Fijan RS, et al. Contact pressures from an instrumented hip endoprosthesis. J Bone Joint Surg Am 1989;71(9):1378–86.
25. Kim WY, Hutchinson CE, Andrew JG, et al. The relationship between acetabular retroversion and osteoarthritis of the hip. J Bone Joint Surg Br 2006;88-B(6):727–9.
26. Ezoe M, Naito M, Inoue T. The prevalence of acetabular retroversion among various disorders of the hip. J Bone Joint Surg Am 2006;88(2):372–9.
27. Nehme A, Trousdale R, Tannous Z, et al. Developmental dysplasia of the hip: Is acetabular

retroversion a crucial factor? Orthopaedics Traumatol Surg Res 2009;95(7):511–9.

28. Mast JW, Brunner RL, Zebrack J. Recognizing acetabular version in the radiographic presentation of hip dysplasia. Clin Orthop Relat Res 2004;418: 48–53.

29. Wassilew GI, Heller MO, Janz V, et al. High prevalence of acetabular retroversion in asymptomatic adults. Bone Joint J 2017;99-B(12):1584–9.

30. Fujii M, Nakashima Y, Yamamoto T, et al. Acetabular retroversion in developmental dysplasia of the hip. J Bone Joint Surg Am 2010;92(4): 895–903.

31. Sponseller PD, Bisson LJ, Gearhart JP, et al. The anatomy of the pelvis in the exstrophy complex. J Bone Joint Surg Am 1995;77(2):177–89.

32. Seringe R, Bonnet JC, Katti E. Pathogeny and natural history of congenital dislocation of the hip. Orthop Traumatol Surg Res 2014;100(1):59–67.

33. Wylie JD, Peters CL, Aoki SK. Natural History of Structural Hip Abnormalities and the Potential for Hip Preservation. JAAOS 2018;26(15):515–25.

34. Pompe B, Daniel M, Sochor M, et al. Gradient of contact stress in normal and dysplastic human hips. Med Eng Phys 2003;25(5):379–85.

35. Ha YC, Yoo JJ, Lee YK, et al. Acetabular component positioning using anatomic landmarks of the acetabulum. Clin Orthop Relat Res 2012;470(12):3515–23.

36. Biedermann R, Tonin A, Krismer M, et al. Reducing the risk of dislocation after total hip arthroplasty: the effect of orientation of the acetabular component. J Bone Joint Surg Br 2005;87(6):762–9.

Physical and Mental Demand During Total Hip Arthroplasty

Kevin Abbruzzese, PhD[a], Alexandra L. Valentino, BS[a],
Laura Scholl, MS[a], Emily L. Hampp, PhD[a],
Zhongming Chen, MD[b], Ryan Smith, MD[c],
Zackary O. Byrd, MD[d], Michael A. Mont, MD[b,e,*]

KEYWORDS

- Total hip arthroplasty • Robotic-assisted • Physical demand • Mental demand

KEY POINTS

- Total hip arthroplasty (THA) is one of the most successful surgical procedures in modern day medicine.
- Robotic-assisted total hip arthroplasty (RATHA) is a technology intended to enhance acetabular component placement accuracy to plan.
- RATHA has shown improved outcomes over manual THA at both short-term and mid-term follow-up.
- THA has been shown to be physically demanding and energy consuming.
- The effect that it may have on surgeons is worthy of investigation.

INTRODUCTION

Computed tomography (CT) scan -based three-dimensional (3D) modeling operative technologies were designed and demonstrated to improve on certain perioperative results of manual total hip arthroplasties (MTHAs).[1–4] Since the advent of robotic-assisted joint arthroplasty, researchers have focused mainly on its effect on patient outcomes.[5] Although total hip arthroplasty (THA) is considered to be one of the most successful surgical procedures in modern day medicine,[6–9] the physically demanding nature of this procedure and the effect that it may have on surgeons has become worthy of investigation as procedures continue to increase.[10–12]

Orthopedic surgery is a physically demanding profession that leads to high rates of musculoskeletal ailments,[13,14] fatigue,[15,16] and burnout[17] among surgeons. Surgeon energy expenditure during THA is similar to that of moderate exercise.[18,19] As physical fatigue has been shown to decrease mental alertness and impair performance,[20–22] it may be prudent to consider factors that can help decrease the physical demand on joint arthroplasty surgeons who may/can perform several THAs on a given day. During robotic-arm assisted THA (RATHA), surgeons use reamers that are held within a haptic boundary, helping them to achieve accurate acetabular implant sizing, alignment, and placement based on their preoperative plan.[23] This also allows for single-stage reaming in RATHA

[a] Department of Orthopaedic Surgery, Stryker, 325 Corporate Drive, Mahwah, NJ 07430, USA; [b] Rubin Institute for Advanced Orthopedics, Sinai Hospital of Baltimore, 2411 W Belvedere Avenue #104, Baltimore, MD 21215, USA; [c] Department of Orthopaedic Surgery, Orthopaedic Institute of Ohio, 801 Medical Drive - Suite A, Lima, OH 45804, USA; [d] Department of Orthopaedic Surgery, Joint Implant Surgeons, 7277 Smiths Mill Road Suite 200, New Albany, OH 43054, USA; [e] Northwell Orthopaedics, Lenox Hill Hospital, 130 East 77th Street, New York, NY 10075, USA
* Corresponding author. Lenox Hill Hospital, 130 East 77th Street, 11th Floor, New York, NY 10075.
E-mail address: rhondamont@aol.com

procedures. This haptic boundary associated with RATHA is just one of many features that may enable surgeons to experience lower levels of mental and physical demand during THA procedures. However, to the best of our knowledge, the impact of this technology on surgeons' physical and mental demand has yet to be examined.[24,25]

As there is a paucity of literature on surgeon physical and mental demand when using a CT-based 3D modeling operative technique, the purpose of this study was to evaluate the physical and mental demand that surgeons experience when performing manual THA compared with its robotic-assisted counterpart. Specifically, we assessed: (1) task duration; (2) biometric parameters (ie, caloric energy expenditure, heart rate); and (3) subjective measures of mental and physical demand during MTHA compared with RATHA.

METHODS
Study Design
A total of six fresh-frozen cadaver specimens were obtained, stored at −20 oC, and then thawed at room temperature for 24 hours before dissection. Each specimen underwent bilateral THA using an MTHA on one hip and an RATHA on the contralateral hip. The surgical procedures were performed by two surgeons who had prior experience with MTHA. For their RATHA experience, one surgeon (Surgeon 1) had previously performed over 20 clinical cases using RATHA, and the other surgeon (Surgeon 2) had minimal prior exposure to RATHA, having performed one RATHA on a cadaveric specimen. Surgeons alternated between MTHA and RATHA, until three of each was completed.

Robotic-Assisted Total Hip Arthroplasty System Operative Details
Cadavers underwent a CT scan, along with the Mako robotic-arm assisted total hip application (Mako Surgical Corp [Stryker], Fort Lauderdale, FL, USA), generate a 3D model of the native hip. The surgeon used this to plan the bone cuts, implant size, and alignment before the procedures. The surgeon used the robotic arm to perform the cuts and stay within the virtual boundaries generated during the planning phase. The system is designed to help surgeons avoid resection of any bone outside of the virtual constraints. This study focused on acetabular reaming and shell impaction as this was the greatest difference between MTHA and RATHA procedures. The task duration times of

acetabular reaming and shell impaction were recorded for all cases.

Biometric Parameters
During the procedures, each surgeon wore a Hexoskin Smart Garment (Carre Technologies, Montreal, Canada). This wearable technology allowed the measurement of biometric parameters including caloric expenditure and heart rate. Using these data, surgeon energy expenditure during acetabular reaming and shell impaction were analyzed.

Subjective Mental and Physical Demand
Following each surgery, the surgeons were asked to perform a modified Surgery Task Load Index (SURG-TLX) questionnaire[26] to compare the physical and mental demands for the overall procedure as well as various individual tasks, including implant planning, exposure, retractor placement, femoral neck resection, broaching, stem tracking, acetabular reaming, and implant trial and placement for MTHA as well as RATHA. All questions were assessed on a scale of 1 to 10, with 1 indicating low and 10 indicating high demand.

Data Analyses
A normality test was performed on all THA tasks and it was determined that data for implant planning, femoral broaching, and implant trial and placement did not have a normal distribution. Therefore, a Mann–Whitney U test was performed to assess median and significant difference values for the questionnaire data based on a nonparametric population. Student's t-tests were used to compare mean and significant difference values for all other tasks of the ergonomic data for MTHA and RATHA based on a parametric normality assessment. Statistically significant results were determined by P-values less than 0.05.

RESULTS
Task Duration
The mean task duration for acetabular reaming and shell impaction was 11 minutes (9–12 minutes) with RATHA and 12 minutes (10–14 minutes) with MTHA. Each surgeon demonstrated reduced task duration during RATHA compared with MTHA, where the task includes reaming and shell impaction (Table 1). For Surgeon 1, mean task time was 12 ± 5 minutes with RATHA and 15 ± 3 minutes with MTHA ($P = .46$). For Surgeon 2, mean task time was 9 ± 3 minutes with RATHA and 10 ± 3 with MTHA. ($P = .66$).

Table 1
Biometric data

	MTHA (n = 3)	Surgeon 1 RATHA (n = 3)	% Change	MTHA (n = 3)	Surgeon 2 RATHA (n = 3)	% Change
Caloric expenditure	100	83.5	−16.5	83.5	75.3	−9.8
Calories per minute	6.8	6.8	−0.7	8.3	8.7	4
Heart rate (beats/min)	85.4	86	0.8	106.9	109.1	2
Mean task duration (min)	15	13	−15.9	10	9	−13.3

Biometric Parameters

Surgeon caloric expenditure was 83.5 ± 0.34 kcal with RATHA and 100 ± 28 kcal with MTHA (P = .49) (Fig. 1). Surgeon 1 demonstrated a 16.5% decrease in caloric expenditure from MTHA (100.0 kcal) to RATHA (83.5 kcal), and Surgeon 2 demonstrated a 9.8% decrease (83.5 kcal to 75.3 kcal). Mean heart rate measurements demonstrated a 1.4% increase with RATHA compared with MTHA, however, this difference did not reach statistical significance (P>.05).

Subjective Mental and Physical Demand

Overall mental demand was 5.5 ± 1.2 (range, 4–7) for MTHA and 4.2 ± 1.2 (range, 3–6) for RATHA (P = .10). Mental demand during acetabular reaming was significantly higher with MTHA (5.7 ± 1.0; range, 4–7) compared with RATHA (3.2 ± 1.5; range, 1–5) procedure (P < .01). Aside from femoral neck resection, the surgeons reported lower mental demand during RATHA for all other individual tasks (P>.05), as shown in Table 1. Mental demands for implant planning, exposure retractor placement, femoral neck resection, broaching, and implant and trial placement are shown in Table 2.

When considering individual surgeons, Surgeon 1 had lower overall mental demand scores when compared with Surgeon 2 for both RATHA (4.0 ± 1.0 vs 4.33 ± 1.53, P = .81) and MTHA (4.67 ± 0.58 vs 6.33 ± 1.15, P = .09).

Mean overall physical demand for MTHA was 5.5 ± 2.6 (range, 2–8) and 4.3 ± 1.6 (range, 2–6) for RATHA (P = .42). Aside from exposure and retractor placement, the surgeons reported lower physical demand during RATHA for all other individual tasks (P>.05), as shown in Table 2. Physical demands for implant planning, exposure and retractor placement, femoral neck resection, broaching and stem tracking, reaming acetabulum, and implant and trial placement are shown in Table 3.

When comparing the individual surgeons, Surgeon 1 had lower overall physical demand scores when compared with Surgeon 2 for both RATHA (3.7 ± 2.1 vs 5.0 ± 1.0, P = .38) and MTHA (4.0 ± 2.6 vs 7.0 ± 1.7, P = .19).

DISCUSSION

Orthopedic surgery is a physically demanding profession that leads to high rates of musculoskeletal ailments,[13,14] fatigue,[15,16] and burnout[17] among surgeons. The purpose of this study was to evaluate the physical and mental demand that surgeons experience when performing MTHA versus RATHA, which is of particular interest given the increasing incidence of THA in the United States, and the potential implications of surgeon fatigue on the clinical outcome of their patients.[10–12] In fact, this increased demand on surgeons has been shown to have a more pronounced effect on patient outcomes in the THA setting compared with total knee arthroplasty (TKA). Peskun and colleagues[15] aimed to determine if the time of day at which total joint arthroplasties are performed had an effect on postoperative patient outcomes. A total of 292 TKAs and 341 THAs were evaluated. It was found that later surgery start time was associated with significantly longer duration of THA (mean difference = 7 min; P = .004), but not TKA (P = .44). In addition, intraoperative periprosthetic femur fractures were associated with later surgery start time for THA (P = .05), but not for TKA (P = .35). These data highlight the importance of evaluating strategies to help reduce the physical and mental demand of THA.

In this study, RATHA demonstrated reduced surgeon energy expenditure compared with manual techniques. The mean task duration for acetabular reaming and shell impaction was faster with RATHA (11 minutes) than with MTHA (12 minutes). Surgeon caloric expenditure was lower with RATHA (83.5 kcal) than with MTHA (100 kcal). Mean overall physical demand

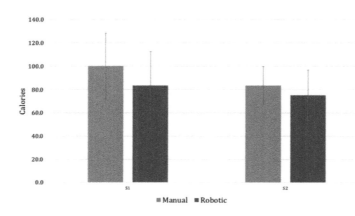

Fig. 1. Average caloric energy expenditure as a function of surgery type for each surgeon during acetabular reaming and acetabular implantation.

for RATHA (4.3) was less than MTHA (5.5). Aside from exposure and retractor placement, the surgeons reported lower physical demand during RATHA for all other individual tasks. Overall mental demand was lower for RATHA (4.2) than for MTHA (5.5). Aside from femoral neck resection, the surgeons reported lower mental demand during RATHA for all other individual tasks. In specific, subjective mental fatigue was significantly reduced during acetabular reaming with RATHA versus MTHA ($P < .05$). One potential reason for these results is that during RATHAs, surgeons use reamers that are held within a haptic boundary that enables the surgeons to ream according to their preoperative plan. This plan also allows for single-stage reaming in RATHA procedures. This feature may enable surgeons to have decreased mental demand when reaming and performing other THA tasks as explored in this study.

This study is not without limitations. The surgeries were performed on cadaveric specimens; therefore, the psychological responses that surgeons experience during clinical procedures may not have been accurately replicated. However, one of the main objectives of this study was to assess the physical demands of THA that are less likely to be influenced by these factors. Our small sample size of 12 THAs may have subjected some of our comparisons to type II errors. Many of the comparisons we evaluated trended toward improved results with RATHA versus MTHA, but did not reach statistical significance. In these cases, it may be inappropriate to accept the null hypotheses before larger-scale investigations are performed. Also, as baseline biometric factors were not accounted for, surgeon-specific differences in resting heart rates and basal metabolic rates may have influenced our results.

Our study also exhibited several strengths. To our knowledge, this is the first attempt to compare the physical and mental demand of MTHA and RATHA techniques. By evaluating various aspects of the procedures separately, we were able to demonstrate which tasks were associated with the highest levels of mental and physical burden. In addition, we used a validated scale to characterize surgeon-associated physical and mental demand.[26]

The physical burden of manual TKA (MTKA) and robotic-assisted total knee arthroplasty

Table 2 Mental demand						
Surgical Approach	Overall Mental Demand	Implant Planning	Exposure and Retractor Placement	Femoral Neck Resection	Femoral Broaching	Reaming Acetabulum	Implant Trial and Placement
MTHA	5.5 ± 1.2 (range, 4–7)	4.0 ± 2.4 (range, 2–7)	4.5 ± 1.4 (range, 3–7)	3.8 ± 1.8 (range, 2–6)	5.0 (range, 4–7)	5.7 ± 1.0 (range, 4–7)	5.0 (range, 3–8)
RATHA	4.2 ± 1.2 (range, 3–6)	3.5 ± 1.5 (range, 2–6)	4.3 ± 2.3 (range, 2–6)	4.0 ± 1.6 (range, 2–6)	4.0 (range, 3–7)	3.2 ± 1.5 (range, 1–5)	4.5 (range, 4–7)

Table 3
Physical demand

Surgical Approach	Overall Mental Demand	Implant Planning	Exposure and Retractor Placement	Femoral Neck Resection	Femoral Broaching	Reaming Acetabulum	Implant Trial and Placement
MTHA	5.5 ± 2.6 (range, 2–8)	3.0 (range, 1–6)	4.0 (range, 3–7)	4.3 ± 2.1 (range, 2–7)	5.2 ± 1.0 (range, 4–6)	5.5 ± 1.2 (range, 4–7)	5.2 ± 1.9 (range, 3–8)
RATHA	4.3 ± 1.6 (range, 2–6)	2.5 (range, 1–4)	4.5 (range, 2–6)	3.5 ± 1.4 (range, 2–5)	5.0 ± 1.2 (range, 4–7)	4.3 ± 2.0 (range, 2–6)	4.8 ± 1.7 (range, 3–8)

(RATKA) has been studied.[5] Scholl and colleagues studied the effect of MTKA versus RATKA on cervical spine static and dynamic postures.[5] In a study of two surgeons performing three MTKAs and three RATKAs each on pairs of cadaveric knees, Scholl and colleagues analyzed flexion–extension at T3 and the occiput, range of motion (ROM) in the flexion–extension angle, repetition rate, and static posture. They found that the mean T3 flexion–extension angle for MTKA cases (19°) was larger than RATKA cases (14°). The mean occiput flexion–extension angle was also larger for MTKA cases (51°) than RATKA cases (36°). Surgeons were found to have spent a significantly greater percentage of time in non-neutral C-spine ROM (greater than 10° flexion–extension angle at T3) during MTKA (78%) than during RATKA (63%) ($P = .02$). They were also found to have spent a significantly greater percentage of time in non-neutral ROM at the occiput during MTKA (100%) than during RATKA (94%) ($P = .00$). The repetition rate, the number of the times T3 and the occiput flexion–extension angle exceeded 10°, at T3 was greater for MTKA (14 reps/min) than RATKA (10 reps/min). The repetition rate at the occiput was also higher for MTKA (18 reps/min) than RATKA (17 reps/min). The percentage of time spent in static posture, where T3 or occiput postures exceed 10° for more than 30 seconds, at T3 was greater for MTKA cases (15%) than for RATKA cases (10%). The percentage of time spent in static occiput posture during MTKA cases (17%) was greater than the percentage of time spent in static occiput posture for RATKA cases (16%). Thus, Scholl and colleagues demonstrated the potential for RATKA to make a difference in a surgeon's cervical ergonomics by reducing physical demand during TKA.

Total hip arthroplasty is a physically demanding procedure that requires surgeons to expend a substantial amount of energy, similar to that of exercise.[18,19] Sharkey and colleagues[19] evaluated surgeon energy expenditure during total joint arthroplasty using an armband calorimeter. The energy expended by a single surgeon was compared between 22 primary THAs and TKAs. It was found that the surgeon's expenditure of energy was significantly greater during THA (340.98 kcal/h) compared with TKA (320.74 kcal/h) ($P < .05$). In our study, the mean energy expenditure for MTHA was higher (453 kcal/h) compared with Sharkey and colleagues' findings. Future studies should evaluate differences in energy expenditure among a larger sample of surgeons in an effort to identify factors that may help reduce the physiologic demands of THA.

Achieving desired positioning of the acetabular component is a key factor for successful outcomes of THA.[27–31] Thus, there can be a great deal of physiologic stress on surgeons during acetabular reaming and implant placement, especially for those who are less experienced. Our results demonstrated a significant reduction in subjective mental fatigue during acetabular reaming with RATHA compared with MTHA ($P < .01$). Similarly, Alexander and colleagues[32] performed a laboratory study to evaluate the accuracy and precision of acetabular component placement with standard fluoroscopic 2-dimensional (2D) projections compared with computer-assisted techniques with 3D CT data. Using the same scale used in our study,[26] the authors demonstrated a significantly lower workload with 3D (19 ± 11) compared with 2D (43 ± 18) techniques ($P < .05$). Although the findings of their laboratory study corroborate our results, further studies are needed for confirmation in a clinical setting.

In conclusion, RATHA demonstrated reduced surgeon energy expenditure compared with MTHA. In addition, RATHA demonstrated reduced mental demand during acetabular reaming compared with MTHA. There may be a relationship between surgeon experience and energy expenditure. Larger scale clinical studies are needed to confirm our findings. The results of our study suggest that compared with manual techniques, robotic assistance for THA may help surgeons reduce physical injury or burnout and improve mental alertness, which may in turn lead to improved patient outcomes.

CLINICS CARE POINTS

- Data suggest robotic-assisted total hip arthroplasty (THA) may reduce surgeon energy expenditure compared with manual total hip arthroplasty.
- Single-stage reaming may lead to decreased mental demand.
- Further investigation on association between surgeon experience and energy expenditure is needed.
- Robotic assistance for THA may reduce physical and mental demand that may lead to an improved surgical experience.

DISCLOSURE

Dr K. Abbruzzese is a Stryker employee. Ms A.L. Valentino is a Stryker employee. Ms L. Scholl is a Stryker employee. Dr E.L. Hampp is a Stryker employee. Dr R. Smith receives research support from Stryker. Dr M.A. Mont is a board or committee member for The Knee Society and The Hip Society, receives research support from National Institutes of Health and is on the editorial board for the Journal of Arthroplasty, Journal of Knee Surgery, Surgical Technology International, and Orthopedics. Dr Mont also receives company support from 3M, Centrexion, Ceras Health, Flexion Therapeutics, Johnson & Johnson, Kolon TissueGene, NXSCI, Pacira, Pfizer-Lily, Skye Biologics, SOLVD Health, Smith & Nephew, Stryker, MirrorAR, Peerwell, US Medical Innovations, and RegenLab. All other authors have no conflict of interest to disclose.

REFERENCES

1. Hepinstall M, Zucker H, Matzko C, et al. Adoption of Robotic Arm-Assisted Total Hip Arthroplasty Results in Reliable Clinical and Radiographic Outcomes at Minimum Two-Year Follow Up. Surg Technol Online 2021. https://doi.org/10.52198/21.sti.38.os1420.
2. Hepinstall MS, Naylor B, Salem HS, et al. Evolution of 3-Dimensional Functional Planning for Total Hip Arthroplasty with a Robotic Platform. Surg Technol Int 2020;37:395–403.
3. Marchand RC, Collins S, Marchand KB, et al. Estimation of Femoral Version During Total Hip Arthroplasty: Surgeon Visual Assessment versus Robotic-Arm Assisted Technology. Surg Technol Int 2020;37:390–4.
4. Hadley CJ, Grossman EL, Mont MA, et al. Robotic-Assisted versus Manually Implanted Total Hip Arthroplasty: A Clinical and Radiographic Comparison. Surg Technol Int 2020;37:371–6.
5. Scholl LY, Hampp EL, Alipit V, et al. Effect of Manual versus Robotic-Assisted Total Knee Arthroplasty on Cervical Spine Static and Dynamic Postures. J Knee Surg 2020. https://doi.org/10.1055/s-0040-1721412.
6. Varacallo M, Chakravarty R, Denehy K, et al. Joint perception and patient perceived satisfaction after total hip and knee arthroplasty in the American population. J Orthop 2018. https://doi.org/10.1016/j.jor.2018.03.018.
7. Varacallo MA, Herzog L, Toossi N, et al. Ten-Year Trends and Independent Risk Factors for Unplanned Readmission Following Elective Total Joint Arthroplasty at a Large Urban Academic Hospital. J Arthroplasty 2017. https://doi.org/10.1016/j.arth.2016.12.035.
8. DeGouveia W, Salem HS, Sodhi N, et al. An Economic Evaluation of Over 200,000 Revision Total Hip Arthroplasties: Is the Current Model Sustainable? Surg Technol Int 2020;37:367–70.
9. Guntaka SM, Tarazi JM, Chen Z, et al. Higher Patient Complexities are Associated with Increased Length of Stay, Complications , and Readmissions After Total Hip Arthroplasty. Surg Technol Int 2021;38.
10. Abdelaal MS, Restrepo C, Sharkey PF. Global Perspectives on Arthroplasty of Hip and Knee Joints. Orthop Clin North Am 2020. https://doi.org/10.1016/j.ocl.2019.11.003.
11. Sloan M, Premkumar A, Sheth NP. Projected volume of primary total joint arthroplasty in the u.s., 2014 to 2030. J Bone Joint Surg Am 2018;100(17):1455–60.
12. Chen Z, Tarazi JM, Salem HS, et al. The Utility of Telehealth in the Recovery From the COVID-19 Pandemic. Surg Technol Int 2021;39:17–21.
13. Davis WT, Sathiyakumar V, Jahangir A, et al. Occupational injury among orthopaedic surgeons. J Bone Joint Surg Am 2013. https://doi.org/10.2106/JBJS.L.01427.
14. Knudsen ML, Ludewig PM, Braman JP. Musculoskeletal pain in resident orthopaedic surgeons: results of a novel survey. Iowa Orthop J 2014;34:190–6.
15. Peskun C, Walmsley D, Waddell J, et al. Effect of surgeon fatigue on hip and knee arthroplasty.

Can J Surg 2012. https://doi.org/10.1503/cjs. 032910.

16. Whitney DC, Ives SJ, Leonard GR, et al. Surgeon Energy Expenditure and Substrate Utilization during Simulated Spine Surgery. J Am Acad Orthop Surg 2019. https://doi.org/10.5435/JAAOS-D-18-00284.

17. Arora M, Diwan AD, Harris IA. Burnout in orthopaedic surgeons: A review. ANZ J Surg 2013. https://doi.org/10.1111/ans.12292.

18. Navalta JW, Manning JW, McCune D, et al. Using Hexoskin Wearable Technology to Obtain Body Metrics in a Trail Hiking Setting. Med Sci Sport Exerc 2015. https://doi.org/10.1249/01.mss. 0000477034.13469.88.

19. Sharkey PF, Danoff JR, Klein G, et al. Surgeon Energy Expenditure During Total Joint Arthroplasty. J Arthroplasty 2007. https://doi.org/10.1016/j.arth. 2006.08.002.

20. Faber LG, Maurits NM, Lorist MM. Mental Fatigue Affects Visual Selective Attention. PLoS One 2012. https://doi.org/10.1371/journal.pone.0048073.

21. van der Linden D, Frese M, Meijman TF. Mental fatigue and the control of cognitive processes: Effects on perseveration and planning. Acta Psychol (Amst) 2003. https://doi.org/10.1016/S0001-6918(02)00150-6.

22. Xu R, Zhang C, He F, et al. How Physical Activities Affect Mental Fatigue Based on EEG Energy, Connectivity, and Complexity. Front Neurol 2018. https://doi.org/10.3389/fneur.2018.00915.

23. Nawabi DH, Conditt MA, Ranawat AS, et al. Haptically guided robotic technology in total hip arthroplasty: A cadaveric investigation. Proc Inst Mech Eng H J Eng Med 2013;227(3):302–9.

24. Hampp EL, Chughtai M, Scholl LY, et al. Robotic-Arm Assisted Total Knee Arthroplasty Demonstrated Greater Accuracy and Precision to Plan Compared with Manual Techniques. J Knee Surg 2019. https://doi.org/10.1055/s-0038-1641729.

25. Mont MA, Cool C, Gregory D, et al. Health care utilization and payer cost analysis of robotic arm assisted total knee arthroplasty at 30, 60, and 90 days. J Knee Surg 2021. https://doi.org/10.1055/s-0039-1695741.

26. Wilson MR, Poolton JM, Malhotra N, et al. Development and validation of a surgical workload measure: The surgery task load index (SURG-TLX). World J Surg 2011. https://doi.org/10.1007/s00268-011-1141-4.

27. Barrack RL, Lavernia C, Ries M, et al. Virtual reality computer animation of the effect of component position and design on stability after total hip arthroplasty. Orthop Clin North Am 2001. https://doi.org/10.1016/S0030-5898(05)70227-3.

28. Charnley J, Cupic Z. The nine and ten year results of the low friction arthroplasty of the hip. Clin Orthop 1973. https://doi.org/10.1097/00003086-197309000-00003.

29. D'Lima DD, Urquhart AG, Buehler KO, et al. The effect of the orientation of the acetabular and femoral components on the range of motion of the hip at different head-neck ratios. J Bone Joint Surg Am 2000. https://doi.org/10.2106/00004623-200003000-00003.

30. Scifert CF, Brown TD, Pedersen DR, et al. A finite element analysis of factors influencing total hip dislocation. Clin Orthop Relat Res 1998. https://doi.org/10.1097/00003086-199810000-00016.

31. Yamaguchi M, Akisue T, Bauer TW, et al. The spatial location of impingement in total hip arthroplasty. J Arthroplasty 2000. https://doi.org/10.1016/S0883-5403(00)90601-6.

32. Alexander C, Loeb AE, Fotouhi J, et al. Augmented Reality for Acetabular Component Placement in Direct Anterior Total Hip Arthroplasty. J Arthroplasty 2020. https://doi.org/10.1016/j.arth. 2020.01.025.

Considerations in the Sickle Cell Patient Undergoing Hip Reconstructive Surgery

Sara J. Sustich, BS, Benjamin M. Stronach, MD,
Jeffrey B. Stambough, MD, C. Lowry Barnes, MD,
Simon C. Mears, MD, PhD*

KEYWORDS

- Sickle cell disease • Total hip arthroplasty • Osteonecrosis • Prosthetic joint infection

---

KEY POINTS

- Osteonecrosis of the femoral head is a common debilitating complication of patients with sickle cell disease (SCD), often requiring total hip arthroplasty at a young age.
- Patients with SCD have unique and dangerous challenges associated with surgery requiring intensive preoperative, intraoperative, and postoperative management.
- Chronic bone changes from SCD can cause intraoperative challenges that result in orthopedic complications and poorer outcomes.

INTRODUCTION

Sickle cell disease (SCD) is the most common congenital hemoglobinopathy in the United States, affecting approximately 100,000 patients. The sickle cell trait originated in West and Central Africa, and due to this, it affects a disproportionate number of Blacks in the United States with a prevalence of 1 in 500.[1] SCD is an autosomal recessive condition typically caused by a single missense mutation on the beta globin gene on chromosome 11. There is a substitution of a nonpolar amino acid in place of a polar amino acid that results in a mutated hemoglobin molecule designated HbS. This molecular structure allows abnormal polymerization in low oxygen conditions, leading to sickling.[2] There are multiple genotypes that can lead to variations of phenotypic SCD, such as hemoglobin SC disease and β-thalassemia.[3,4] Both are hemoglobinopathies that, when combined with the sickle cell gene, cause a less severe disease than homozygous SS disease.[3] SCD causes anemia through intravascular hemolysis and decreased

hematopoiesis.[4] Additionally, sickled RBCs get trapped in microvasculature, leading to vaso-occlusion and tissue ischemia. The microcirculation in bone is a common site for RBC sickling, leading to many orthopedic manifestations of the disease including osteonecrosis. This process can occur as medullary infarcts or periarticular osteonecrosis of the femoral head (ONFH), knee, humeral head, or talus. ONFH is a common sequela of SCD, with an estimated prevalence of up to 50% in patients with SCD aged 35 years.[5,6] Hip pain associated with osteonecrosis has been documented as a significant limiting factor in patients' lives with adverse effects on activity, function, and quality of life.[7] Multiple procedures have been used in an effort to preserve the femoral head to include core decompression, osteotomy, and vascularized fibular grafting. There has been some success with these procedures in the early stages of osteonecrosis before head collapse. The goal of core decompression is to improve blood flow to the femoral head through decreasing intraosseous pressure.[8] Osteotomy aims to redistribute

---

Department of Orthopaedic Surgery, University of Arkansas for Medical Sciences, 4301 West Markham Street, Slot 531, Little Rock, AR 72205, USA
* Corresponding author.
E-mail address: SCMears@uams.edu

Orthop Clin N Am 53 (2022) 421–430
https://doi.org/10.1016/j.ocl.2022.06.006
0030-5898/22/© 2022 Elsevier Inc. All rights reserved.

weight-bearing area away from the necrotic regions of the femoral head.[9] Vascularized fibular grafting has had success in preventing progression and collapse likely attributed to the preserved blood supply allowing incorporation of the graft with the recipient bone.[9] These are joint-preserving methods that are important options for the young SCD population, who will likely need multiple arthroplasties in their lifetime. Unfortunately, these procedures typically do not always prevent progression and collapse in patients with this chronic disease, which then necessitates further intervention. Total hip arthroplasty (THA) is the mainstay treatment of symptomatic ONFH, especially those with advanced disease to include femoral head collapse and secondary osteoarthritis (Fig. 1). However, THA in the face of SCD can be a technically challenging procedure associated with high rates of complication and revision.[3,6,10] Additionally, SCD puts patients at risk for serious postoperative complications such as infection, excessive blood loss, sickle cell crisis, and acute chest syndrome. The objective of this article is to discuss the perioperative management and medical implications associated with SCD in the context of THA.

PATHOLOGIC CONDITION

The pathologic condition of ONFH in SCD is not entirely understood but several mechanisms are proposed including vaso-occlusion, thrombosis, and microvascular ischemia stemming from the pathologic sickled structure of erythrocytes.[11] Sickled RBCs have difficulty passing through small vessels and are therefore more likely to form a clot with resultant downstream ischemia. Another proposed mechanism is that adhesion of RBCs to vascular endothelium leads to occlusion of the vasculature. Finally, it is theorized that hemoglobin released during hemolysis consumes nitric oxide, a strong vasodilator, with resultant local vasoconstriction as nitric oxide concentrations decrease. These 3 proposed mechanisms of action are associated with compromised blood supply that increases the risk for osteonecrosis (Fig. 2).

Most patients with SCD are diagnosed with ONFH at early stages using history, physical examination, and radiologic imaging. Symptoms associated with ONFH include groin pain, especially during ambulation, and decreased range of motion. Untreated ONFH in SCD naturally progresses to degenerative arthritis and collapse of the femoral head.[10,11] Hernigou and colleagues followed 121 patients, all initially with asymptomatic ONFH.[12] After a mean follow-up of 14 years, 75% (91 hips) of patients had significant joint degeneration requiring hip replacement. The progression to collapse at 5-year follow-up was 10%, 55%, and 100% for Ficat stage 0, I, and II, respectively. At 10-year follow-up, 30% and 80% of Ficat stage 0 and I hips had progressed to collapse. Mean time to femoral head collapse from the onset of pain was around 5 years with a consensus that surgical intervention is ultimately necessary when a patient with SCD develops ONFH.[10,11]

PREOPERATIVE CONSIDERATIONS

Patients with SCD are prone to complications, both medical and surgical, when THA is

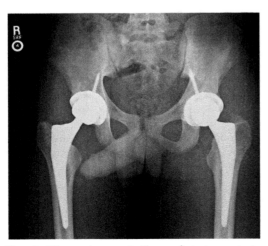

Fig. 1. Hip replacement X-ray. Anterior-posterior radiograph of pelvis in a patient with SCD.

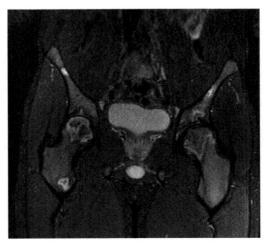

Fig. 2. Avascular necrosis of femoral head (MRI). MRI showing bilateral avascular necrosis of the femoral head.

performed. The increased risk for complication should be properly communicated with the patient when discussing surgical options. An integrated multidisciplinary team approach with professionals well-versed in the care of patients with SCD is important to address the risks across the different organ systems. Postoperative complications can be minimized through optimizing the patient medical condition preoperatively (Table 1). It is recommended to create a surgical risk assessment based on the procedure; blood loss potential; and patient's history of stroke, sickle crisis, acute chest syndrome, adverse reactions to anesthesia, surgical complications, transfusion and transfusion-related reactions as well as nonsickle cell-related comorbidities.[13,14] Hernigou and colleagues found that surgical risk was the only preoperative predictor of complications in patients with SCD with major orthopedic surgery being categorized as medium risk.[15] The physical capacity of the patient with SCD to undergo surgery must also be thoroughly investigated. Preoperative interventions can reduce the risk of sickle cell-related complications primarily through prevention of RBC sickling. The first step is to avoid conditions that promote sickling to include acidosis, dehydration, hypoxia, infection, vasoconstriction, venostasis, and hypothermia. The relative risk of sickle-associated complications can be reduced by managing oxygenation, hydration, blood loss, and fluid balance before, during, and after surgery.

Preoperative transfusion can be used with the goal of decreasing the percentage of HbS and improving oxygen carrying capacity, through increasing total Hgb. However, this is not a standardized protocol for patients with SCD undergoing THA and there is insufficient evidence to support a standard recommendation. Additionally, the amount of transfusion is not standardized and varies among providers. Vichinsky and colleagues showed there was no advantage of an aggressive transfusion protocol (HbS concentration less than 30% and total hemoglobin greater than 10 mg/dL) compared with a simple conservative transfusion approach (total hemoglobin greater than 10 mg/dL).[14] There was no evident difference in postoperative complication rates between the randomized transfusion groups. Additionally, there has been evidence of increased total blood loss associated with preoperative transfusions.[15] The risks associated with transfusion can be classified as minor (febrile, nonhemolytic reaction) and major (severe alloimmunization, delayed hemolytic transfusion reaction, infection, increased blood viscosity, and iron overload).[15,16] Alloimmunization is common among patient with SCD who chronically receive transfusions, with reported ranges of 7% to 58% for this condition, depending on patient age and number of previous transfusion.[13,17] Vichinsky and colleagues found that there was an increased risk of alloimmunization with aggressive transfusions, another reason why many centers prefer a simple conservative transfusion protocol.[18] Many patients can tolerate their steady state of anemia without the need for transfusion. Amar and colleagues recommended no preoperative transfusion if patient's Hbg is greater than 8g and is close to their steady state.[19] A preoperative transfusion could be given if patient's Hbg is lesser than 7g or is significantly less than their steady state.[19] Overall, decisions around transfusion should involve the hematologist with consideration that no transfusion in a chronically well-controlled patient with SCD is an equally valid option.

POSTOP MANAGEMENT

Patients with SCD are at increased risk for postoperative complications, making this a critical time for optimized medical management to prevent morbidity and mortality. Complication rates have been reported to be as high as 50% in patients with SCD undergoing THA.[14] Although complication rates have improved during the last several decades, they remain higher than the general population. Perfetti and colleagues found that

Table 1	
Preoperative management recommendations	
Preoperative Considerations	
Maintain normothermia (warming blanket, blood/fluid warmer, heat lamp, ambient room temperature)	Assess need for transfusion with hematologist, using conservative measures when transfusion is deemed appropriate
Provide IV fluids if requiring prolonged fasting before surgery and consider shortened fasting window for clear liquids	Maintain adequate oxygenation at SpO_2 100%

patients with SCD undergoing THA had 2.5 times more complications (2.17× minor, 2.53× major) when compared with patients without SCD. Major complications included death, myocardial infarction, pulmonary embolism, stroke, pneumonia, and acute renal failure, whereas minor complications include deep vein thrombosis, deep infection, implant dislocation, sepsis, UTI, wound hemorrhage, and superficial wound infection.[5]

The major cause of mortality in this population is secondary to pulmonary complications associated with sickle cell crisis and acute chest syndrome. These processes are sickle cell-specific complications that occur due to deoxygenation that causes RBC sickling and a subsequent cascade of vascular occlusion, ischemia, and pain. This physiologic response can be caused or exacerbated by the stress of surgery. Rates of vaso-occlusive crisis vary between 3.8% and 13% in studies,[14,15,20,21] whereas rates of acute chest syndrome are 1.9% to 15% with a mortality rate reported as high as 15%.[14] The goal of preoperative management is to prevent these complications from occurring; however, it is always a possibility under optimal management and should be monitored postoperatively. Management should include adequate hydration and appropriate analgesia with cautious attention to opioid respiratory depression. Appropriate oxygenation should be maintained with Po_2 greater than 95 mm Hg for the first 24 to 48 hours postoperatively.[22]

In patients with SCD, the most common complication associated with THA is blood loss requiring transfusion. Average blood loss in SCD undergoing THA is a higher amount than the general population with reported values averaging 1150 mL.[10,18,20,22,23] Excess blood loss is managed with postoperative transfusion with associated potential for transfusion-related complication. Patients with SCD typically have a history of multiple transfusions, which increases the risk of forming alloantibodies with 20% to 30% being alloimmunized.[3] Prevention of reaction is best done with phenotypic matching of ABO, Rhesus (Cc, D, Ee) and Kell as well as screening for antibodies before surgery.[24] Transfusion reactions occur in 4% to 12% of patients with SCD receiving transfusions.[4,14] These reactions range from febrile nonhemolytic reaction to severe alloimmunization with massive intravascular hemolysis.[15]

PAIN CONTROL

SCD patients have chronic pain associated with vaso-occlusive crises and the musculoskeletal ramifications of the disease process. They often require recurrent opiate treatment that can lead to drug tolerance and potential for addiction. Nevertheless, opiates are first-line treatment of postoperative pain, in part because of their diverse routes of delivery, the number of agents available, and their ability to be titrated.[16] Long-acting opioid agonists can be used in combination with short-acting agonists for breakthrough pain. Pain medication can additionally be placed on continuous administration with patient-controlled pump.[13,16,25,26] Due to life-long narcotic requirements, patients with SCD often require larger doses to obtain adequate pain control.[16,25,26] As with all narcotic use, special attention should be given to opiate-induced respiratory depression because this can be a potential instigator for sickling events. It is recommended to develop a long-term pain management plan with the hematology team before surgery and to consult the pain management service for appropriate considerations in the acute perioperative period.

The use of multimodal pain medications can combat pain while keeping the doses of each medication, and related side effects, to a minimum. Methadone is a long-acting opioid, which may be useful in patients with tolerance to opiates. Tramadol can also be a useful agent because it acts on central opioid receptors as well as catecholamine and serotonin receptors that are thought to alter patient's perception of pain.[16] Nonopioid analgesics can minimize the opioid dose necessary for adequate pain control thus reducing the risk of respiratory depression. Nonsteroidal anti-inflammatories (NSAIDs) are effective for inflammatory pain from vaso-occlusion, whereas acetaminophen primarily acts centrally to combat mild-to-moderate pain.[16] It is important to evaluate the renal function of the patient with SCD before the use of NSAIDs because many have chronic kidney disease due to SCD.[16] We recommend conferring with the treating hematologist in regards to the use of NSAIDs and other pain-management strategies before surgery. It is also important to ensure the anesthesia team is aware the patient has SCD to ensure adequate pain control with the anesthetic event and in the postoperative period. This may include a combination of regional, spinal, and general anesthesia.

Suboptimal pain management for patients with SCD is prevalent due to the fear of creating dependency as well as stigmatization of sickle cell patients with chronic pain by the medical field.[16] It is important to acknowledge and address pain in these patients as legitimate and is unethical to not do so. Of additional importance, excess pain and associated undue stress and anxiety on the body can induce sickling with associated sequelae and a further increase in pain.

Many of these patients have some baseline narcotic tolerance and require larger doses of opioids for pain control beyond what the orthopedic surgeon is comfortable with providing, so preoperative planning with hematology and pain management and anesthesia teams can be of significant benefit to provide pain control and prevent crisis for the patient.

SURGICAL CONSIDERATIONS

Patients with SCD require THA at younger ages, on average in their mid 30s, compared with the general population with an average age in the mid 60s.[5] Symptoms associated with ONFH include groin pain, especially during ambulation, and decreased range of motion. These symptoms have a larger influence on this younger and more active population, with one study finding that the most limiting factor in the life of these young patients with SCD is hip pain and associated limitation of activity and function.[10] There are feared complications associated with THA in patients with SCD as well as the concern for survivorship and inevitable implant revision. However, THA can provide significant improvement in quality of life for these patients that typically outweighs the risks.[27]

Many different procedures have been attempted for ONFH outside of THA to include core decompression, femoral osteotomy, hemiarthroplasty, resection arthroplasty, and arthrodesis.[3] The last 4 procedures are typically not recommended and rarely practiced in the United States for ONFH. However, core decompression is a surgical option for early stage ONFH with the goal of delaying the need for THA by relieving elevated intraosseous pressure and encouraging new bone growth[3] (Fig. 3). Core decompression is a less invasive procedure, has lower complication rates, and has shorter hospitalization time compared with THA.[14] This procedure relieves symptomatic pain with one study showing an improvement rate of 85%.[28] However, ONFH secondary to SCD shows poor clinical response to core decompression compared with ONFH due to other causes.[29] Additionally, there are no long-term prospective studies assessing the efficacy of core decompression making it somewhat controversial for surgical management in SCD.

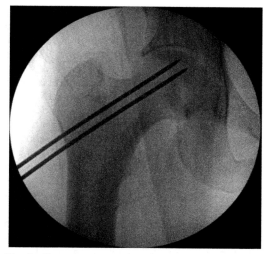

Fig. 3. Core decompression during. A: Intraoperative anterior-posterior radiograph during a core decompression of right hip for avascular necrosis.

Often, the femoral head involvement is too large for decompression because subchondral collapse and articular cartilage delamination has already occurred by the time the patient presents for the treatment (Fig. 4). Hernigou and colleagues found that at presentation, all sickle cell-induced osteonecrosis lesions involved greater than 40% of the femoral head.[3,12] Finally, although core decompression relieves

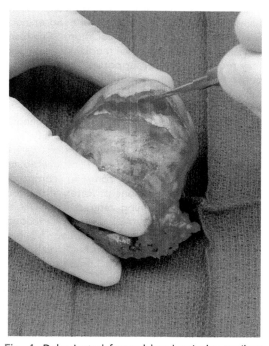

Fig. 4. Delaminated femoral head articular cartilage due to osteonecrosis secondary to SCD.

pain associated with ONFH, it does not address the underlying pathophysiology; repeated ischemic events that are common in SCD will potentially lead to further osteonecrotic insults and eventual femoral head collapse.[30]

The pathophysiology of SCD in relation to bone present technical challenges for THA. Chronic anemia, as well as repeated vaso-occlusive events, stimulates bone marrow hyperplasia with resultant widening of the medullary canal with patchy sclerosis and thinning of the trabeculae and cortices.[7] Bone remodeling can also result in a narrow femoral canal (Fig. 5). These abnormalities create challenges with intramedullary reaming and acetabular prosthesis fixation with frequent complications of fracture and perforation. Preoperative planning and intraoperative care must be taken to avoid such complications.

Eccentric reaming and femoral perforation are common complications associated with reaming and prothesis insertion with rates of femoral perforation between 2.9% and 5.8% (Fig. 6). Preparation of the canal can be done by using incrementally sized reamers.[24] To avoid overpreparation of the medullary canal, studies suggest using a drill bit under radiographic imaging to prepare the femoral bone for the placement of a guidewire through which a flexible reamer can then be used to open the femoral canal.[3,7,22] Acetabular protrusio is common in SCD and can make hip dislocation difficult, potentially necessitating in situ femoral head or neck osteotomy to aid with dislocation.[3] Protrusio can also limit the extent of medial reaming and may require structural support of the acetabular implant.[3] Poor bone quality also makes the acetabulum more susceptible to fracture during implant impaction.

Orthopedic complications are frequently encountered due to poor bone quality.[6,7,15] Aseptic loosening requiring revision varied among studies with loosening of acetabular component being more common compared with the femoral component. Rates of femoral and acetabular loosening ranged from 0% to 21.7%[6,15,20,31] and 0% to 21.1%,[6,15,31,32] respectively, with follow-up times between 3.8 and 14.6 years. Cementless implants had significantly lower rates of loosening compared with cemented prostheses. Deep infection requiring revision ranged from 0% to 14.5%,[6,15,20,32] and overall revision rates ranged from 0% to 22.2%.[6,15,31,32] The use of cemented versus cementless implants has been an ongoing debate with multiple studies advocating for each technique. One suggested advantage for

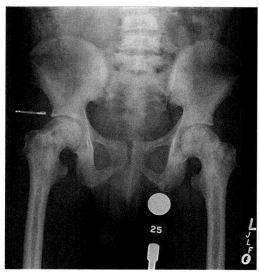

Fig. 5. Sclerotic canal and avascular necrosis of femoral head (X-ray). Anterior-posterior radiograph of pelvis showing sclerotic canals and avascular necrosis of the femoral heads.

cemented implants is that necrotic bone has a limited potential for bone in growth, which is needed for biologic fixation in cementless implants.[15] Cemented implants provide initial rigid fixation and can minimize blood loss through tamponade of the highly vascularized marrow. Less preparation of the femoral canal is required for cementation potentially decreasing the risk of femoral perforation and fracture.[3] It is theorized that the use of cement causes thermal necrosis in already diseased bone predisposing patients to these long-term complications.

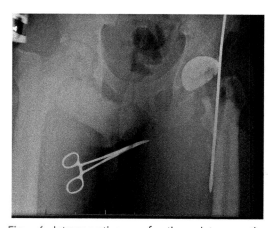

Fig. 6. Intraoperative perforation. Intraoperative anterior-posterior radiograph during THA of left hip showing perforation of medullary canal during eccentric reaming status-post bilateral THA.

Hernigou and colleagues are strong advocates for cemented implants and report the highest success rate among cemented implant studies with aseptic loosening rates of 7% for the acetabular cup and 5% for the femoral components. They attribute their lower rate of stem loosening to the technique of using the largest possible rectangular stem with a minimal cement mantle, described as the "French Paradox."[15] The deep infection rate in this study was also comparatively low at 3% attributable to the use of antibiotics within the cement, a recommendation they endorse with cemented implant use in this population.

There are no prospective studies directly comparing the use of cemented versus cementless implants in THA for SCD. However, recent studies have shown more favorable results with the use of cementless implants. Biologic fixation achieved with cementless implants has a lower rate of aseptic loosening and revision when compared with cemented fixation.[4,33] This is important for the SCD population requiring THA, who are young with a lifetime chronic disease, with a goal of avoiding the need for further surgery.[4,21,23] The surgeon may consider restricting activity postoperatively to low levels to allow bone ingrowth and minimize the risk of aseptic loosening.[33] Additionally, the use of screws for cementless acetabular components may be used to provide additional fixation that may not be achieved with press-fit alone.[3] Cementless implants require more intense canal preparation with a higher potential for intraoperative complications of perforation and fracture compared with cemented implants.[34] Finally, there can be greater intraoperative blood loss with cementless implants due to the lack of initial tamponade found with cement use. Jeong and colleagues found more than half a liter higher blood loss for cementless implants (2000 mL) in comparison with cemented implants (1390 mL).[3,21,35] Although no direct comparative studies exist, results from current literature strongly endorse the use of cementless implants for THA in the SCD population.[36]

OUTCOMES

The goal of hip arthroplasty is to resolve pain and regain functionality, notably important for this young and active patient population. Hernigou and colleagues found complete resolution of pain in 64% of patients with the other 36% having only occasional discomfort, along with improved function scores and hip range of motion, in patients with SCD undergoing THA for ONFH.[15] Azam and colleagues had similar findings with significant improvement in quality of life scores THA in this population, even with a high frequency of postoperative complications.[7]

Medical and orthopedic complications are common in the postoperative setting in the SCD population with a 2.5 times risk for complication compared with patients without SCD.[5] Perioperative blood loss was the most frequent complication with average blood loss ranging between 950 and 1420 mL.[14,15,20,22,23] The need for postoperative transfusion is significantly increased in SDC patients (52%–62%) compared with their non-SCD counterparts (25%) with an associated increase of intraoperative blood loss.[5,20,37] A conservative transfusion goal is to keep the hemoglobin greater than 10 mg/dL to decrease cardiopulmonary complications while also minimizing complications due to the transfusion itself.[24] We recommend evaluating the long-term preoperative hemoglobin trend for the specific patient, along with assessment of vital signs and symptoms of anemia, to determine when transfusion is required because patients with SCD are adapted to a state of chronic anemia. Wound hematomas are another postoperative complication associated with excessive blood loss often requiring evacuation.[7,15] Rates ranged from 1.3% to 10.4% with one study showing lower rates of hematoma formation among patients who received low molecular weight heparin for thromboembolic prophylaxis compared with warfarin.[15]

The average age for patients with SCD undergoing THA is 37 years, compared with the average age of THA being 65 years in the non-SCD population. Patients with SCD are more likely to be Black (90% compared with 6% in the non-SCD population) with a slight female predominance. Osteonecrosis was the most common underlying diagnosis necessitating THA in 87% of patients with SCD compared with 11% without SCD. Patients with SCD had a significantly longer hospital stay, staying on average 42% longer than patients without SCD, 6.92 and 3.83 days, respectively. Patients with SCD were more likely to have Medicaid with medical costs 19% higher than their non-SCD counterparts, $51,240 compared with $37,802. When the data was restricted to patients without SCD with a diagnosis of osteonecrosis, the results were similar.[5]

INFECTION PREVENTION

Postoperative infection is a big concern with patients with SCD due to the potential for osteomyelitis in infarcted bone and due to their relative immune deficiency due to asplenia.[38] Prosthetic joint and wound infection rates after THA range from 3% to 20% with deep infection being an important cause of implant removal and revision.[15,23,27,35]

Recommendations for infection prevention include preoperative management of potential infection sources. Remote sites of infection have potential to seed the prosthesis causing secondary infection.[4] Locations include chronic stasis ulcers as well as gallbladders containing gallstones.[15,24] Additionally, preoperative laboratories should be performed to ensure white blood cell count, erythrocyte sedimentation rate, and c-reactive protein levels are at adequate levels.[24] The erythrocyte sedimentation rate in patients with SCD is typically elevated due to the presence of sickled red blood cells causing a delay in the sedimentation rate. Due to previously infarcted bone along with high rates of childhood osteomyelitis, patients with SCD tend to be colonized with latent staphylococcal and *Salmonella* organisms. Intraoperative antibiotic use along with culture of femoral head and histologic examination of surgical specimens are recommended to detect if the patient is harboring bacteria in order to prevent secondary infection.[15,20,24] First-generation or second-generation cephalosporins are recommended to be continued for 2 to 3 days postoperatively. Antibiotics should be continued for at least a month if culture results are positive and may need to be adjusted to maximize the sensitivity profile of cultured organisms.[3,15] We recommend consulting infectious disease colleagues regarding treatment in this setting. Additionally, cement-containing antibiotics should be used when a cemented implant is chosen. One study suggested the use of systemic antibiotics in combination with local antibiotics within cemented implants had a longer prophylactic effect and was more efficient than either local or systemic antibiotic treatment alone.[15,39]

Prosthetic joint infection is a major cause of revision with THA in the SCD population. Late prosthetic infections are often due to recurrent bacteremia with hematogenous spread and seeding of the prosthesis most commonly from staphylococcal and Gram-negative organisms.[4] Late hematogenous infection is difficult to predict or prevent. In one study, there were 10 instances of late infection (3%), all requiring revision, which occurred at an average of 11 years after the index THA.[15]

SUMMARY

ONFH is a common complication of SCD that can be debilitating, especially to the relatively younger population. The sickling of RBCs creates unique challenges associated with surgery and requires preoperative and postoperative management with a multidisciplinary approach. It is important to maintain adequate hydration, oxygenation, temperature, and Hgb levels to decrease postoperative complications. Sclerosing of the medullary canal along with vascularization of the marrow creates surgical challenges intraoperatively that can result in complications such as perforation and aseptic loosening of the implant. Patients can suffer from postoperative complications to include excessive blood loss to acute sickle crisis to acute chest syndrome.

There are many conservative and surgical options to treat ONFH in the patients with SCD, including pain management and core decompression. However, due to the progressive nature of the disease, THA, despite its increased risks compared with patients without SCD, is the definitive treatment to improve pain, functionality, and quality of life.

CLINICS CARE POINTS

- Osteonecrosis of the hip is common in patients with sickle cell disease.
- Hip replacement is challenging from both a technical and medical perspective.
- A team approach is needed to obtain good outcomes.

DISCLOSURE

The authors have nothing to disclose.

REFERENCES

1. Vaishya R, Agarwal AK, Edomwonyi EO, et al. Musculoskeletal Manifestations of Sickle Cell Disease: A Review. Cureus 2015. https://doi.org/10.7759/cureus.358.
2. Sundd P, Gladwin MT, Novelli EM. Pathophysiology of Sickle Cell Disease. Annu Rev Pathol Mech Dis 2019;14. https://doi.org/10.1146/annurev-pathmechdis-012418-012838.
3. Jeong GK, Ruchelsman DE, Jazrawi LM, et al. Total hip arthroplasty in sickle cell hemoglobinopathies. Am Acad Orthopaedic Surgeons

2005;13(3). https://doi.org/10.5435/00124635-200505000-00007.

4. Kamath AF, McGraw MH, Israelite CL. Surgical management of osteonecrosis of the femoral head in patients with sickle cell disease. World J Orthopedics 2015;6(10). https://doi.org/10.5312/wjo.v6.i10.776.

5. Perfetti DC, Boylan MR, Naziri Q, et al. Does sickle cell disease increase risk of adverse outcomes following total hip and knee arthroplasty? A nationwide database study. J Arthroplasty 2015;30(4):547–51.

6. Farook MZ, Awogbade M, Somasundaram K, et al. Total hip arthroplasty in osteonecrosis secondary to sickle cell disease. Int Orthop 2019;43(2). https://doi.org/10.1007/s00264-018-4001-0.

7. Azam MQ, Sadat-Ali M. Quality of Life in Sickle Cell Patients After Cementless Total Hip Arthroplasty. J Arthroplasty 2016;31(11). https://doi.org/10.1016/j.arth.2016.04.025.

8. Cohen-Rosenblum A, Cui Q. Osteonecrosis of the Femoral Head. Orthop Clin North Am 2019;50(2): 139–49.

9. Korompilias Av, Lykissas MG, Beris AE, et al. Vascularised fibular graft in the management of femoral head osteonecrosis: Twenty years later. J Bone Joint Surg - Ser B 2009;91(3). https://doi.org/10.1302/0301-620X.91B3.21846.

10. Hernigou P, Habibi A, Bachir D, et al. The natural history of asymptomatic osteonecrosis of the femoral head in adults with sickle cell disease. J Bone Joint Surg - Ser A 2006;88(12). https://doi.org/10.2106/JBJS.E.01455.

11. Issa K, Naziri Q, Maheshwari Av, et al. Excellent results and minimal complications of total hip arthroplasty in sickle cell hemoglobinopathy at mid-term follow-up using cementless prosthetic components. J Arthroplasty 2013;28(9). https://doi.org/10.1016/j.arth.2013.03.017.

12. Patel Y, Szczech B, Patel S, et al. Management strategies for total hip arthroplasty in sickle cell patients. J Long-Term Effects Med Implants 2014;24(2–3). https://doi.org/10.1615/JLongTermEffMedImplants.2014010493.

13. Hernigou P, Bachir D, Galacteros F. The natural history of symptomatic osteonecrosis in adults with sickle-cell disease. J Bone Joint Surg - Ser A 2003;85(3). https://doi.org/10.2106/00004623-200303000-00016.

14. Oyedeji CI, Welsby IJ. Perioperative Man Age Ment of Sickle Cell Dis Ease | 405 Optimizing Man Age Ment of Sickle Cell Dis Ease in Patients under Go Ing Sur Gery. Available at: http://ashpublications.org/hematology/article-pdf/2021/1/405/1851532/405oyedeji.pdf.

15. Vichinsky EP, Neumayr LD, Haberkern C, et al. The perioperative complication rate of orthopedic surgery in sickle cell disease: Report of the national sickle cell surgery study group. Am J Hematol 1999;62(3). https://doi.org/10.1002/(SICI)1096-8652(199911)62:3<129::AID-AJH1>3.0.CO;2.

16. Hernigou P, Zilber S, Filippini P, et al. Total THA in adult osteonecrosis related to sickle cell disease. Clin Orthopaedics Relat Res 2008;466. https://doi.org/10.1007/s11999-007-0069-3.

17. Khurmi N, Gorlin A, Misra L. Perioperative considerations for patients with sickle cell disease: a narrative review. Can J Anesth 2017;64(8). https://doi.org/10.1007/s12630-017-0883-3.

18. Vichinsky EP, Earles A, Johnson RA, et al. Alloimmunization in Sickle Cell Anemia and Transfusion of Racially Unmatched Blood. N Engl J Med 1990;322(23). https://doi.org/10.1056/nejm199006073222301.

19. Vichinsky EP, Haberkern CM, Neumayr L, et al. A Comparison of Conservative and Aggressive Transfusion Regimens in the Perioperative Management of Sickle Cell Disease. N Engl J Med 1995;333(4). https://doi.org/10.1056/nejm199507273330402.

20. Ould Amar K, Rouvillain JL, Loko G. Perioperative transfusion management in patients with sickle cell anaemia undergoing a total hip arthroplasty. Is there a role of red-cell exchange transfusion? A retrospective study in the CHU of Fort-de-France Martinique. Transfus Clinique Biologique 2013; 20(1). https://doi.org/10.1016/j.tracli.2012.11.001.

21. Ilyas I, Alrumaih HA, Rabbani S. Noncemented Total Hip Arthroplasty in Sickle-Cell Disease: Long-Term Results. J Arthroplasty 2018;33(2). https://doi.org/10.1016/j.arth.2017.09.010.

22. Hickman JM, Lachiewicz PF. Results and complications of total hip arthroplasties in patients with sickle-cell hemoglobinopathies: Role of cementless components. J Arthroplasty 1997;12(4). https://doi.org/10.1016/S0883-5403(97)90198-4.

23. Kalacy A, Ozkan C, Togrul E. Revision hip arthroplasty in sickle cell disease. Ann Saudi Med 2007; 27(2). https://doi.org/10.4103/0256-4947.51522.

24. Acurio MT, Friedman RJ. Hip arthroplasty in patients with sickle-cell haemoglobinopathy. J Bone Joint Surg - Ser B 1992;74(3). https://doi.org/10.1302/0301-620x.74b3.1587879.

25. Hernigou P, Housset V, Pariat J, et al. Total hip arthroplasty for sickle cell osteonecrosis: guidelines for perioperative management. EFORT Open Rev 2020;5(10). https://doi.org/10.1302/2058-5241.5.190073.

26. Adjepong KO, Otegbeye F, Adjepong YA. Perioperative management of sickle cell disease. Mediterr J Hematol Infect Dis 2018;10(1). https://doi.org/10.4084/MJHID.2018.032.

27. Okpala I, Tawil A. Management of pain in sickle-cell disease. J R Soc Med 2002;95(9). https://doi.org/10.1258/jrsm.95.9.456.

28. Styles LA, Vichinsky EP. Core decompression in avascular necrosis of the hip in sickle-cell disease.

Am J Hematol 1996;52(2). https://doi.org/10.1002/(SICI)1096-8652 (199606)52:2<103::AID-AJH6>3.0.CO;2-Y.

29. Hsu JE, Wihbey T, Shah RP, et al. Prophylactic decompression and bone grafting for small asymptomatic osteonecrotic lesions of the femoral head. HIP Int 2011;21(6). https://doi.org/10.5301/HIP.2011.8760.

30. Moran MC. Osteonecrosis of the hip in sickle cell hemoglobinopathy. Am J Orthop 1995;24(1).

31. AlOmran AS. Choice of implant in total hip arthroplasty for sickle cell disease patients. Eur Orthopaedics Traumatol 2010;1(1). https://doi.org/10.1007/s12570-010-0006-x.

32. Gulati Y, Sharma M, Bharti B, et al. Short term results of cementless total hip arthroplasty in sicklers. Indian J Orthopaedics 2015;49(4). https://doi.org/10.4103/0019-5413.159659.

33. Fassihi SC, Lee R, Quan T, et al. Total Hip Arthroplasty in Patients With Sickle Cell Disease: A Comprehensive Systematic Review. J Arthroplasty 2020;35(8). https://doi.org/10.1016/j.arth.2020.04.014.

34. Kenanidis E, Kapriniotis K, AnagnOstis P, et al. Total hip arthroplasty in sickle cell disease: A systematic review. EFORT Open Rev 2020;5(3):180–8.

35. Clarke HJ, Jinnah RH, Brooker AF, et al. Total replacement of the hip for avascular necrosis in sickle cell disease. J Bone Joint Surg - Ser B 1989;71(3). https://doi.org/10.1302/0301-620x.71b3.2722941.

36. Severyns M, Gayet LE. Aseptic osteonecrosis of the femoral head in patients with sickle cell anemia. Morphologie 2021;(349):105. https://doi.org/10.1016/j.morpho.2020.08.002.

37. Gu A, Agarwal AR, Fassihi SC, et al. Impact of sickle cell disease on postoperative outcomes following total hip arthroplasty. HIP Int 2021. https://doi.org/10.1177/11207000211052224.

38. Neonato MG, Guilloud-Bataille M, Beauvais P, et al. Acute clinical events in 299 homozygous sickle cell patients living in france. Eur J Haematol 2000;65(3). https://doi.org/10.1034/j.1600-0609.2000.90210.x.

39. Espehaug B, Engesaeter LB, Vollset SE, et al. Antibiotic prophylaxis in total hip arthroplasty. J Bone Joint Surg - Ser B 1997;79. https://doi.org/10.1302/0301-620X.79B4.7420.

Trauma

A Review on Management of Insufficiency Fractures of the Pelvis and Acetabulum

Colin K. Cantrell, MD*, Bennet A. Butler, MD

KEYWORDS

- Acetabular fracture • Pelvic fracture • Fragility fracture • Insufficiency fracture • Osteoporosis

---

KEY POINTS

- Pharmacologic treatments for osteoporosis, the most prevalent risk factor, include vitamin D, calcium, bisphosphonates, and parathyroid hormone.
- Although conventional classifications of pelvic ring fractures such as the Young-Burgess and Tile classification systems are used, the fragility fractures of the pelvis classification may better characterize injuries and help guide treatment.
- Acetabular fractures in the elderly population demonstrates extensive anterior column comminution and severe comminution and marginal impaction of posterior wall fractures.
- Nonoperative treatment is the preferred method of treatment in most insufficiency fractures of the pelvis and acetabulum.
- Operative fixation of the acetabulum using percutaneous or minimally invasive methods to provide stable column support for total hip arthroplasty provides good outcomes when an anatomic reduction may not be possible or the patient cannot tolerate an extensive surgical approach.

INTRODUCTION

Insufficiency fractures, also termed fragility or osteoporotic fractures, of the pelvis and acetabulum are fractures that occur in abnormally weakened bone with an absence of trauma or more commonly from a low-energy mechanism with force atypical of pelvic injuries such as a ground level fall.[1] These fractures were first described in 1982 by Lourie who described spontaneous sacral fractures in 3 elderly patients.[2] These fractures are associated with increased functional disability and morbidity, along with a 1-year mortality rate reported as high as 27%.[3,4] In this review, the authors explore the epidemiology, risk factors, diagnosis, and treatment of pelvic and acetabular insufficiency fractures.

EPIDEMIOLOGY

Pelvic insufficiency fractures occur primarily in elderly patients with a reported average age of 69 years in one series.[5] Melton and colleagues examined the incidence of pelvic fractures of over a 10-year period and found an overall incidence of 37 per 100,000 person years, which increased in men aged 75 to 84 years (63.9 per 100,000) and women aged 75 to 84 years (249.5 per 100,000). When examining ages greater than 85 years, men demonstrated an incidence of 220.3 per 100,000, whereas women demonstrated an incidence of 446.3 per 100,000.[5] Kannus and colleagues noted an increase in the incidence of pelvic fractures of patients aged 60 years or older by 23% per year from 1970 to 1997.[6] The incidence of

---

Department of Orthopaedic Surgery, Northwestern University Feinberg School of Medicine, 676 North Saint Clair, Suite 1350, Chicago, IL 60611, USA
* Corresponding author.
E-mail address: colincantrellmd@gmail.com

Orthop Clin N Am 53 (2022) 431–443
https://doi.org/10.1016/j.ocl.2022.06.007
0030-5898/22/© 2022 Elsevier Inc. All rights reserved.

osteoporotic pelvic fractures is predicted to continue to increase by 60% to 100% by 2030.[7,8]

Acetabulum insufficiency fractures, similar to pelvic fractures, are also increasing in incidence in patients with increasing ages. A consecutive series of operatively treated acetabulum fractures from 1980 to 2007 demonstrated a 30% increase in the proportion of acetabular fractures in patients ages 60 years or older.[9] Of note, almost 50% of the aforementioned fractures were noted to be the result of a low-energy fall. Two other retrospective reviews out of Sweden and Australia noted 10% and 11% incidences of geriatric acetabular fractures over a 10-year period, respectively.[10,11]

RISK FACTORS

Any condition that weakens bone or decreases bone density may predispose a patient to an insufficiency fracture such as osteopenia, or more commonly, osteoporosis. Osteoporosis is the most prevalent predisposing condition in patients with pelvic insufficiency fractures. A Singh index of 4 or less indicating osteoporosis was found in 93% of patients with low-energy pelvis fractures.[3] Furthermore, Breuil and colleagues found that more than half of patients who had an insufficiency fracture of the pelvis had a prior diagnosis of osteoporosis and had sustained a prior fracture, yet only one-third had received treatment of their osteoporosis.[12] A biomechanical study has demonstrated that cortical porosity of 20% can decrease bone strength.[13] In patients older than 65 years, the average cortical porosity is 46%. Muscles, which normally provide a protective effect to the bone by absorbing some mechanical stress, are often atrophied in the elderly, diminishing this potentially protective effect.[14]

Another risk factor for insufficiency fractures includes pelvic radiation, which damages local circulation impeding bone turnover and remodeling.[15] Baxter and colleagues found a significantly higher 5-year rate of fracture in patients who underwent pelvic irradiation, whereas Housman and colleagues also found a 30% higher incidence of pelvic fractures in men with prostate cancer treated with radiation.[16,17] Total hip arthroplasty has been identified as a risk factor for rami and acetabular fractures due to preoperative osteopenia from relative immobilization followed by increased activity after their arthroplasty procedure.[18,19] Rheumatoid arthritis is a risk factor for insufficiency fracture of the pelvis due to osteopenia resulting from chronic corticosteroid use.[20]

HISTORY AND PHYSICAL EXAMINATION

Evaluation of pelvic and acetabular fragility fractures warrants history and physical examination coupled with imaging studies. Patients often complain of hip or groin pain, particularly with anterior pelvic ring or acetabular injuries, and may also endorse buttock or back pain, which is more common in sacral and posterior pelvic ring injuries.[21] The most identified mechanism of injury is a ground level fall but may occur after no specific trauma or inciting event.[3,22] Patients will often experience pain with ambulation, noting an immediate refusal to bear weight or a constant decline in mobility over a short course of time.

Physical examination may reveal tenderness to palpation over the groin, pubic symphysis, or sacrum. Difficulty initiating hip flexion on the affected side is often seen, noting the leg feels "heavy."[23] Less commonly, pain with log roll or axial loading may be demonstrated. Most patients will be neurovascularly intact in the lower extremities.

DIAGNOSIS

Diagnosis of pelvic or acetabular insufficiency fractures can be difficult and requires an index of suspicion, as many patients present with vague low back or pelvic pain and loss of independent mobility without history of significant trauma.[24] These symptoms are usually exacerbated by weight-bearing and relieved by rest. Given the absence of trauma or presence of only minor trauma, diagnosis can sometimes be significantly delayed.[25]

Initial imaging evaluation of suspected pelvic or acetabular insufficiency fracture begins with anteroposterior (AP) plain radiograph. If pelvic ring injury is identified on the AP radiograph, inlet and outlet radiographs are obtained. Conversely, if an acetabular fracture is identified, 3 Judet views (AP pelvis, iliac oblique, and obturator oblique) are obtained.[26] Although these initial radiographs often identify pubic rami fractures, the posterior elements of the injury may be missed. In a series of 177 patients with pubic rami fractures, 96.8% of patients had an injury to the posterior pelvic ring.[27]

The next imaging modality used in evaluation of the pelvis and acetabulum is the computed tomography (CT) scan. Grasland and colleagues looked at 16 patients with sacral insufficiency fractures where only 50% were identified on plain radiograph. Nine patients underwent CT scan, and sacral fracture was identified in all patients.[28] When insufficiency fractures are clinically suspected but not diagnosed on the aforementioned imaging modalities, MRI may be indicated. MRI has been shown to be superior to CT scan for detecting insufficiency fractures with sensitivities of 99% and 69%, respectively.[29] Henes and colleagues confirmed this finding with a prospective study where 96.3% of fractures were diagnosed on MRI versus 77% on CT.[30]

Lastly, bone scans or PET/CT can identify insufficiency fractures of the pelvis. Bone scans were previously the advanced imaging technique of choice. Some patterns of uptake in these scans, such as the "Honda sign" for sacral insufficiency fracture, may be diagnostic, with a positive predictive value up to 92% and sensitivity of 94%.[31,32] The "Honda sign" is transverse uptake in the sacral body with vertical uptake in the sacral alae bilaterally, forming an H-like shape. Conversely, the "Honda sign" was only demonstrated on 63% of patients with sacral insufficiency fractures.[31] In addition, sacroiliac joints in normal patients may demonstrate uptake. For these reasons and possibly greater familiarity, CT and MRI have replaced bone scans as the second-line imaging modalities.

CLASSIFICATION
Pelvic Ring
Pelvic ring injuries are commonly classified using the Young-Burgess classification system.[33] Patients presenting with insufficiency fractures of the pelvic ring most commonly have lateral compression (LC) type patterns resulting from ground level falls.[34] Melton and colleagues found that LC type 1 or 2 patterns were present in 95% of pelvis fragility fractures in their series.[5] Another widely accepted classification system of pelvic ring system is that of Marvin Tile, which was adopted by the Association for the Study of Internal Fixation/Orthopedic Trauma Association.[35] Whereas the Young-Burgess system classifies injuries based on the disruptive force, the Tile system focuses on the stability and direction of instability of the pelvic ring.

Understanding that fragility fractures of the pelvic ring are primarily bony injuries in nature and do not always fit into conventional classifications systems, Rommens and colleagues proposed a new classification for fragility fractures of the pelvis (FFPs).[36] This classification system is categorized from types I to IV based on an increasing degree of instability (Fig. 1). FFP type I lesions are solely anterior injuries with type Ia corresponding to unilateral anterior disruption and type Ib corresponding to bilateral

anterior disruption. Increased instability is noted in FFP type II lesions. Type IIa is a nondisplaced and isolated unilateral sacral fracture; type IIb are pubic, and ischial rami fractures are combined with crush injury of the ventral sacral ala without displacement; and type IIc injuries are a combination of rami fractures and a nondisplaced sacral ala fracture with dorsal and ventral sacral disruption. Type III lesions are increasingly unstable and are subdivided based on the localization of the dorsal injury with IIIa traversing the posterior iliac bone, IIIb through the sacroiliac joint with complete anterior ring disruption, and IIIc with complete unilateral sacral disruption with complete anterior rami disruption. Type IV lesions demonstrate the highest degree of instability. The complete dissociation from the iliolumbar spine and the pelvic ring is the distinguishing characteristic of FFP type IV lesions. Type IVa contains bilateral iliac fractures, IVb are bilateral and complete sacral ala fractures, and IVc has combinations of different dorsal pelvic instabilities, which include the following:

- Transiliac instability on one side combined with a transsacral instability on the other side
- Transsacral instability on one side combined with transiliosacral on the other side
- Transiliac instability on one side with a transiliosacral instability on the other side

The prevalence of pure FFP type Ia and Ib injuries is less common in the elderly with a prevalence ranging from 3.2% to 41%.[27,37] Type IIb and IIc morphologies, corresponding to LC type 1 injuries of the Young-Burgess classification, result from the typical mechanism of injury, ground level falls.[33] FFP type IIIa injuries are similar to LC-II pelvic ring injuries or type B2 Tile injuries. Rommens and colleagues noted that type II injuries were primarily seen in the acute phase where type III were typically seen after 4 to 6 weeks of pain, demonstrating that injuries may move from a lower degree of instability to a category of higher instability.[36]

Acetabulum
Fractures of the acetabulum are classified according to the classification system defined by Letournel.[38] Although elderly patients can present with any of the fracture patterns in Letournel's classification system, low-energy osteoporotic acetabular fractures most commonly include a comminuted anterior column fracture with disruption of the medial wall

FFP Type I - anterior pelvic ring fracture only

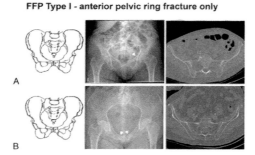

FFP Type III - displaced unilateral posterior pelvic ring fracture

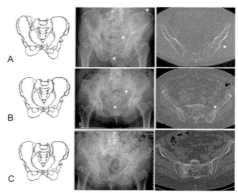

FFP Type II - non-displaced posterior pelvic ring fracture

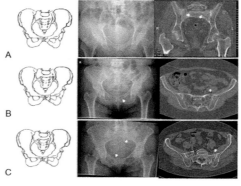

FFP Type IV - displaced bilateral posterior pelvic ring fracture

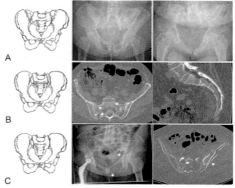

Fig. 1. The 4 types of fragility fractures of the pelvis (FFP), including type I fractures involving the anterior pelvic ring only, type II nondisplaced posterior pelvic ring fractures, type III displaced unilateral posterior pelvic ring fractures, and type IV displaced bilateral posterior pelvic ring fractures. The letters A, B, and C correspond with the subcategories of each fracture type as defined in the text. (*From* Rommens PM, Hofmann A. Comprehensive classification of fragility fractures of the pelvic ring: recommendations for surgical treatment. Injury. 2013 Dec;44 [12]:1733-44. Epub 2013 Jul 18.)

of the acetabulum, also known as the quadrilateral plate.[39] Furthermore, Ferguson and colleagues noted that comminuted anterior column fractures were significantly more common in elderly patients than the young.[9] In this cohort, a separate quadrilateral plate component was noted in 50%, whereas roof impaction was seen in 40%. These radiological features have been established as predictors of poor outcomes. More severe comminution and marginal impaction are seen in elderly posterior wall fractures, and they are more likely to sustain a hip dislocation. Although the associated both column is the most common fracture pattern in this group, the anterior column posterior hemitransverse (ACPHT) acetabular fracture pattern has been dubbed the "classic osteopenic acetabular fracture," as it displays many of the aforementioned features common to geriatric acetabular fractures.[40,41]

MANAGEMENT
Acute Phase
Severe hemorrhage has been documented in cases of low-energy geriatric pelvic fractures.[34,42–46] For this reason, these low-energy injuries demand similar assessment and attention as other pelvic ring injuries. A review of 328 low-energy pelvic ring fractures found that 8 (2.4%) developed severe hemorrhage requiring embolization.[34] The mean hemoglobin decrease in these patients was 4.0 g/dL and stabilized in all patients postembolization.

Several factors are thought to contribute to hemorrhage in these low-energy geriatric fractures. Arteriosclerosis increases as patients age, decreasing compliance and increasing fragility of the vessels, predisposing them to rupture. These sclerotic arteries may impair vasospasm. Elderly patients are also more likely to be taking anticoagulants or other coagulopathic medications for a variety of reasons, increasing their bleeding times and volume of hemorrhage after a trauma. In addition, lack of muscle tone may impair tamponade effects.[24]

Nonoperative Treatment

Nonoperative treatment of pelvic and acetabular insufficiency fractures is preferrable in cases in which the patient is expected to have an acceptable result without incurring the risks of surgery. There are certain debated criteria that orthopedic surgeons use to determine which patients undergo nonoperative treatment. Pelvic ring injuries and acetabular fractures are, in most circumstances, exclusive injuries and are treated as such when determining the course of treatment.

Nonoperative Pelvic Ring

Nonoperative management is the mainstay of treatment of most pelvic ring insufficiency fractures. These fractures are managed with progressive mobilization and serial radiographs if the fractures are determined to be stable. The goal of mobilization in these patients is to prevent the complications of immobility that are increased in prevalence and severity in the elderly. If deemed stable fracture patterns, weight-bearing as tolerated is allowed immediately with a large portion of patients using assistive devices. In a series of 148 patients aged 65 years or older with a pelvic fracture, more than half required personal assistance for mobility and all required assistive devices at discharge.[3] Repeat radiographs (AP/inlet/outlet) are traditionally taken 1 week, 4 to 6 weeks, 3 months, 6 months, and 1-year postinjury.

Average length of hospital stays range from 14 to 45 days for these injuries.[4,12,47] Koval reported that 95% of their patients were able to return home but did not comment on further assistance required.[47] Other studies suggest a much greater loss of independence. Taillandier and colleagues demonstrated that only 59% of previously self-sufficient patients recovered self-sufficiency at 1 year.[4] Of all the patients who resided at home in the Breuil series, only 31% returned home on discharge from the hospital, whereas assistance required with activities of daily living increased from 18% preinjury to 60% at final follow-up.[12] Morris and colleagues further collaborated these findings in their independent preinjury cohort, with only 13% returning home independently and 63% returning home with assistance and the final 24% requiring nursing homes.[3]

Nonoperative Acetabulum

Acetabulum fractures in the elderly present unique challenges in management. Nonoperative criteria for any acetabular fractures are minimal displacement, maintained stability of the hip joint, and a concentric reduction of the femoral head.[23] Understanding that significant displacement and comminution is often present in fragility fractures of the acetabulum, the primary goal of treatment is to maintain or restore the relationship with the femoral head and the weight-bearing dome. In injuries where this relationship is not disrupted, a nonoperative treatment strategy is used.

Patients deemed appropriate for nonoperative management may begin toe-touch weight-bearing, which assists with balance but prevents fracture displacement or joint subluxation that may occur with full weight-bearing. Almost all patients in this group will require a walker or another assistive device, given the difficulty with this weight-bearing restriction. Butterwick and colleagues discussed a protocol for nonsurgical management that consisted of therapy-assisted toe touch weight-bearing for 6 weeks.[48] Patients are prescribed venous thromboembolism prophylaxis and fall prevention is paramount. Radiographs are obtained at 2, 6, and 12 weeks. They note that bedrest is specifically contraindicated, given the severe morbidity and mortality associated. Mears and colleagues indicated that minimally displaced acetabular fractures treated nonoperatively may become asymptomatic with full weight-bearing in as few as 4 to 8 weeks.[39]

Another consideration of determining nonoperative management is secondary congruence. Secondary congruence is a circumstance in both column acetabular fractures, which arises when the femoral head maintains its congruency with the articular fragments of the acetabulum despite medial displacement. According to a biomechanical assessment, both column fractures with secondary congruence have increased stress concentrations in the dome of the acetabulum.[49] Despite this, clinical studies have shown that these patients have minimal pain, high functional scores at time of union, and an acceptably low rate of complications.[50]

Nonoperative Pharmacologic

Patients presenting with an osteoporotic fragility fracture have a 1.8 to 2.0 relative risk of incurring a second fragility fracture.[51] A thorough laboratory workup should be performed to evaluate for reversible causes of osteoporosis such as hyperthyroidism, hypothyroidism, vitamin D deficiency, and hypogonadism.

Vitamin D/calcium

Many geriatric patients are vitamin D deficient. For this reason, Vitamin D and calcium supplementation is a common mainstay of osteoporotic treatment. There is a decreased risk of fragility fracture in patients receiving vitamin D and calcium supplements.[52] Current International Osteoporosis Foundation recommends vitamin D dosing for patients aged 50 years or older to be 800 to 1000 IU per day.[53] Current recommendation for calcium dosing for men ages 51 to 71 years is 1000 mg/d and men 71+ years and women 51+ years is 1200 mg/d.[53]

Bisphosphonates

Antiresorptive agents, that is, bisphosphonates, are often used in the treatment of osteoporosis. Bisphosphonates inhibit osteoclasts, decreasing bone resorption and turnover.[54] Randomized trials have demonstrated a reduction in the risk of hip and spine fractures in osteoporotic women.[55,56] This risk reduction can be appreciated within 6 months of therapy initiation.[57] Although the long-term benefit in fracture reduction is well established, the effect in the acute fracture setting is still under investigation. The most common adverse reaction to bisphosphonates is gastrointestinal distress followed by the less common side effects of renal damage, osteonecrosis of the jaw, and atypical subtrochanteric femur fracture.[58]

Human recombinant parathyroid hormone

Teriparatide, recombinant parathyroid hormone (PTH), increases bone density, cortical thickness, and bone strength while reducing fracture risk[59,60]; this is accomplished by increasing the number of osteoblasts by both stimulating formation and preventing apoptosis.[59] A randomized trial in treatment of osteoporotic pelvic fractures with PTH demonstrated a faster healing time, reduction in pain, and faster functional improvements when compared with placebo.[61] PTH has been linked with osteosarcoma and is not recommended in patients with a history of osteosarcoma or conditions associated with skeletal malignancy.

Operative Pelvic Ring

Few absolute operative indications for pelvic insufficiency fractures exist: open fractures, displaced H- or U-type sacral fractures with cauda equina syndrome, and locked pubic symphysis. If a patient is unable to mobilize secondary to

pain or gait alterations, operative fixation may stabilize the fracture enough to alleviate pain and enhance mobilization.[62] Delayed operative fixation to correct symptomatic nonunion or malunion may be used also. Operative treatment options include open reduction internal fixation, percutaneous fixation, or sacroplasty.

Posterior pelvic ring

Internal fixation options of the posterior pelvic ring consist of iliosacral screws, transiliac transsacral screws, spinopelvic fixation, transiliac rod or plate, and transsacral plate. Iliosacral screws were designed and function primarily for injuries to the sacroiliac joint. Failure of these screws was noted in sacral fractures, particularly vertically oriented fractures in zone 2 of the sacrum.[63] Transsacral screws demonstrate decreased displacement and increased force to failure in sacral fractures when compared with iliosacral screws.[64] A series of 19 patients with pelvic insufficiency fractures who underwent fixation with trans-iliac-sacral-bar demonstrated quick pain relief in all patients, improved mobility, and no neurologic complications.[65]

A review of geriatric sacral-U insufficiency fractures demonstrated an incidence of 16.7% in their low-energy pelvic ring fracture cohort.[66] These fractures were stabilized with 2 transiliac transsacral screws in 81% of patients. The other 3 patients had pelvic dysmorphism and were treated with bilateral sacroiliac screws of various configurations. All patients had debilitating pain and were unable to ambulate before surgery. All but 2 were ambulatory on postoperative day 1. Rommens and colleagues advocated for iliolumbar fixation in FFP type IVb fractures.[36]

Osteoporotic bone can lead to radiographic visualization difficulties, making safe screw insertion difficult with standard fluoroscopy. In addition, understanding safe corridors is paramount in all transsacral screw placement. An anatomic study assessing safe corridors of transsacral screw placement found that in patients without sacral dysmorphism, 96% had an acceptable transsacral screw corridor in S1, followed by 93% in S2, and 7% in S3; this contrasts with patients with sacral dysmorphism where only 63% had safe S1 corridors, 97% in S2, and 14% in S3.[67]

Anterior pelvic ring

Fixation of the posterior ring is prioritized over the anterior ring due to most of the weight-bearing being through the posterior lumbopelvic region. Once this fixation has occurred, fixation can occur in the anterior pelvis, the patient can undergo stress examination under anesthesia, or forego anterior fixation. Fixation options in the anterior pelvic ring include retrograde or antegrade ramus screws, external fixation, and other plate and rod constructs. Rommens and colleagues treated 65 elderly patients with 76 retrograde ramus screws and had found no difference in implant loosening or nonunion when compared with those placed in younger patients with high-energy mechanisms.[68] Screws in patients with FFP were more often implanted percutaneously and had lower rates of infection but higher incidence of postoperative hematoma.

Nonunion

Nonunions may occur after fragility fracture of the pelvis. In a review of 44 nonunions treated with in situ fixation, 82% healed after initial fixation.[69] Eight patients did not heal after their initial fixation. Six of these patients had prior radiation therapy and 7 healed after additional surgery. However, 30% of patients who achieved union still endorsed pain at 1 year.

Cement augmentation

Opinion in the literature regarding cement augmentation with screw fixation is varied. Some recommend screw fixation alone due to the concern that cement augmentation would inhibit the ability for incorporation of native bone and restoration of physiologic load transmission.[70] Cement also may prevent evaluation of fracture healing on follow-up radiographs. On the contrary, other studies have argued that it is difficult to generate compression with screw fixation alone.[22,71,72] A systematic review by König and colleagues reviewed cement augmentation of sacroiliac screws in pelvic fragility fractures and found that augmented screws were biomechanically stronger in terms of pull out strength and construct stiffness.[73] However, no clinically significant benefit has been demonstrated. They noted various methods of application of cement including insertion through the cannulation of the screw and application on the tip of the screw.

Sacroplasty

Sacroplasty was first described for the treatment of metastatic lesions of S1 in 2000.[74] Extending the principles of vertebroplasty, the proposed concept was that filling the sacral defect with polymethylmethacrylate (PMMA) cement would reduce micromotion and pain. Garant described the first case report of sacroplasty as a treatment of a pelvic insufficiency fracture in 2002.[75] The patient was bedridden with multiple spinal compression fractures as well as a sacral fracture and underwent vertebroplasty and sacroplasty and was able to sit up and bear weight on postoperative day 1 and pain free at 9 months.

Frey and colleagues conducted a prospective study of 52 patients evaluating complications and midterm outcomes of percutaneous sacroplasty for sacral insufficiency fractures.[76] These patients, with an average age of 75.9 years, has no improvement with conservative care for 34.5 days. After undergoing the procedure, visual analogue score improved from 8.1 to 3.6 at 30 minutes. All patients reported 75% to 100% satisfaction. Thirteen percent of patients were pain free 30 minutes postprocedure and 25% pain free at 2 weeks. Of note, all sacral fractures treated in this group were zone 1, with the concern that in zone 2 and 3 fractures, there could be a risk for cement leakage into the presacral space, spinal canal, or sacral foramen. Two separate literature reviews on sacroplasty for the treatment of pelvic insufficiency fractures found a high portion of immediate pain reduction as well as lasting pain relief for more than 1 year postsacroplasty with relatively few complications.[77,78]

Although the aforementioned studies have indicated that sacroplasty is safe and effective, others have expressed concerns about the biomechanics. PMMA is excellent at resisting compression as seen in vertebral bodies but poor at resisting shear loads that are seen by the sacrum. This cement does not restore the stiffness to baseline in an osteoporotic pelvis.[79] In a biomechanical study comparing sacroplasty, unilateral iliosacral fixation, and transsacral screw fixation, all techniques were found to be effective at decreasing motion of the sacrum.[71] There was a greater increase in motion following cyclical loading in the sacroplasty group, followed by the short iliosacral screw group.

Operative Acetabulum

Tile originally suggested that osteosynthesis of geriatric acetabular fractures should be abandoned because of poor bone quality.[80] However, Letournel reported that 76% patients older than 60 year with acetabular fractures treated by open reduction and internal fixation (ORIF) had good to excellent outcomes.[81] Achieving a reduction less than 3 mm of intraarticular incongruity is key to obtaining a good clinical result.[82] Achieving an anatomic reduction has proved to be difficult in the geriatric population, with only 44% and 58% of reductions being anatomic in 2 separate studies.[82,83] Absolute indications for operative management of osteopenic acetabular fractures include open fractures, hip joint instability, and intraarticular loose bodies. Hip joint incongruity and intraarticular displacement greater than 2 to 3 mm are associated with an increased risk of early posttraumatic arthritis.

Surgical options include open reduction internal fixation, percutaneous internal fixation, and early total hip arthroplasty (THA). Of note, patients treated operatively or nonoperatively have the potential to progress to posttraumatic arthritis becoming a candidate for delayed total hip arthroplasty.

Percutaneous fixation

Percutaneous fixation of acetabular fractures may minimize risks of postoperative infection and blood loss to ultimately offer potentially quicker recovery.[84] Percutaneous fixation was popularized by the development of the techniques for column fixation using large cannulated 6.5- or 7.3-mm screws.[85] In Gary and colleagues' review of 80 geriatric acetabular fractures, 56% were displaced associated both column or ACPHT fractures.[84] Twenty-five percent underwent percutaneous reduction, whereas 75% required "mini-open" access to the quadrilateral plate via a portion of the lateral window. Twenty-five percent underwent conversion to THA at a mean of 1.4 years postoperatively, and loss of reduction with medialization of the femoral head was noted in 6%. In a later study, Gary and colleagues examined functional outcomes with the Short Musculoskeletal Functional Assessment (SMFA) at a mean of 6.8 years postoperatively.[86] No significant difference in SMFA scores was found between those who retained their native hip and the population norms for patients older than 60 years. Although the outcomes of this technique seem comparable with those after formal ORIF, the literature supporting this comparison is sparse. Specific contraindications to this technique include posterior wall fractures with joint instability and lack of expertise with percutaneous column fixation.[48]

Open reduction internal fixation

It has been noted that anatomic reduction is more difficult in the elderly population with acetabular fractures.[82,83] Anglen and colleagues demonstrated that patients with the Gull sign, superomedial dome impaction, was predictive of inadequate reduction, early loss of reduction, and early joint space narrowing.[87] To address various characteristics of elderly acetabular fractures, numerous techniques have been developed. Laflamme and Herbert-Davies used the anterior intrapelvic approach to address the superomedial dome impaction.[88] The femoral head usually returned to its original position following anterior column reduction. The quadrilateral fragment was then hinged open, allowing direct visualization of the impacted surface, which was subsequently reduced with a periosteal elevator. A satisfactory reduction was obtained in 78% of patients.

Although the ilioinguinal approach is appropriate for many acetabular fracture patterns in the elderly, the potential for substantial blood loss exists. To attempt to minimize the approach, Jeffcoat and colleagues used 2 lateral windows in patients with a mean age of 67 years.[89] In comparison to patients treated with a conventional ilioinguinal approach, the patients undergoing 2 lateral windows had decreased blood loss and operative time while maintaining similar outcomes and THA conversion rates.

A systematic review of 8 studies on acetabular fractures in patients aged 55 years and older found similar failure rates, measured by conversion to tTHA, between formal open reduction internal fixation (22%) and percutaneous fixation (25%).[90] Acceptable reduction (<3 mm) was found in 86% but anatomic reduction achieved in only 45%. Of note, the mortality rate in the percutaneous group was 31% compared with 15% in the ORIF group; however, the percutaneous group was significantly older at 74.4 years versus 69.5 years ($P < .001$).

Acute total hip arthroplasty

Indications for acute THA for acetabular fracture generally include poor prognostic factors such as nonreconstructible comminution, femoral head lesions, impaction of greater than 40% of the dome, femoral head and/or neck fractures, and preexisting severe degenerative arthritis.[91] Rigid stabilization of the fracture allowing good stability of the acetabular component promotes both fracture healing and long-term stability of the implant. The primary goal of reduction in this scenario is not to achieve an anatomy reduction but reduce the columns to provide sufficient stability for cup impaction. Anterior column and iliac wing fixation with braided cerclage cabling of the acetabulum and quadrilateral plate to prevent protrusion was described by Mears and colleagues and Mouhsine and colleagues.[92,93] The "Combined Procedure" with acetabular stabilization and subsequent acetabular component implantation has become increasingly popular.[94] A systematic review comparing THA and ORIF

(THA + ORIF) versus ORIF alone noted less operative time and increased blood loss in the THA + ORIF group, but there was no significant difference in complications or mortality.[90] Lin and colleagues reported on 33 patients with acetabular fractures treated with THA and demonstrated a 94% implant survival rate.[95]

Delayed total hip arthroplasty

Delayed THA, offered in the setting of posttraumatic arthritis following operative or nonoperative treatment, initially yielded high loosening rates with cemented acetabular components but has improved with press fit cups.[96,97] Bellabarba and colleagues noted a Kaplan-Meyer 10-year survival rate of 97% of 30 patients with cementless acetabular components.[98] In this study, comparison between acute and delayed THA has demonstrated similar component survival at 3 years with 99% for acute and 97% for delayed THA.

MORBIDITY AND MORTALITY

Insufficiency fractures of the pelvis and acetabulum are associated with decreased mobility, loss of independence, and significant mortality.[23] Morris and colleagues found that in a series of 148 patients aged 65 years or older with a pelvic fracture, more than half (51.1%) required personal assistance for mobility and all required assistive devices at discharge.[3] Adverse events during hospitalization are also frequent in these patients. A review of outcomes of 60 patients noted 52.5% of patients suffered an adverse event, with urinary tract infections (50%) being the most common followed by bed sores (33%) and mental status changes including depression or altered cognitive function (18%).[12] Before injury, 82.5% of this cohort was living independently. Only 31% returned home on discharge, with 66% being discharged to a geriatric inpatient rehabilitation setting. Almost 50% of these patients had lost autonomy at final follow-up. These findings are reinforced in a study by Taillandier and colleagues who noted that only 58.5% of previously self-sufficient patients returned to this status postdischarge and only 39% returned to preinjury level of function at 1 year postinjury.[4]

Mortality related to pelvic insufficiency fractures can be very high. Hill and colleagues reviewed 273 patients admitted to the hospital with pubic rami fractures and noted 1- and 5-year survival rates of 87% and 46%, respectively.[99] Dementia proved to be a significant risk factor for mortality with 1- and 5-year survival rates lowered to 80% and 28% in this cohort. Morris and colleagues noted a 1-year mortality rate of 27%, with a subsequent annual mortality rate of 10% after the first year.[3] A review of geriatric acetabular fractures noted mortality rates at 2.3% at 30 days, 8.1% at 6 months, and up to 25% at 1 year depending on the presence of other injuries.[100]

SUMMARY AND RECOMMENDATIONS (CLINICS CARE POINTS)

- Insufficiency fractures of the pelvis and acetabulum are common injuries and are increasing as the population ages.
- Osteoporosis is the most prevalent risk factor, and workup for causes of osteoporosis is warranted.
- Pharmacologic treatments for osteoporosis include vitamin D, calcium, bisphosphonates, and parathyroid hormone.
- Plain radiographs are the standard initial imaging evaluation of these fractures, followed by CT and/or MRI.
- Although conventional classifications of pelvic ring fractures such as the Young-Burgess and Tile classification systems are used, the FFP classification may better characterize injuries and help guide treatment.
- The Letournel classification is the standard classification of acetabular fractures, with certain features more prevalent in the elderly population including extensive anterior column and quadrilateral plate comminution and multifragmentary posterior wall fractures with impaction.
- Nonoperative treatment is the preferred method of treatment in most insufficiency fractures of the pelvis and acetabulum.
- Operative fixation of the acetabulum using percutaneous or minimally invasive methods to provide stable columnar support provides good outcomes when an anatomic reduction may not be possible or the patient cannot tolerate an extensive surgical approach.
- Acute and delayed THA provide similar outcomes after acetabular fracture.
- Fragility fractures of the pelvis and acetabulum impart significant morbidity and mortality in the elderly.

DISCLOSURE

The authors have nothing to disclose.

REFERENCES

1. Matcuk GR, Mahanty SR, Skalski MR, et al. Stress Fractures: pathophysiology, clinical presentation, imaging features, and treatment options. Emerg Radiol 2016;23:365–75.
2. Lourie H. Spontaneous osteoporotic fracture of the sacrum. An unrecognized syndrome of the elderly. JAMA 1982;248(6):715–7.
3. Morris R, Sonibare A, Green D, et al. Closed pelvic fractures: characteristics and outcomes in older patients admitted to medical and geriatric wards. Postgrad Med J 2000;76(900):646.
4. Taillandier J, Langue F, Alemanni M, et al. Mortality and functional outcomes of pelvic insufficiency fractures in older patients. Joint Bone Spine 2003; 70:287–9.
5. Melton LJ III, Sampson JM, Morrey BF, et al. Epidemiologic features of pelvic fractures. Clin Orthop Relat Res 1981;155:43–7.
6. Kannus PP, Palvanen MM, Miemi SS, et al. Epidemiology of osteoporotic pelvic fractures in elderly people in Finland: sharp increase in 1970-1997 and alarming projections for the new millennium. Osteoporos Int 2000;11(5):443–8.
7. Kannus P, Palvanen M, Parkkari J, et al. Osteoporotic pelvic fractures in elderly women. Osteoporos Int 2000;16(10):1304–5.
8. Burge R, Dawson-Hughes B, Solomon DH, et al. Incidence and economic burden of osteoporosis-related fractures in the United States, 2005-2025. J Bone Miner Res 2007;22(3):465–75.
9. Ferguson TA, Patel R, Bhandari M, et al. Fractures of the acetabulum in patients aged 60 years and older: an epidemiological and radiological study. J Bone Joint Surg Br 2010;92(2):250–7.
10. Ragnarsson B, Jacobsson B. Epidemiology of pelvic fractures in a Swedish county. Acta Orthop Scand 1992;63:297–300.
11. Boufous S, Finch C, Lord S, et al. The increasing burden of pelvic fractures in older people, New South Wales, Australia. Injury 2005;36:1323–9.
12. Breuil V, Roux CH, Testa J, et al. Outcome of osteoporotic pelvic fractures: an underestimated severity. Survey of 60 cases. Joint Bone Spine 2008;75(5):585–8.
13. Zebaze RM, Ghasem-Zadeh A, Bohte A, et al. Intracortical remodeling and porosity in the distal radius and post-mortem femurs of women: a cross-sectional study. Lancet 2010;375(9727):1729–36.
14. Iundusi R, Scialdoni A, Arduini M, et al. Stress fractures in the elderly: different pathogenetic features compared with young patients. Aging Clin Exp Res 2013;25(Suppl 1):S89–91.
15. Moreno A, Clemente J, Crespo C, et al. Pelvic insufficiency fractures in patients with pelvic irradiation. Int J Radiat Oncol Biol Phys 1999;44(1):61–6.
16. Baxter NN, Habermann EB, Tepper JE, et al. Risk of pelvic fractures in older women following pelvic irradiation. JAMA 2005;294(20):2587–93.
17. Housman D, Savage C, Zelefsky M, et al. Pelvic fracture after radiation therapy for localized prostate cancer: a population-based study. Int J Rad Onc Biol Phys 2010;78(3):S64.
18. Smith D, Zuckerman JD. Bilateral stress fractures of the pubic rami following THA- an unusual case of groin pain. Bull NYU Hosp Jt Dis 2010;68(1):43–5.
19. Kanaji A, Ando K, Nakagawa M, et al. Insufficiency fracture in the medial wall of the acetabulum after total hip arthroplasty. J Arthroplasty 2007;22(5):763–7.
20. Abtahi S, Driessen JHM, Burden AM, et al. Concomitant use of oral glucocorticoids and proton pump inhibitors and risk of osteoporotic fractures among patients with rheumatoid arthritis: a population-based cohort study. Ann Rheum Dis 2020;80:423–31.
21. Gotis-Graham I, McGuigan L, Diamond T, et al. Sacral insufficiency fractures in the elderly. J Bone Joint Surg Br 1994;76:882–6.
22. Sembler-Soles GL, Ferguson TA. Fragility fractures of the pelvis. Curr Rev Musculoskelet Med 2012;5:222–8.
23. Humphrey CA, Maceroli MA. Fragility Fractures Requiring Special Considerations: Pelvic Insufficiency Fractures. Clin Geriatr Med 2014;30:373–86.
24. O'Connor TJ, Cole PA. Pelvic Insufficiency Fractures. Geriatr Orthop Surg Rehabil 2014;5(4):178–90.
25. Finiels H, Finiels PJ, Jacquot JM, et al. Fractures of the sacrum caused by bone insufficiency. Meta-analysis of 508 cases. Presse Med 1997;26(33):1568–73.
26. Judet R, Judet J, Letournel E. Fractures of the acetabulum. Classification and surgical approaches for open reduction. J Bone Joint Surg Am 1964;46A:1615–38.
27. Scheyerer MJ, Osterhoff G, Wehrle S, et al. Detection of posterior pelvic injuries in fractures of the pubic rami. Injury 2012;43(8):1326–9.
28. Grasland A, Pouchot J, Mathieu A, et al. Sacral insufficiency fractures: an easily overlooked cause of back pain in elderly women. Arch Intern Med 1996;156(6):668–74.

29. Cabarrus MC, Ambekar A, Lu Y, et al. MRI and CT of insufficiency fractures of the pelvis and proximal femur. AJR AM J Roentgenol 2008;191(4):995–1001.

30. Henes FO, Nuchtern JV, Groth M, et al. Comparison of diagnostic accuracy of magnetic resonance imaging and multidetector computed tomography in the detection of pelvic fractures. Eur J Radiol 2012;81(9):2337–42.

31. Fujii M, Abe K, Hayashi K, et al. Honda sign and variants in patients suspected of having a sacral insufficiency fracture. Clin Nucl Med 2005;30(3):165–9.

32. Joshi P, Lele V, Gandhi R, et al. Honda sign on 18-FDG PET/CT in a case of lymphoma leading to incidental detection of sacral insufficiency fracture. J Clin Imaging Sci 2012;2:29.

33. Young JW, Burgess AR, Brumback RJ, et al. Pelvic fractures: value of plain radiography in early assessment and management. Radiology 1986;160(2):445–51.

34. Krappinger D, Kammerlander C, Hak DJ, et al. Low-energy osteoporotic pelvic fractures. Arch Orthop Trauma Surg 2010;130(9):1167–75.

35. Tile M. Pelvic ring fractures: should they be fixed? J Bone Joint Surg Br 1988;70:1–12.

36. Rommens PM, Hofmann A. Comprehensive classification of fragility fractures of the pelvic ring: Recommendations for surgical treatment. Injury 2013;44(12):1733–44.

37. Lau TW, Leung F. Occult posterior pelvic ring fractures in elderly patients with osteoporotic pubic rami fractures. J Orthop Surg (Hong Kong) 2010;18:153–7.

38. Letournel E. Acetabular fractures: classification and management. Clin Orthop 1980;151:81–106.

39. Mears DC. Surgical treatment of acetabular fractures in elderly patients with osteoporotic bone. J Am Acad Orthop Surg 1999;7:128–41.

40. Culemann U, Holstein JH, Kohler D, et al. Different stabilization techniques for typical acetabular fractures in the elderly—a biomechanical assessment. Injury 2010;41(4):405–10.

41. Hessmann MH, Nijs S, Rommens PM. [Acetabular fractures in the elderly. Results of a sophisticated treatment concept]. Unfallchirurg 2002;105(10):893–900.

42. Coupe NJ, Patel SN, McVerry S, et al. Fatal haemorrhage following a low-energy fracture of the pubic ramus. J Bone Joint Surg Br 2005;87(9):1275–6.

43. Henning P, Brenner B, Brunner K, et al. Hemodynamic instability following an avulsion of the corona mortis artery secondary to a benign pubic ramus fracture. J Trauma 2007;62(6):E4–17.

44. Loffroy R, Yeguiayan JM, Guiu B, et al. Stable fracture of the pubic rami: a rare cause of life-threatening bleeding from the inferior epigastric artery managed with transcatheter embolization. CJEM 2008;10(4):392–5.

45. Macdonald D, Tollan C, Robertson I, et al. Massive haemorrhage after a low-energy pubic ramus fracture in a 71-year-old woman. Postgrad Med J 2006;82(972):e25.

46. Meyers TJ, Smith WR, Ferrari JD, et al. Avulsion of the pubic branch of the inferior epigastric artery: a cause of hemodynamic instability in minimally displaced fractures of the pubic rami. J Trauma 2000;49(4):750–3.

47. Koval KJ, Aharonhoff GB, Schwartz MC, et al. Pubic rami fracture: a benign pelvic injury? J Orthop Trauma 1997;11(1):7–9.

48. Butterwick D, Papp S, Gofton W, et al. Acetabular fractures in the elderly: evaluation and management. J Bone Joint Surg Am 2015;97(9):758–68.

49. Levine RG, Renard R, Behrens FF, et al. Biomechanical consequences of secondary congruence after both-column acetabular fracture. J Orthop Trauma 2002;16(2):87–91.

50. Gansslen A, Hildebrand F, Krettek C. Conservative treatment of acetabular both column fractures: Does the concept of secondary congruence work? Acta Chir Orthop Traumatol Cech 2012;79(5):411–5.

51. Klotzbuecher CM, Ross PD, Landsman PB, et al. Patients with prior fractures have an increased risk of future fractures: a summary of the literature and statistical synthesis. J Bone Miner Res 2000;15(4):721–39.

52. Larsen ER, Mosekilde L, Foldspang A. Vitamin D and calcium supplementation prevents osteoporotic fractures in elderly community dwelling residents: a pragmatic population-based 3-year intervention study. J Bone Miner Res 2004;19(3):370–8.

53. International Osteoporosis Foundation. Clinicians guide to the prevention and treatment of osteoporosis. Switzerland, 2019.

54. Rodan GA, Fleisch HA. Bisphosphonates: mechanisms of action. J Clin Invest 1996;97(12):2692–6.

55. Black DM, Cummings SR, Karpf DB, et al. Randomized trial of effect of alendronate on risk of fracture in women with existing vertebral fractures. Fracture intervention trial research group. Lancet 1996;348(9041):1535–41.

56. McClung MR, Geusens P, Miller PD, et al. Effect of risedronate on the risk of hip fracture in elderly women. Hip intervention program study. N Engl J Med 2001;344(5):333–40.

57. Harrington JT, Ste-Marie LG, Brandi ML, et al. Risedronate rapidly reduces the risk for nonvertebral fractures in women with postmenopausal osteoporosis. Calcif Tissue Int 2004;74(2):129–35.

58. Liberman UA, Weiss SR, Broll J, et al. Effect of oral alendronate on bone mineral density and the incidence of fractures in postmenopausal osteoporosis. The alendronate phase III osteoporosis treatment study group. N Engl J Med 1995; 333(22):1437–43.

59. Body JJ, Gaich GA, Scheele WH, et al. A randomized double-blind trial to compare the efficacy of teriparatide [recombinant human parathyroid hormone (1-34]] with alendronate in postmenopausal women with osteoporosis. J Clin Endocrinol Metab 2002;87(10):4528–35.

60. Dempster DW, Cosman F, Kurland ES, et al. Effects of daily treatment with parathyroid hormone on bone microarchitecture and turnover in patients with osteoporosis: a paired biopsy study. J Bone Miner Res 2001;16(10):1846–53.

61. Piechl P, Holzer LA, Maier R, et al. Parathyroid hormone 1-84 accelerates fracture-healing in pubic bones of elderly osteoporotic women. J Bone Joint Surg Am 2011;93(17):1583–7.

62. Barei DP, Shafer BL, Beingessner DM, et al. The impact of open reduction internal fixation on acute pain management in unstable pelvic ring injuries. J Trauma 2010;68:949–53.

63. Griffin DR, Starr AJ, Reinert CM, et al. Vertically unstable pelvic fractures fixed with percutaneous iliosacral screws: does posterior injury pattern predict fixation failure? J Orthop Trauma 2006;20(1 Suppl):S30–6.

64. Tabaie SA, Bledsoe JG, Moed BR. Biomechanical comparison of standard iliosacral screw fixation to transsacral locked screw fixation in a type C zone II pelvic fracture model. J Orthop Trauma 2013; 27(9):521–6.

65. Vanderschot P, Kuppers M, Sermon A, et al. Trans-iliac-sacral-iliac-bar procedure to treat insufficiency fractures of the sacrum. Indian J Orthop 2009;43(3):245.

66. Pulley BR, Cotman SB, Fowler TT. Surgical Fixation of Geriatric Sacral U-Type Insufficiency Fractures: A Retrospective Analysis. J Orthop Trauma 2018;32(12):617–22.

67. Hwang JS, Reilly MC, Shaath MK, et al. Safe Zone Quantification of the Third Sacral Segment in Normal and Dysmorphic Sacra. J Orthop Trauma 2018;32(4):178–82.

68. Rommens PM, Graafen M, Arand C, et al. Minimal-invasive stabilization of anterior pelvic ring fractures with retrograde transpubic screws. Injury 2020;51(2):340–6.

69. Mears DC, Velyvis JH. In situ fixation of pelvic nonunions following pathologic and insufficiency fractures. J Bone Joint Surg Am 2002;84-A(5):721–8.

70. Tsiridis E, Upadhyay N, Giannoudis P. Sacral insufficiency fractures: current concepts of management. Osteoporos Int 2006;17(12):1716–25.

71. Mears SC, Sutter EG, Wall SJ, et al. Biomechanical comparison of three methods of sacral fracture fixation in osteoporotic bone. Spine (Phil Pa 1976) 2010;35(10):E392–5.

72. Tjardes T, Paffrath T, Baethis H, et al. Computer assisted percutaneous placement of augmented iliosacral screws: a reasonable alternative to sacroplasty. Spine (Phil PA 1976) 2008;33(13):1497–500.

73. König A, Oberkircher L, Beeres FJP, et al. Cement augmentation of sacroiliac screws in fragility fractures of the pelvic ring- A synopsis and systematic review of the current literature. Injury 2019;50(8): 1411–7.

74. Dehdashti AR, Martin JB, Jean B, et al. PMMA cementoplasty in symptomatic metastatic lesions of the S1 vertebral body. Cadriovasc Intervent Radiol 2000;23(3):235–7.

75. Garant M. Sacroplasty: a new treatment for sacral insufficiency fracture. J Vasc Interv Radiol 2002; 13(12):1265–7.

76. Frey ME, Depalma MJ, Cifu DX, et al. Percutaneous sacroplasty for osteoporotic sacral insufficiency fractures: a prospective, multicenter, observational pilot study. Spine J 2008;8(2): 367–73.

77. Bayley E, Srinivas S, Boszczyk BM. Clinical outcomes of sacroplasty in sacral insufficiency fractures: a review of the literature. Eur Spine J 2009;18(9):1266.

78. Gupta AC, Yoo AJ, Stone J, et al. Percutaneous sacroplasty. J Neurointerv Surg 2012;4(5):385–9.

79. Waites MD, Mears SC, Richards AM, et al. A biomechanical comparison of lateral and posterior approaches to sacroplasty. Spine (Phil Pa 1976) 2008;33(20):E735–8.

80. Tile M. Fractures of the pelvis and acetabulum. 2nd edition. Baltimore: Williams & Wilkins; 1995.

81. Letournel E. The treatment of acetabular fractures through the ilioinguinal approach. Clin Orthop Relat Res 1993;292:62–76.

82. Matta JM. Fractures of the acetabulum: accuracy of reduction and clinical results in patients managed operatively within three weeks after the injury. J Bone Joint Surg Am 1996;78(11): 1632–45.

83. Miller AN, Prasarn ML, Lorich DG, et al. The radiological evaluation of acetabular fractures in the elderly. J Bone Joint Surg Br 2010;92(4):560–4.

84. Gary JL, Lefaivre KA, Gerold F, et al. Survivorship of the native hip joint after percutaneous repair of acetabular fractures in the elderly. Injury 2011; 42(10):1144–51.

85. Starr AJ, Reinert CM, Jones AL. Percutaneous fixation of the columns of the acetabulum: a new technique. J Orthop Trauma 1998;12(1):51–8.

86. Gary JL, VanHal M, Gibbons SD, et al. Functional outcomes in elderly patients with acetabular

fractures treated with minimally invasive reduction and percutaneous fixation. J Orthop Trauma 2012; 26(5):278–83.

87. Anglen JO, Burd TA, Hendricks KJ, et al. The "Gull sign": a harbinger of failure for internal fixation of geriatric acetabular fractures. J Orthop Trauma 2003;17(9):625–34.

88. Laflamme GY, Herbert-Davies J. Direct reduction technique for superomedial dome impaction in geriatric acetabular fractures. J Orthop Trauma 2014;28(2):e39–43.

89. Jeffcoat DM, Carroll EA, Huber FG, et al. Operative treatment of acetabular fractures in an older population through a limited ilioinguinal approach. J Orthop Trauma 2012;26(5):284–9.

90. Daurka JS, Pastides PS, Lewis A, et al. Acetabular fractures in patients aged >55 years: a systematic review of the literature. Bone Joint J 2014;96-B(2): 157–63.

91. Mears DC, Velyvis JH. Acute total hip arthroplasty for selected displaced acetabular fractures: two to twelve-year results. J Bone Joint Surg Am 2002; 84(1):1–9.

92. Mears DC, Shirahama M. Stabilization of an acetabular fracture with cables for acute total hip arthroplasty. J Arthroplasty 1998;13(1):104–7.

93. Mouhsine E, Garofalo R, Borens O, et al. Acute total hip arthroplasty for acetabular fractures in the elderly: 11 patients followed for 2 years. Acta Orthop Scand 2002;73(6):615–8.

94. Herscovici D Jr, Lindvall E, Bolhofner B, et al. The combined hip procedure: open reduction internal fixation combined with total hip arthroplasty for the management of acetabular fractures in the elderly. J Orthop Trauma 2010;24(5):291–6.

95. Lin C, Caron J, Schmidt AH, et al. Functional outcomes after total hip arthroplasty for the acute management of acetabular fractures: 1- to 14-year follow-up. J Orthop Trauma 2015;29(3):151–9.

96. Romness DW, Lewallen DG. Total hip arthroplasty after fracture of the acetabulum. Long-term results. J Bone Joint Surg Br 1990;72(5):761–4.

97. Weber M, Berry DJ, Harmsen WS. Total hip arthroplasty after operative treatment of an acetabular fracture. J Bone Joint Surg Am 1998; 80(9):1295–305.

98. Bellabarba C, Berger RA, Bentley CD, et al. Cementless acetabular reconstruction after acetabular fracture. J Bone Joint Surg Am 2001;83(6):868–76.

99. Hill RM, Robinson CM, Keating JF. Fractures of the pubic rami, epidemiology and 5-year survival. J Bone Joint Surg Br 2001;81-B:1141–4.

100. Bible JE, Wegner A, McClure JM, et al. One-year mortality after acetabular fractures in elderly patients presenting to a level-one trauma center. J Orthop Trauma 2014;28(3):154–9.

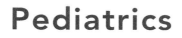

Pediatrics

Osteochondritis Dissecans Lesions of the Pediatric and Adolescent Knee

John Roaten, MD*, Borna Guevel, MA, MB, BChir, MRCS,
Benton Heyworth, MD, Mininder Kocher, MD, MPH

KEYWORDS

- OCD • Pediatric • Adolescent • Cartilage • Osteochondritis dissecans • Knee

KEY POINTS

- Osteochondritis dissecans of the knee is the result of a focal idiopathic alteration of subchondral bone that may result in disruption of the articular cartilage and lead to premature osteoarthritis.
- It has a variable presentation and is mostly a juvenile disease with preadolescent and adolescent age group predilection.
- Diagnosis is based on history, physical examination, and imaging with MRI thought to be essential in diagnosing the stage and stability of the lesion.
- Goals of treatment are to promote subchondral bone healing and preservation of the overlying articular cartilage to prevent fissure, fracture, dissection, and ultimately joint arthritis.
- Treatment can vary from activity modification and observation of natural healing to arthroscopic drilling with or without fixation. Unsalvageable lesions may require arthrotomy, excision and autogenous or allograft osteochondral implantation, or chondral resurfacing techniques.

INTRODUCTION

First described by Franz König[1] in his 1886 classic German article, "Ueber freie Körper in den Gelenken," which translates in English to "On Loose Bodies in the Joint," osteochondritis dissecans (OCD) is primarily a subchondral, subarticular bone disease that can secondarily affect the overlying chondral surface. It has more recently been defined by the ROCK study group,[2] which is composed of high-volume OCD surgeons, musculoskeletal radiologists, physical therapists, and researchers as "a focal, idiopathic alteration of subchondral bone with risk for instability and disruption of adjacent articular cartilage that may result in premature osteoarthritis."[3] The process of disease development must be distinguished from osteochondral fractures that result secondary to a traumatic event that disrupts previously healthy bone and cartilage. Furthermore, it must be recognized that OCD lesions can be acutely disrupted, and features of OCD must be evaluated with history taking and imaging to distinguish them from osteochondral fractures.

Although many joints can be affected, it is most often monoarticular, with the knee being the most common site.

The hallmark of OCD is that symptoms do not always correlate with disease severity. It is an acquired condition with variable presentation, most in its juvenile form, ages 6 to 16 years, and can often be asymptomatic, whereas others may report focal pain or mild vague pain deep in the knee with activities, with variable degrees of joint swelling or mechanical symptoms. It is also reported to be found incidentally on radiographs in patients with knee pain related to other causes.

OCD of the knee is mostly a juvenile disease with preadolescent and adolescent age group

Department of Orthopedic Sports Medicine, Boston Children's Hospital, 300 Longwood Avenue, Boston, MA 02446, USA
* Corresponding author.
E-mail address: john.roaten@childrens.harvard.edu

Orthop Clin N Am 53 (2022) 445–459
https://doi.org/10.1016/j.ocl.2022.05.001
0030-5898/22/© 2022 Elsevier Inc. All rights reserved.

predilection. Although OCD of the knee can present in an adult knee, many investigators believe it to simply be an undiagnosed case or delayed presentation of juvenile OCD.[4] Even still, de novo cases of adult OCD have been reported.[5] Although abnormal bone vascularity is a more common etiologic factor proposed, OCD is still considered by most experts an idiopathic process and likely multifactorial. Konig[1] thought the process to be related to inflammatory changes, whereas multiple other investigators proposed repetitive microtrauma as the inciting event, subsequently leading to subchondral bone contusion and abnormal blood flow and resultant osteonecrosis.[6–9] Along these lines, the theory of OCD development in its classic location in the medial femoral condyle has been reasoned to arise in part from repetitive impingement from a prominent medial tibia spine.[10,11] Other offered causes include single-event macrotrauma,[12] genetic causes,[13] and more recently, a disturbance of secondary ossification process of epiphyseal growth,[14] as evidenced in histologic studies showing formation of uncalcified cartilage within the lesion. Blanke and colleagues suggested instability of the anterior horn of the meniscus as a cause of OCD lesions, and with arthroscopic stabilization of the meniscus, 80% of patients had complete healing of the OCD on MRI at 12 months.[15] Patient-specific biomechanical factors including obesity,[16] lower extremity malalignment,[17] and soft tissue imbalances, as well as metabolic factors such as underlying vitamin D deficiencies have all been implicated by researchers.[18]

The cause of OCD is clearly incompletely understood and likely multifactorial in a rapidly growing pediatric patient.

Goals of treatment are to promote subchondral bone healing and preservation of the overlying articular cartilage and prevention of fissure or fracture, dissection, and ultimately joint arthritis.

Treatment can vary from observation of natural healing, often pursued in younger patients with stable lesions, directed by limitations on impact activities, weight-bearing, and bracing. Although older patients with more advanced lesions are often treated with arthroscopic drilling, with or without fixation and possible bone grafting. Whenever possible, retention of native chondral surface is paramount for joint preservation in salvageable lesions. Ultimately, some unstable and/or unsalvageable lesions require arthrotomy, excision and autogenous or allograft osteochondral implantation, or other chondral resurfacing techniques.

The purpose of this review is to provide a current outline of the epidemiology and anatomy, diagnosis, classification, and staging; discuss nonoperative management strategies; review operative treatment for stable and unstable as well as cartilage resurfacing and salvage procedures for failed OCD fixation and unsalvageable osteochondral defects.

EPIDEMIOLOGY AND ANATOMY

In one of the largest epidemiology studies on OCD of the knee, Kessler and colleagues, reviewing more than 1 million children, concluded the incidence of OCD of the knee in ages 6 to 19 years was 9.5 per 100,000 per year. Gender discrepancies existed, showing in boys the incidence was 15.4 per 100,000 and in girls 3.3 per 100,000.[19] The average age of OCD was 13 years with no reported cases arising in children ages 2 to 5 years. In addition, children ages 12 to 19 years had 3.3 times greater risk of developing OCD of the knee than ages 6 to 11 years. Regarding racial predilection, blacks had the highest odds ratio compared with non-Hispanic whites, Hispanics, Asian and Pacific Islanders, and other ethnicities.[19] Although men seem to have a higher incidence of OCD of the knee compared with women, some investigators have shown a trend of increasing female incidence, relating it to their increasing participation in sports.[5,7]

The knee is the most common location for OCD development, with other less common sites including the ankle and elbow, followed by shoulder and hip.[19]

In the knee, Kessler and colleagues[19] showed 63.6% of OCD lesions develop within the medial femoral condyle, most often in the lateral aspect of the medial femoral condyle in the coronal plane and central or posterior in the sagittal plane. In 32.5%, the lesion developed in the lateral femoral condyle, with these often presenting as larger lesions, at a more advanced stage. Kessler also demonstrated 7.3% of patients from this study had bilateral knee lesions, differing from a prior report by Cooper and colleagues, who calculated 29% of 108 consecutive cases presented with bilateral lesions.[20] Other locations include the patella, lateral femoral trochlea, central femoral trochlea, and lateral tibia plateau, in decreasing order of incidence.[21] There does not seem to be a laterality dominance of OCD development, with similar numbers of left versus right lesions.[22]

DIAGNOSIS, CLASSIFICATION, AND STAGING

Diagnosis of OCD should be on the differential diagnosis in adolescents and teenagers with knee pain and should be diagnosed based on history, physical examination, and radiographs. MRI can be essential in diagnosis but is also critical in determining the stage, and therefore stability, of the lesion. It should therefore be included in the preliminary workup after diagnosis of OCD is made. A visible OCD and bony loose body on a knee radiograph represents an obviously unstable lesion; otherwise, further classification of lesion stability, such as that proposed by Guhl[23] or more recently the ROCK study group, is done at time of arthroscopy.

Cahill further delineated femoral condylar OCD classification based on lesion location on anteroposterior (AP) (medial to lateral zones) and lateral (anterior to posterior) radiographs of the knee.[5]

Clinical presentation of OCD of the knee can be variable in degree of pain or dysfunction and stage of the lesion. OCD can be discovered on radiograph incidentally after unrelated knee injury and, when asymptomatic, may require no intervention, especially if stable and in a location with low joint contact pressures. Often, stable lesions present as vague pain or limping, often free from joint swelling, whereas unstable lesions may present with pain and joint swelling or mechanical symptoms such as locking or catching of the joint with motion, especially if dissection of the progeny fragment from its origin has occurred and a loose body is present. Symptoms at any stage are often amplified by impact activities such as running, jumping, and sports participation.

Physical examination too can vary from point tenderness over the lesion with trochlear lesions palpated in knee extended and those more condylar and posterior palpated with deeper degrees of knee flexion. Pain from trochlear and patellar lesions may be elicited by compression of the patellofemoral joint. The presence of joint effusion should be examined, as this may represent an unstable OCD lesion. This effusion may be from a reactive synovitis, a dialysate of plasma in more chronically evolving lesions, and possibly frank hemarthrosis after acute shear injuries.

Imaging

Common imaging studies that are used for diagnosis and staging of OCD consist of radiographs and MRI. Bone scintigraphy and computed tomography scans are less commonly used due to exposure to radiation concerns in the pediatric population but can be useful in characterizing lesions and the healing in response to treatment. The common knee radiographic series to evaluate OCD are the AP, lateral, sunrise, and notch views, the latter being particularly helpful in viewing the more posterior femoral condyle, which is a common area for OCD in the knee. More anterior condylar lesions are seen more clearly on the AP view. Discretion must be given to distinguish anatomic normal variants including secondary ossification centers near the posterior condyles and changes seen in the normally developing epiphyseal bone in children younger than 6 years and rapidly growing adolescents, such as boys younger than 13 years and girls younger than 11 years. Often in this age group, the subchondral bone deep to the thick epiphyseal cartilage can seem corrugated with irregular borders or as islands of bone. Assessment of features seen on T2-weighted MRI such as hyperintense bone marrow edema adjacent to the area of subchondral bone in question may facilitate distinction of normal development from OCD lesions.

Although radiographic assessment of healing has been shown to be suboptimal,[24] follow-up surveillance most commonly is done with serial radiographs, whereas repeat MRI may be necessary if response to treatment suggests poor healing or progression of the lesion is evident.

After diagnosis has been made, pretreatment MRI of the lesion should be completed to most accurately characterize and appropriately stage the lesion based on the features seen within the subchondral bone and status of the adjacent cartilage. Characteristics more readily apparent on MRI are the extent of subchondral bone enhancement, architectural features such as size and depth of the lesion, and presence of cystic changes within the subchondral bone that may lend to increasing degrees of lesion instability. Although there are multiple classification systems described, the most commonly applied MRI-based classification system was developed by Hefti and colleagues in 1999[25] (Fig. 1). This system divides OCD lesions into progressive stages of severity, 1 through 5, based on features in the MRI. However, an assortment of additional criteria may be considered beyond those articulated by Hefti and colleagues For example, stable lesions (Hefti stages 1 and 2) should be distinguished from unstable lesions (Hefti 3–5) by the presence of nondisrupted lesional cartilage to the adjacent cartilage and the continuity of the subchondral

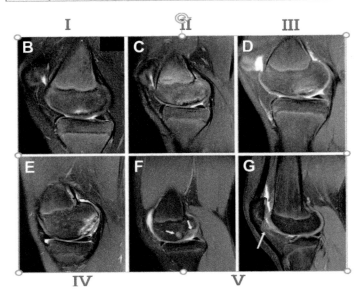

Stage	**Explanation**
1	Signal change in subchondral bone without clear lesion margins
2	Clear lesion margins, but without clear linear high signal (fluid-like) pattern signal between fragment and adjacent bone
3	Clear linear high signal (fluid-like) pattern signal between some areas of lesion and adjacent bone, but not surrounding entire fragment (i.e. not seen in all sequences/images involving lesion)
4	Clear linear high signal (fluid-like) pattern signal between entire in-situ fragment and adjacent bone (i.e. seen in all sequences/images involving lesion)
5	Detached fragment/loose body

Fig. 1. Hefti classification of osteochondritis dissecans (OCD) lesions. (A) Describing the staging of OCD lesions based on MRI findings. (B–F) Sagittal T2-weighted MRI scans demonstrating the features of condylar. Hefti stage 1 (see Fig. 1B), stage 2 (C), stage 3 (D), stage 4 (E), and stage 5 (F) lesions. The stage 5 lesion in F is associated with an osteochondral defect (*right arrow*) and a subchondral cyst (*left arrow*). (G) Different sagittal T2-weighted MRI scan of the knee in the same patient shown in F, demonstrating a loose OCD fragment (*arrow*). ([A] *Adapted from* Table 1 of Hefti, F., et al., Osteochondritis dissecans: a multicenter study of the European Pediatric Orthopedic Society. Journal of Pediatric Orthopedics, 1999. 8(4):p. 231-245; and [B] *From* Heyworth BE, Kocher MS. Osteochondritis Dissecans of the Knee. *JBJS Rev.* Jul 2015;3(7) https://doi.org/10.2106/jbjs.Rvw.N.00095; with permission.)

bone plate. In these more stable type of in situ lesions, it should follow that there will be a paucity of high-intensity fluidlike signal behind the lesion or deep to the chondral surface, lending a lower likelihood that the cartilage has been breached. Unstable features include loss of a low signal bone plate continuity immediately below the cartilage, obvious chondral breech, and varying degrees of fluid signal deep to the lesion, deep fissuring, or delamination of overlying cartilage suggesting imminent breach of fluid deep to the lesion, if not already present. Further degrees of unstable features include elongated, linear signal surrounding the entire progeny bone fragment that are hyperintense fluidlike signal or hyper-intense cystlike lesions (CLLs).

More recently, Hussain and colleagues proposed an MRI-based, 3-group approach to staging and diagnosis of knee OCD and compared the reliability of that approach with that of the more complex (5-group) Hefti classification.[26] In doing so, they graded lesions as follows. Grade 1 is characterized by intact cartilage

without a breach. Grade 2 cartilage is breech but the lesion is stable and nondisplaced. In grade 3, they included all lesions with cartilage breach and some degree of instability and deemed unstable by presence of a fluid signal between the parent and progeny bone fragment, hinged lesion with partial displacement, and lesions that are fully displaced. Their results suggested a near-perfect intrarater reliability for their novel 3-group classification system of 98% compared with Hefti intrarater reliability of 88%. By simplifying the grouping and combining the groups included in grade 3 lesions, it may be more reliable for surgeons to identify unstable lesions that require fixation versus drilling alone. They concluded that subsequent studies on validation and clinical utility are needed.

Regardless of the classifications systems, assessment for the presence of symptoms, chondral integrity and lesion stability, and degree of displacement are vital to guide treatment. These features can be ascertained on MRI alone. However, arthroscopic assessment of these factors should further guide treatment with the surgeon being prepared for multimodal strategies to obtain stability, restore biology, and promote healing.

TREATMENT

Nonoperative Treatment

Nonoperative treatment is the preferred primary approach in stable OCD lesions of the knee in skeletally immature patients.[7,27] Type of nonsurgical treatment and length of treatment have been debated but most investigators agree a period of 3 months, regardless of modality, be allowed to assess degree of and therefore potential for healing. Rates of healing vary greatly in the literature for nonsurgical treatment of juvenile osteochondritis dissecans (JOCD).

Options for treatment include immobilization, limited weight-bearing, and activity restrictions with the American Academy of Orthopaedic Surgeons guidelines in 2010 unable to recommend for or against any particular method.[28]

In 1952, van Demark reported reasonable revascularization of 2 children treated for knee OCD when restricted weight-bearing was used for a minimum of 6 months.[29] By 1985, Cahill argued that because JOCD was a fracture, any method of fracture treatment should be used, except joint immobilization.[30] Other investigators have agreed that immobilization is detrimental to chondrocyte health and contributes to quadriceps atrophy and knee stiffness.[9,31] Full immobilization seems to have fallen out of favor in more contemporary treatment algorithms. Gauzy and colleagues demonstrated healing of 30 of 31 knees in 24 children, mean age 11.4 years, with a protocol of activity modification alone, until the children were pain-free.[32] Fullick and colleagues, in a comparative study, showed more promise with the use of an unloader brace rather than crutches or activity modification alone.[27]

Although it has been shown that younger patient with stable lesions healed more frequently, there are reported higher rates of failure of JOCD lesions to heal with nonsurgical treatment.

Atypical lesion location such as those in the non–weight-bearing portion of the lateral femoral condyle are less likely to heal with nonop treatment, as they are 15 times more likely to be unstable compared with lesion on the medial femoral condyle, as shown by Samora and colleagues.[33] This evidence could serve as guidance when counseling patient and families and may be an indication for pursuing immediate or earlier surgical treatment.

In a retrospective cross-sectional study by Krause and colleagues, after 6 months of nonop treatment of stable JOCDs with activity restrictions alone and until a pain-free state was reached, 67% of 76 JOCD lesions showed no sign of progression toward healing or increased signs of instability.[34] Assessing for predictors of healing in that study, the investigators showed, in a multivariate logistic regression model used to predict healing at 12 months, that the presence of a cystlike lesion 2.6 mm provided only 39% probability of healing. If no CLL was present deep to the subchondral plate, then probability increased to 80%. After 12 months, if no healing was evident or progression observed, surgery was undertaken; this also serves to highlight the difficulty in treating JOCD, as often families do not wish to undergo 12 months of activity restrictions if an earlier surgery can return them to activities sooner.

Other studies have shown greater than or equal to 50% healing success with nonop treatment.[35–37] Wall and colleagues[29] in a study of skeletally immature patient who received 6 months of nonop treatment demonstrated 66% healing of 47 lesions. A nomogram was created from a logistic regression model suggesting larger lesion surface area and presence of mechanical symptoms such as giving-way, clicking, or locking to be predictive of poor healing rates, whereas younger age was not.

Larger scale, comparative, controlled trials would be needed to better elucidate best nonoperative strategies for the treatment of JOCD of the knee.

OPERATIVE TREATMENT OF STABLE OSTEOCHONDRITIS DISSECANS

Failed nonop treatment (3–6 months) or lesions with poor healing potential such as those with closed peri-genu physes in the skeletally mature adolescents and teens are indications for surgical treatment. Failed nonop treatment can be defined as persistent symptoms (pain, effusion, or mechanical symptoms) or failure of the OCD lesion to show progression toward healing on serial radiographs or MRI scans. Masquijo and Kothari[22] proposed an algorithm for treatment based on stability of the lesion and integrity of the articular surface (Fig. 2). The first line of surgical treatment of stable OCD lesions is drilling of the lesion. The 2 principal techniques for condylar drilling include transarticular drilling and retroarticular drilling. Transarticular drilling is performed across the articular surface in a retrograde fashion with arthroscopic guidance, whereas retroarticular drilling is drilling through nonarticular epiphyseal bone in an antegrade

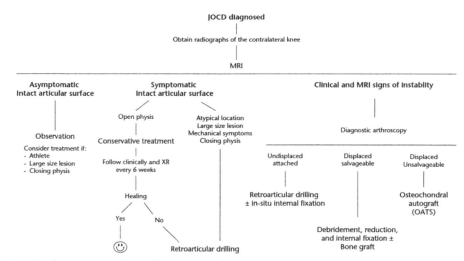

Fig. 2. Algorithm for treatment of juvenile osteochondritis dissecans (JOCD). (*From* Masquijo J, Kothari A. Juvenile osteochondritis dissecans (JOCD) of the knee: current concepts review. *EFORT Open Rev.* May 2019;4(5):201–212. https://doi.org/10.1302/2058-5241.4.180079; with permission.)

fashion into the lesion and uses fluoroscopic, electromagnetic,[38] or open MRI[38] guidance. Other techniques have been offered such as intercondylar notch drilling[39] as to minimize disruption of intact articular surface. All share a common principal of using a Kirschner wire (K wire) to penetrate and disrupt the sclerotic margins of the OCD lesion to establish tunnels between the healthy, adjacent cancellous bone and the diseased subchondral bone of the lesion. The intention is to establish a conduit for bleeding and thus healing factors and ossification of the lesion. Healing with this treatment on average takes 4 to 6 months in most series.[36,40–44] All drilling techniques are combined with diagnostic arthroscopy to evaluate the lesion and palpate its degree of stability, inspecting for gross fragment motion or chondral fissures at its margin. Varying degrees of stability may be encountered with this assessment and can further guide decision-making if fixation of the lesion may also be needed.

Multiple studies have demonstrated excellent healing rates with drilling for stable lesions. Earlier reports by Bradley and Dandy, using the transarticular technique, reported healing in 9 of 11 children within 12 months postoperatively.[45] Other investigators have reported excellent healing rates with this technique, with poorer results occurring in patients with chondral fissuring and closed distal femur physes, advancing the concept that additional fixation should be considered when evidence of lesion instability is present, particularly for more skeletally mature patients.[40,46,47]

Kocher and colleagues, in a large series of transarticular OCD drilling of 30 knees in patients 8.5 years to 16.1 years (average 12.3 years) who had failed nonop treatment for at least 6 months, showed healing of all lesions at an average of 4.4 months, with improvement of Lysholm score from 58 to 93.[41]

Lee and Mercurio[48] in a report on 5 lesions, one of which was in the lateral femoral condyle and another in the talus, provided the first description of outcomes using the retroarticular technique and included bone grafting of the lesion. All lesions healed by 6 months, with one patient remaining partially symptomatic at 6 months but with significant improvement.

Larger series in skeletally immature patients have shown a majority healing response of OCD lesions with resolution of symptoms by Donaldson and Wojtys,[49] Adachi and colleagues,[50] and Ojala and colleagues.[51]

Edmonds and colleagues showed a return to activities at 2.8 months after retroarticular drilling in all 59 children treated with this technique for JOCD of the knee.[42] Seventy percent of the lesions in this study showed radiographic healing at average time of 11.9 months.

Relative advantages of transarticular drilling are that it is technically simpler with no need for fluoroscopy and allows for direct visualization of the drilling passes and their spacing relative the size and margins of the lesion. There are some unknown concerns, however, as to the long-term implications of disrupting the articular chondral surface, which can be lessened by a degree by first pressing the tip of the wire through the chondral surface to underlying bone before drilling, which is anticipated to leave more linear rather than circular distortion of the articular continuity. With this technique, the chondral surface would heal with fibrocartilage, rather than hyaline cartilage. Advantages of the retroarticular technique are that it avoids disruption of intact articular cartilage, thereby allowing for greater number of passes with a larger wire and also the potential for cannulated bone grafting. In a systematic review, Gunton and colleagues[44] showed no statistically significant difference in the 2 techniques in terms of patient outcomes. Retroarticular drilling led to radiographic healing of 86% of 111 lesions at a mean time of 5.6 months, whereas transarticular drilling resulted in healing of 91% of 94 lesions at 4.5 months.

OPERATIVE TREATMENT OF UNSTABLE OSTEOCHONDRITIS DISSECANS

For stable lesions that have failed drilling procedures and for unstable lesions that remain in situ, fixation of the lesions is generally the next step in treatment. Instability of the lesion can range from in situ lesions with micro- or macro-instability and gross instability with dissection and loose body. Adjuvant techniques often included with fixation are drilling of the lesion and bone grafting deep to the progeny fragment; this might be done arthroscopically or via parapatellar arthrotomy, with autogenous or allograft bone, and with variable types of fixation implants.[52] All techniques use the concepts of restoring the articular surface, use of rigid fixation, enhancement of the vascularity to the osseous portions of the lesion, and early joint mobilization.[30]

If subchondral bone access can be obtained, for example, in a trap door lesions, the fibrous or necrotic bone deep to the lesion can be excised and bone graft material can fill the void, providing structure and biology critical to healing.

There are a variety of fixation implants available (Table 1). In 1990, in a series of 17 skeletally immature patients, Anderson and colleagues described fixation with one or multiple K wires combined with debridement and bone grafting.[4] Sixteen of the seventeen lesions were healed at an average of 8 months. The use of K wires,

Table 1
Surgical methods for the treatment of unstable knee osteochondritis dissecans

| Method | Methods of Internal Fixation for Useable OCD of the Knee | |
	Advantages	Disadvantages
Metallic devices		
Kirschner wire	Cost, availability, ease of placement	Exit site morbidity, lack of compression, need for removal, bending
Cannulated screws	Good fixation, multiple size options	Increase damage to articular surface from screw head, need for removal, backing out
Variable-pitch screws	Good fixation, "headless" countersinking	Possible need for removal
Bioabsorbable devices		
Pins/rods/pins	Size, planes of fixation, less stress shielding	Breakage, loss of fixation, foreign body immune response
Screws	Good fixation, obviate hardware removal	Breakage, loss of fixation, foreign-body immune
Biological devices		
Mosaicplasty	Native tissue, graft across interface, obviate hardware removal	Possible donor site fracture, bone peg loosening, technically more challenging
Bone sticks	Native tissue, graft across interface, obviate hardware removal	Donor site morbidity, loss of fixation, technique in its infancy technically more challenging

Nathan L. Grimm, Christopher K. Ewing, Theodore J. Ganley, The Knee: Internal Fixation Techniques for Osteochondritis Dissecans, Clinics in Sports Medicine, 33(2), 2014, 313–319, https://doi.org/10.1016/j.csm.2013.12.001.

however, has fallen out of favor due to their lack of compressive forces, tendency to bend, and possibility of migration. As an alternative, the use of screw fixation has become more popular, given the lower profile, rigid fixation with compressive forces provided. Different screw options have evolved including small, solid, flat-head screws (often countersunk deep to the chondral surface), variable pitch screws,[53–55] and cannulated, partially threaded screws.[56] The goal of solid fixation and minimizing implant-related complications, such as potential for loosening and migration, prominence to the chondral surface and the chondral wear that can then ensue, should be considered when choosing fixation of OCD lesions.

Healing rates with variable pitch and cannulated screws have been reported to be 90% with near-normal functional knee scores.[53–56]

Most metallic screws have the potential to become prominent if lesion healing leads to chondral settling or if lesions fail to heal and progress. Smaller or fragmented progeny bone fragments make the use of metallic screws less desirable, as it is difficult to bury the implant and achieve intended compression and rigid fixation. It remains somewhat controversial whether such implants require routine removal, unless abrasion on the opposing surface becomes apparent, in which case it is required. Because of this concern and the desire to avoid further surgery after fixation of OCD lesions, recently, implants made from bioabsorbable materials, such a polylactide (PLA) and polyglycolide (PGA), are being used with greater frequency. Variable descriptive terms have been assigned to these types of implants, including pins, rods, tacks, nails, darts, and screws.

Another advantage of nonmetal, bioabsorbable implants are that they generate less implant-related artifact if repeat MRI is needed after fixation.

Disadvantages documented in case reports of bioabsorbable implants are sterile abscess formation, synovitic reactions to the foreign material, implant breakage during or after insertion, and migration.[57–60] PGA has been reported to degrade by 3 months after implantation potentially rendering the lesion unstable if not healed by that time, which we know it often to be 6 months or greater. PLA degrades as much as 6 years after implantation and may pose a threat to the opposing chondral surface if lesion settling or implant migration were to occur. More recent advances combine the 2 substances to maximize benefits of fixation while minimizing each implant's risk of complications.[61]

Other reports have shown high healing rates, low implant-related complications, and improved knee functional scores with the use of bioabsorbable implants.[61,62]

Kocher and colleagues reported on 26 skeletally immature knee OCD lesions that underwent fixation of instability with one or more of 4 different fixation methods: variable pitch screws (n = 11); bioabsorbable tacks (n = 10); partially threaded, cannulated screws (n = 3); or bioabsorbable pins (n = 3). Healing occurred in 84.6% (22 lesions) at an average of 6 months and mean functional knee scores of 80% to 85% with no significant difference according to lesion location, stage, and fixation method.[63] Tabaddor and colleagues reported no implant-related complication using bioabsorbable implants used for fixation of 24 unstable OCD lesions with healing rates in 16 or 17 lesions based on postoperative MRI and in 22 of 24 based on postoperative radiographs.[61]

Both metal and bioabsorbable implant length must be accounted for during implantation to avoid injury to the distal femur physis, which can be as shallow as 20 to 25 mm from the articular surface in some locations.[64]

Autogenous purely osseous or osteochondral bone pegs or bone sticks is a category of stabilization techniques that has also been performed as an alternative to implant fixation with good results. Navarro and colleagues[65] and Slough and colleagues[66] in retrospective series using bone stick fixation reported satisfactory results in 91% of 11 patients at 4-year follow-up and 80% of 10 patients at 2.9-year follow-up, respectively.

CARTILAGE RESURFACING AND SALVAGE TECHNIQUES

Chondral resurfacing and salvage procedures are most commonly done after failed fixation surgery of unstable OCD lesions or residual defects from dissection of OCD lesions with loose fragments that are unsalvageable. Because this is often encountered after attempted fixation of OCD fragments, the chondral surface or underlying bone fragment often is degenerated, macerated, fragmented, or otherwise in such poor condition that fixation is not possible or healing rate is expected to be very low (Fig. 3). Such procedures often are considered as an index procedure for chronically dissected OCD lesions with a residual defect.

Although reports exist showing good healing of Hefti stage V lesions after fixation,[63] lesions that dissect greater than 6 to 12 weeks from attempted

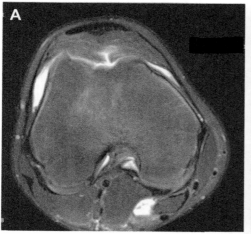
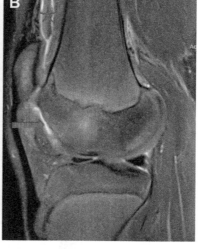

13 yr old male, large trochlea OCD – chronic, unsalvageable

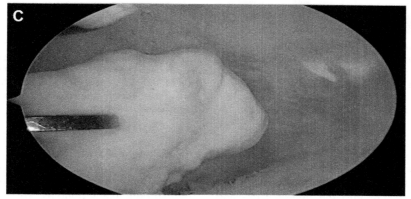

Fig. 3. Example of chronic loose body from a trochlear OCD that had no bone on the undersurface, irregular borders, and macerated edges and had enlarged due to synovial fluid intravasation (A–C). Red star indicates a large osteochondral loose body in the suprapatellar pouch and the red arrow indicates the origin of the loose body and residual defect on the lateral trochlea of the femur.

fixation may have detrimentally necrotic or sclerotic changes to the progeny bone and/or there has been an increase in size of the progeny fragment due to synovial fluid intravasation that may substantially decrease the chances of successful fixation. In these circumstances or those after failed fixation or intralesional degeneration such that the fragment is incongruous, more advanced cartilage salvage techniques are often used (Fig. 4). These techniques include single autogenous osteochondral plug transfer or multiple plugs (mosaicplasty), osteochondral allograft transplantation, or autogenous cultured chondrocyte implantation. The timing and the degree to which a young patient must be symptomatic before undergoing these more involved techniques is variable and controversial. In a long-term follow-up study by Anderson and colleagues[67] poor results were

seen in patients who underwent OCD fragment excision alone, highlighting the importance of more aggressive resurfacing procedures for unsalvageable lesions before the onset of degenerative changes. It has also been noted in multiple studies that younger patients who undergo these salvage procedures for unsalvageable OCD lesions have better outcomes than their older counterparts.[68,69] Moreover, unaddressed OCD defects can be associated with meniscus tears, especially those lesions located on the tibia plateau.[70]

AUTOLOGOUS CHONDROCYTE IMPLANTATION

Autogenous chondrocyte transplantation (ACI) is a 2-stage technique where a cartilage biopsy is obtained from nonarticulating area often

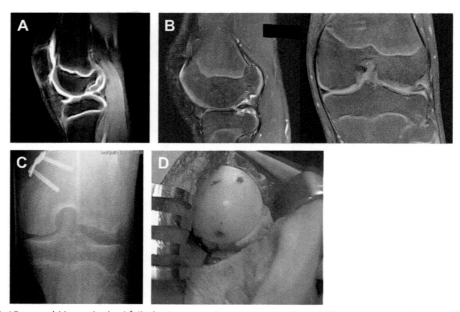

Fig. 4. A 15-year-old boy who had failed prior operative attempts such as drilling, autogenous bone grafting, and fixation. He was indicated for an osteochondral allograft due to the size of the lesion and poor containment. (A) Initial sagittal plane MRI with high signal intensity deep to the progeny fragment indicating lesion instability. Initial treatment was autogenous bone grafting, drilling, and internal fixation. (B) Coronal and sagittal MRI before osteochondral allograft implantation. (C) AP radiograph demonstrating the lateral femoral condyle lesion and previously placed guided growth implant. (D) Osteochondral allograft implant after fixation.

within the notch or superior, peripheral condyles of the femur, which is then grown ex vivo and implanted at an interval of growth no sooner than 6 weeks later into the defect. First- and second-generation ACO is done by placing a patch (periosteal—Gen I, or bovine—Gen II) over the lesion and injecting culture chondrocytes deep to this graft. Third-generation technique involves matrix-induced culture growth of the chondrocytes (MACI), in which the chondrocytes are grown on a collagen matrix and implanted in this manner, obviating graft suture and injection (Fig. 5). At implantation, the lesion to receive the implant is debrided sharply at its periphery and deep to the calcified cartilage layer, hemostasis is achieved, and the MACI implant is placed into the defect and then glued (fibrin) in place. In Gen I technique, a periosteum patch is used, and it is important to ensure the cambium layer of the patch is placed on the deep surface. Suture fixation should ensure a water-tight seal, which can be tested with saline injection before chondrocyte culture injection.

Multiple studies looking at the outcomes of ACI in adolescent patients exist. Most recently, Carey and colleagues[71] in a 10- to 25-year follow-up study with a mean follow-up of 19 years and average follow-up age of 43 years,

of ACI done for unsalvageable OCD lesions done between 1990 and 2005, showed that although most of the patients underwent a second surgery (many done as "second look" procedures as part of study protocol), when defining failure as revision of the ACI graft or joint arthroplasty, the survivorship of ACI for OCD was 87% at 10 years, 85% at 15 years, 82% at 20 years. Years prior, Macmull and colleagues[72] demonstrated 84% good or excellent results at 5.5 years in 31 adolescent patients with a mean age of 16.3 years. Although some feel ACI is limited to purely chondral lesions with minimal bone loss, it has been applied with good results in OCD lesions with depths greater than or equal to 8 mm, using a bilayer collagen membrane technique (sandwich technique).[73,74] This technique involves placing morselized cancellous bone graft to fill the defect that is covered with a collagen membrane, superficial to which the cultured chondrocytes are placed and in turn covered with a second collagen membrane, creating the ACI sandwich. Minas and colleagues[75] evaluated the outcomes of this sandwich technique of ACI combined with autogenous bone grafting in 24 patients from 2001 to 2013 to a historical control group that underwent autogenous bone grafting alone

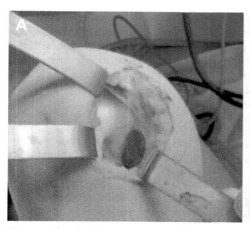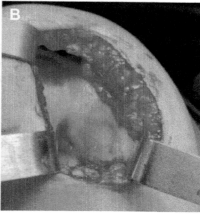

Fig. 5. A 14-year-old girl with a prior loose body removal, drilling procedure of a medial femoral condylar OCD, and cartilage biopsy. She was indicated for matrix-induced autogenous chondrocyte implantation. (A) After templated resection of the lesion. (B) After tourniquet deflation to ensure subchondral hemostasis and MACI implantation.

from 1995 to 2002. The procedure was done by a single surgeon for symptomatic lesions greater than 8 mm. The groups were matched in terms of age, sex, side of the operated knee, body mass index, lesion type, lesion size, lesion depth, lesion location, or the need for realignment osteotomy. They showed a 62% failure rate in the ABG alone group versus 13% in the ACI sandwich group.

OSTEOCHONDRAL AUTOGRAFT TRANSFER SYSTEM

Mosaicplasty techniques, including the osteochondral autograft transfer system (OATS; Arthrex, Naples, Florida), are often used for contained, smaller (2.5 cm sq or smaller) lesions. This system provides transfer of both cartilage and subchondral bone from areas of the knee that do not articulate, often from the lateral femoral condyle lateral to the trochlea and anterior to the articulation with the tibia at its meniscal margin. Lesions are indicated for this if they are not so large that 1 or 2 autogenous plugs are adequate to fill the lesion without compromising the donor site and infringing on its articulating boundaries, although the contralateral knee can provide additional graft options. It has been shown that mosaicplasty may be a better long-term solution for such lesions compared with microfracture alone. Gudas and colleagues[76] demonstrated this in a study of 50 adolescent and teenage JOCD lesions of the femoral condyle treated in a randomized method to either microfracture or OATS. They found good or excellent results in both groups

at 1 year in terms of subjective and objective outcomes but reassessment at beyond 4 years showed the OATS group to maintain 83% excellent results, whereas the microfracture group declined to 63%. In addition, there were 41% failures in the microfracture group and none in the OATS group, with a direct correlation between defect size and poor outcome in the microfracture group that was not observed in the OATS group, showing that even with larger lesions, OATS provided better outcomes. Furthermore, the patients in the microfracture group returned to their preinjury level 14% of the time at 4.2 years, whereas those in the OATS group did so at 81%.

FRESH CADAVERIC OSTEOCHONDRAL ALLOGRAFT

An alternative to mosaicplasty, for larger, uncontained lesions, is the use of osteochondral allograft transplantation that has been developed with promising success; this involves the procurement of fresh (nonfrozen) allograft bulk tissue donors, such as an entire femoral condyle from which a custom-sized graft can be obtained and implantation into a defect, providing both the chondral resurface and the supportive subchondral bone (see Fig. 4). The advantages of this approach avoid the donor site morbidity seen with mosaicplasty and the ability to address larger lesions with a single operation. There remains, however, a concern regarding long-term maintenance of graft incorporation and the phenomenon of creep substitution with the use of these graft options.

Lyon and colleagues[77] reported on the use of fresh osteochondral allograft transplantations in 11 children, average age 15.2 years, with a mean follow-up of 2 years, in which all grafts achieved radiographic incorporation with a return to sport activities between 9 and 12 months post-operatively. Murphy and colleagues[78] reported in a larger series of 43 pediatric and adolescent knees that underwent this procedure, average age 16 years, that graft survivorship was 90% at 10 years with good functional scores. In that study, however, only 60% of all procedures were done for OCD, and of those patients, 35% underwent secondary surgery with patients with OCD representing 4 of the 5 allograft revision procedures done. These revisions were done at an average of 2.7 years after the index procedure.

More recently, in perhaps one of the largest studies to date, Daud and colleagues[68] reported on 244 patients between 1972 and 2018 who underwent fresh cadaveric osteochondral allograft (FOCA) for unsalvageable knee OCDs. Mean patient age was 37.8 years (range 10–75 years) and mean follow-up was 9 years (range 1.0–29.8 years). With survivorship as the primary outcome, failure was defined as conversion to total knee arthroplasty, revision allograft or graft removal, knee fusion, and amputation. Measured secondary outcomes were the functional modified Hospital for Special Surgery Score (mHSS) and radiographic assessment of arthritis using the Kellgren-Lawrence grading scale. Graft survivorship was evaluated at 5-year intervals from 5 to 30 years, and a stepwise decline was noted (insert graph with results). Thirty-eight percent (93 grafts) resulted in failure at an average of 11 years (0.5–38 years), and the mean mHSS score improved significantly, from 68.7 (range, 19–91) preoperatively to 80.3 (range, 52–100) at the time of the latest follow-up. Multivariate analysis revealed that graft location (ie, medial-sided or multiple grafts) and increased age were significantly negatively associated with survival. Ten-year survival was greater than 80% in patients younger than 50 years but less than 40% in patients older than 60 years.

Leon and colleagues[69] also showed promising results of FOCA in a similar patient population (average age 28 years) when combined with realignment osteotomy and found that persistent postoperative malalignment occurred more frequently in failed grafts (28.6% vs 4.3%; $P = .023$) and was a risk factor for graft failure, highlighting the need to identify and treat malalignment if FOCA is being considered.

Although several techniques seem to be feasible as salvage options for unsalvageable OCD lesions, one theoretic advantage of ACI as an index procedure is that OATS and osteochondral allograft transplants still remain a viable secondary option in the setting of failed ACI, whereas the reverse is less likely to be true.

SUMMARY

Symptomatic knee OCD lesions in the pediatric and adolescent population are an increasingly common presentation and should be considered when a young patient presents with knee pain. Treatment varies depending on the history, examination, and lesion type (size, site, stability). Nonoperative management is the first line of treatment of stable OCD lesions. For unstable OCD lesions operative management in the form of fixation is indicated. Should fixation fail salvage treatment options such as ACI or OATS are available but further multicenter research in these techniques are needed to determine the preferred treatment option.

CLINICS CARE POINTS

- It is important to assess for features of OCD in history taking, such as a previous pain deep in the knee with activities or joint swelling and mechanical symptoms, to distinguish them from osteochondral fractures.

- Physical examination in symptomatic patient reveals point tenderness at point of lesion with pain from trochlear and patellar lesions elicited by compression of the patellofemoral joint. The presence of a joint effusion may represent an unstable OCD lesion.

- MRI in addition to knee radiographs is an important aspect of imaging workup and helps determine stage and stability. Notch view knee radiographs are particularly helpful in viewing the posterior femoral condyle, which is a common area for OCD in the knee.

- Nonoperative treatment, such as partial weight-bearing and activity modification, is the primary approach in stable OCD lesions of the knee in skeletally immature patients, with a minimum of 3 months of observation of healing required before deciding on any further intervention.

- Failure of nonoperative treatment is defined as persistent symptoms (pain, effusion, or mechanical symptoms) or failure of the OCD lesion to progress toward healing on imaging.

- Failed nonoperative treatment or lesions with poor healing potential in skeletally mature adolescents and teens are indications for surgical treatment. The first line of treatment is drilling with a K wire to disrupt the margins of the OCD lesion and establish tunnels with healthy, adjacent cancellous bone. Healing takes on average 4 to 6 months.

- For stable lesions that have failed drilling procedures and for unstable lesions, operative fixation of the lesions is generally the next step in treatment.

- Should fixation fail then chondral resurfacing and salvage procedures such as osteochondral allograft transplantation are considered.

DISCLOSURE

J. Roaten: nothing to disclose. B. Guevel: nothing to disclose. B. Heyworth: has received other financial or material support from AlloSource and Vericel Corp and education and hospitality payments from Kairos Surgical and Arthrex; M. Kocher: has received consulting fees from Smith & Nephew, Ossur, OrthoPediatrics, and Best Doctors and royalties from OrthoPediatrics.

REFERENCES

1. König F. The classic: On loose bodies in the joint. 1887. Clin Orthop Relat Res 2013;471(4):1107–15.
2. Edmonds EW, Polousky J. A review of knowledge in osteochondritis dissecans: 123 years of minimal evolution from König to the ROCK study group. Clin Orthop Relat Res 2013;471(4):1118–26.
3. Edmonds EW, Shea KG. Osteochondritis dissecans: editorial comment. Clin Orthop Relat Res 2013;471(4):1105–6.
4. Anderson AF, Lipscomb AB, Coulam C. Antegrade curettage, bone grafting and pinning of osteochondritis dissecans in the skeletally mature knee. Am J Sports Med 1990;18(3):254–61.
5. Cahill BR. Osteochondritis dissecans of the knee: treatment of juvenile and adult forms. J Am Acad Orthop Surg 1995;3(4):237–47.
6. Shea KG, Jacobs JC Jr, Carey JL, et al. Osteochondritis dissecans knee histology studies have variable findings and theories of etiology. Clin Orthop Relat Res 2013;471(4):1127–36.
7. Kocher MS, Tucker R, Ganley TJ, et al. Management of osteochondritis dissecans of the knee: current concepts review. Am J Sports Med 2006;34(7):1181–91.
8. HAT F. Osteo-chondritis dissecans. Br J Surg 1933;21:67–82.
9. Smillie IS. Treatment of osteochondritis dissecans. J Bone Joint Surg Br 1957;39-b(2):248–60.
10. Cavaignac E, Perroncel G, Thépaut M, et al. Relationship between tibial spine size and the occurrence of osteochondritis dissecans: an argument in favour of the impingement theory. Knee Surg Sports Traumatol Arthrosc 2017;25(8):2442–6.
11. Chow RM, Guzman MS, Dao Q. Intercondylar notch width as a risk factor for medial femoral condyle osteochondritis dissecans in skeletally immature patients. J Pediatr Orthop 2016;36(6):640–4.
12. Shea KG, Jacobs JC Jr, Grimm NL, et al. Osteochondritis dissecans development after bone contusion of the knee in the skeletally immature: a case series. Knee Surg Sports Traumatol Arthrosc 2013;21(2):403–7.
13. Mubarak SJ, Carroll NC. Familial osteochondritis dissecans of the knee. Clin Orthop Relat Res 1979;140:131–6.
14. Laor T, Zbojniewicz AM, Eismann EA, et al. Juvenile osteochondritis dissecans: is it a growth disturbance of the secondary physis of the epiphysis? AJR Am J Roentgenol 2012;199(5):1121–8.
15. Blanke F, Feitenhansl A, Haenle M, et al. Arthroscopic meniscopexy for the treatment of nontraumatic osteochondritis dissecans in the knee joint of adult patients. Cartilage 2020;11(4):441–6.
16. Kessler JI, Jacobs JC Jr, Cannamela PC, et al. Childhood obesity is associated with osteochondritis dissecans of the knee, ankle, and elbow in children and adolescents. J Pediatr Orthop 2018;38(5):e296–9.
17. Gonzalez-Herranz P, Rodriguez ML, de la Fuente C. Femoral osteochondritis of the knee: prognostic value of the mechanical axis. J Child Orthop 2017;11(1):1–5.
18. Maier GS, Lazovic D, Maus U, et al. Vitamin D deficiency: the missing etiological factor in the development of juvenile osteochondrosis dissecans? J Pediatr Orthop 2019;39(1):51–4.
19. Kessler JI, Nikizad H, Shea KG, et al. The demographics and epidemiology of osteochondritis dissecans of the knee in children and adolescents. Am J Sports Med 2014;42(2):320–6.
20. Cooper T, Boyles A, Samora WP, et al. Prevalence of Bilateral JOCD of the Knee and Associated Risk Factors. J Pediatr Orthop 2015;35(5):507–10.
21. Wall EJ, Heyworth BE, Shea KG, et al. Trochlear groove osteochondritis dissecans of the knee patellofemoral joint. J Pediatr Orthop 2014;34(6):625–30.
22. Masquijo J, Kothari A. Juvenile osteochondritis dissecans (JOCD) of the knee: current concepts review. EFORT Open Rev 2019;4(5):201–12.
23. Guhl JF. Arthroscopic treatment of osteochondritis dissecans. Clin Orthop Relat Res 1982;167:65–74.
24. Parikh SN, Allen M, Wall EJ, et al. The reliability to determine "healing" in osteochondritis dissecans from radiographic assessment. J Pediatr Orthop 2012;32(6):e35–9.

25. Hefti F, Beguiristain J, Krauspe R, et al. Osteochondritis dissecans: a multicenter study of the European Pediatric Orthopedic Society. J Pediatr Orthop B 1999;8(4):231–45.

26. Hussain ZB, Mathew ST, Feroe AG, et al. Novel magnetic resonance imaging classification of osteochondritis dissecans of the knee: a reliability study. J Pediatr Orthop 2021;41(6): e422–6.

27. Fullick RME ME, Shearer D, Ganley TJ, Flynn JM, Agrawal N, Kocher MS. Comparison of three nonoperative treatments for juvenile osteochondritis dissecans of the knee. . Presented as a podium presentation at the 77th Annual Meeting of the American Academy of Orthopaedic Surgeons, New Orleans, LA. 2010 Mar 9–13 2010.

28. Chambers HG, Shea KG, Anderson AF, et al. American Academy of orthopaedic surgeons clinical practice guideline on: the diagnosis and treatment of osteochondritis dissecans. J Bone Joint Surg Am 2012;94(14):1322–4.

29. Wall EJ, Vourazeris J, Myer GD, et al. The healing potential of stable juvenile osteochondritis dissecans knee lesions. J Bone Joint Surg Am 2008; 90(12):2655–64.

30. Cahill B. Treatment of juvenile osteochondritis dissecans and osteochondritis dissecans of the knee. Clin Sports Med 1985;4(2):367–84.

31. Hughston JC, Hergenroeder PT, Courtenay BG. Osteochondritis dissecans of the femoral condyles. J Bone Joint Surg Am 1984;66(9):1340–8.

32. Sales de Gauzy J, Mansat C, Darodes PH, et al. Natural course of osteochondritis dissecans in children. J Pediatr Orthop B 1999;8(1):26–8.

33. Samora WP, Chevillet J, Adler B, et al. Juvenile osteochondritis dissecans of the knee: predictors of lesion stability. J Pediatr Orthop 2012;32(1):1–4. https://doi.org/10.1097/BPO.0b013e31823d8312.

34. Krause M, Hapfelmeier A, Möller M, et al. Healing predictors of stable juvenile osteochondritis dissecans knee lesions after 6 and 12 months of nonoperative treatment. Am J Sports Med 2013;41(10): 2384–91.

35. Cahill BR, Phillips MR, Navarro R. The results of conservative management of juvenile osteochondritis dissecans using joint scintigraphy. A prospective study. Am J Sports Med 1989;17(5):601–5 [discussion: 605-6].

36. Cepero S, Ullot R, Sastre S. Osteochondritis of the femoral condyles in children and adolescents: our experience over the last 28 years. J Pediatr Orthop B 2005;14(1):24–9.

37. Pill SG, Ganley TJ, Milam RA, et al. Role of magnetic resonance imaging and clinical criteria in predicting successful nonoperative treatment of osteochondritis dissecans in children. J Pediatr Orthop 2003;23(1):102–8.

38. Hoffmann M, Schröder M, Petersen JP, et al. Arthroscopically assisted retrograde drilling for osteochondritis dissecans (OCD) lesions of the knee. Knee Surg Sports Traumatol Arthrosc 2012; 20(11):2257–62.

39. Kawasaki K, Uchio Y, Adachi N, et al. Drilling from the intercondylar area for treatment of osteochondritis dissecans of the knee joint. Knee 2003;10(3): 257–63.

40. Anderson AF, Richards DB, Pagnani MJ, et al. Antegrade drilling for osteochondritis dissecans of the knee. Arthroscopy 1997;13(3):319–24.

41. Kocher MS, Micheli LJ, Yaniv M, et al. Functional and radiographic outcome of juvenile osteochondritis dissecans of the knee treated with transarticular arthroscopic drilling. Am J Sports Med 2001; 29(5):562–6.

42. Edmonds EW, Albright J, Bastrom T, et al. Outcomes of extra-articular, intra-epiphyseal drilling for osteochondritis dissecans of the knee. J Pediatr Orthop 2010;30(8):870–8.

43. Boughanem J, Riaz R, Patel RM, et al. Functional and radiographic outcomes of juvenile osteochondritis dissecans of the knee treated with extra-articular retrograde drilling. Am J Sports Med 2011;39(10):2212–7.

44. Gunton MJ, Carey JL, Shaw CR, et al. Drilling juvenile osteochondritis dissecans: retro- or transarticular? Clin Orthop Relat Res 2013;471(4): 1144–51.

45. Bradley J, Dandy DJ. Results of drilling osteochondritis dissecans before skeletal maturity. J Bone Joint Surg Br 1989;71(4):642–4.

46. Aglietti P, Buzzi R, Bassi PB, et al. Arthroscopic drilling in juvenile osteochondritis dissecans of the medial femoral condyle. Arthroscopy 1994;10(3): 286–91.

47. Louisia S, Beaufils P, Katabi M, et al. Transchondral drilling for osteochondritis dissecans of the medial condyle of the knee. Knee Surg Sports Traumatol Arthrosc 2003;11(1):33–9.

48. Lee CK, Mercurio C. Operative treatment of osteochondritis dissecans in situ by retrograde drilling and cancellous bone graft: a preliminary report. Clin Orthop Relat Res 1981;158:129–36.

49. Donaldson LD, Wojtys EM. Extraarticular drilling for stable osteochondritis dissecans in the skeletally immature knee. J Pediatr Orthop 2008;28(8):831–5.

50. Adachi N, Deie M, Nakamae A, et al. Functional and radiographic outcome of stable juvenile osteochondritis dissecans of the knee treated with retroarticular drilling without bone grafting. Arthroscopy 2009;25(2):145–52.

51. Ojala R, Kerimaa P, Lakovaara M, et al. MRI-guided percutaneous retrograde drilling of osteochondritis dissecans of the knee. Skeletal Radiol 2011;40(6): 765–70.

52. Grimm NL, Ewing CK, Ganley TJ. The knee: internal fixation techniques for osteochondritis dissecans. Clin Sports Med 2014;33(2):313–9.

53. Wombwell JH, Nunley JA. Compressive fixation of osteochondritis dissecans fragments with Herbert screws. J Orthop Trauma 1987;1(1):74–7.

54. Thomson NL. Osteochondritis dissecans and osteochondral fragments managed by Herbert compression screw fixation. Clin Orthop Relat Res 1987;(224):71–8.

55. Makino A, Muscolo DL, Puigdevall M, et al. Arthroscopic fixation of osteochondritis dissecans of the knee: clinical, magnetic resonance imaging, and arthroscopic follow-up. Am J Sports Med 2005. https://doi.org/10.1177/0363546505274717.

56. Cugat R, Garcia M, Cusco X, et al. Osteochondritis dissecans: a historical review and its treatment with cannulated screws. Arthroscopy 1993;9(6):675–84.

57. Dervin GF, Keene GC, Chissell HR. Biodegradable rods in adult osteochondritis dissecans of the knee. Clin Orthop Relat Res 1998;(356):213–21.

58. Fridén T, Rydholm U. Severe aseptic synovitis of the knee after biodegradable internal fixation. A case report. Acta Orthop Scand 1992;63(1):94–7.

59. Scioscia TN, Giffin JR, Allen CR, et al. Potential complication of bioabsorbable screw fixation for osteochondritis dissecans of the knee. Arthroscopy 2001;17(2):E7.

60. Tuompo P, Arvela V, Partio EK, et al. Osteochondritis dissecans of the knee fixed with biodegradable self-reinforced polyglycolide and polylactide rods in 24 patients. Int Orthop 1997;21(6):355–60.

61. Tabaddor RR, Banffy MB, Andersen JS, et al. Fixation of juvenile osteochondritis dissecans lesions of the knee using poly 96L/4D-lactide copolymer bioabsorbable implants. J Pediatr Orthop 2010;30(1):14–20.

62. Weckström M, Parviainen M, Kiuru MJ, et al. Comparison of bioabsorbable pins and nails in the fixation of adult osteochondritis dissecans fragments of the knee: an outcome of 30 knees. Am J Sports Med 2007;35(9):1467–76.

63. Kocher MS, Czarnecki JJ, Andersen JS, et al. Internal fixation of juvenile osteochondritis dissecans lesions of the knee. Am J Sports Med 2007;35(5):712–8.

64. Ladenhauf HN, Jones KJ, Potter HG, et al. Understanding the undulating pattern of the distal femoral growth plate: Implications for surgical procedures involving the pediatric knee: A descriptive MRI study. Knee 2020;27(2):315–23.

65. Navarro R, Cohen M, Filho MC, et al. The arthroscopic treatment of osteochondritis dissecans of the knee with autologous bone sticks. Arthroscopy 2002;18(8):840–4.

66. Slough JA, Noto AM, Schmidt TL. Tibial cortical bone peg fixation in osteochondritis dissecans of the knee. Clin Orthop Relat Res 1991;(267):122–7.

67. Anderson AF, Pagnani MJ. Osteochondritis dissecans of the femoral condyles. Long-term results of excision of the fragment. Am J Sports Med 1997;25(6):830–4.

68. Daud A, Safir OA, Gross AE, et al. Outcomes of Bulk Fresh Osteochondral Allografts for Cartilage Restoration in the Knee. J Bone Joint Surg Am 2021;103(22):2115–25.

69. León SA, Mei XY, Safir OA, et al. Long-term results of fresh osteochondral allografts and realignment osteotomy for cartilage repair in the knee. Bone Joint J 2019;101-b(1_Supple_A):46–52.

70. Croman M, Kramer DE, Heyworth BE, et al. Osteochondritis dissecans of the tibial plateau in children and adolescents: a case series. Orthop J Sports Med 2020;8(8). 2325967120941380.

71. Carey JL, Shea KG, Lindahl A, et al. Autologous Chondrocyte Implantation as Treatment for Unsalvageable Osteochondritis Dissecans: 10- to 25-Year Follow-up. Am J Sports Med 2020;48(5):1134–40.

72. Macmull S, Parratt MT, Bentley G, et al. Autologous chondrocyte implantation in the adolescent knee. Am J Sports Med 2011;39(8):1723–30.

73. Vijayan S, Bartlett W, Bentley G, et al. Autologous chondrocyte implantation for osteochondral lesions in the knee using a bilayer collagen membrane and bone graft: a two- to eight-year follow-up study. J Bone Joint Surg Br 2012;94(4):488–92.

74. Bartlett W, Gooding CR, Carrington RW, et al. Autologous chondrocyte implantation at the knee using a bilayer collagen membrane with bone graft. A preliminary report. J Bone Joint Surg Br 2005;87(3):330–2.

75. Minas T, Ogura T, Headrick J, et al. Autologous chondrocyte implantation "sandwich" technique compared with autologous bone grafting for deep osteochondral lesions in the knee. Am J Sports Med 2018;46(2):322–32.

76. Gudas R, Simonaityte R, Cekanauskas E, et al. A prospective, randomized clinical study of osteochondral autologous transplantation versus microfracture for the treatment of osteochondritis dissecans in the knee joint in children. J Pediatr Orthop 2009;29(7):741–8.

77. Lyon R, Nissen C, Liu XC, et al. Can fresh osteochondral allografts restore function in juveniles with osteochondritis dissecans of the knee? Clin Orthop Relat Res Apr 2013;471(4):1166–73.

78. Murphy RT, Pennock AT, Bugbee WD. Osteochondral allograft transplantation of the knee in the pediatric and adolescent population. Am J Sports Med 2014;42(3):635–40.

The Insidious Effects of Childhood Obesity on Orthopedic Injuries and Deformities

Breann Tisano, MD[a], Kendall Anigian, MD[a],
Nyssa Kantorek, BS[b], Yves J. Kenfack, BS[b],
Megan Johnson, MD[c], Jaysson T. Brooks, MD[c],*

KEYWORDS

• Obesity • Children • Orthopedics • Overweight • Scoliosis • Perthes • Trauma • Sports

---

KEY POINTS

- The adolescent growth spurt is a critical time to amass bone density and obesity, through the effect of increased insulin and leptin levels via the RANK pathway, results in decreased bone mass and bone quality.
- In the nonoperative treatment of scoliosis, increased BMI negatively impacts both brace wear compliance and effectiveness. Obese adolescents present more often with a curve of surgical magnitude and are at an increased risk of surgical site infections.
- Obesity has been associated with childhood pathology of the lower extremity including slipped capital femoral epiphysis (SCFE), Legg–Calvé Perthes (LCP), Blount's, and flatfoot. There is a clearly established association between metabolic syndrome and SCFE, with increased risk up to 17 times greater in obese children compared with those with normal BMI. Obesity is associated with increased prevalence among those with LCPD compared with those without but is also seen to be protective against the need for surgical intervention.
- Acute injury also disproportionately affects the lower extremities in obese children-both with sporting activities and higher mechanism trauma. Increased BMI has been associated with increased complexity of bony and soft tissue injuries.

INTRODUCTION

Childhood obesity is a worldwide epidemic with a 60% global increase in overweight and obese children of preschool age in 2010 as compared with 1990.[1] In the United States, these statistics are even more alarming, with the percentage of children aged 2 to 19 years old who are obese tripling to 17% between the 1970s and the year 2010.[2,3] Clinicians caring for children with musculoskeletal injuries and deformities are not doing so within a vacuum. These patients and potentially their outcomes are likely being affected by the obesity epidemic surrounding them. The purpose of this article is to review the insidious and not so insidious effects of childhood obesity on the presentation, prevalence, and outcomes of various orthopedic injuries and deformities.

---

[a] Department of Orthopaedic Surgery, UT-Southwestern, 1801 Inwood Road, Dallas, TX 75390, USA; [b] UT-Southwestern School of Medicine, 5323 Harry Hines Blvd, Dallas, TX 75390, USA; [c] Department of Orthopaedic Surgery, Scottish Rite for Children/UT-Southwestern, 2222 Welborn Street, Dallas, TX 75219, USA
* Corresponding author.
E-mail address: jaysson.brooks@tsrh.org

DISCUSSION

The Orthopedic Basic Science of Childhood Obesity

Obesity in children has a deleterious effect on bone physiology and overall bone health. Forty percent of bone mineral accrual occurs within 2 years of the adolescent growth spurt.[4–6] Obesity has been shown to have a negative effect on attaining peak bone mass, 90% of which is obtained by the age of 18.[4,7,8] Even though obese children have larger bones, the endocrine changes and nutritional deficiencies caused by obesity leads to an overall lower ratio of overall bone mass in relationship to the patient's weight.[4,5,9–12] Obesity, specifically visceral/abdominal obesity, leads to the development of metabolic syndrome, which leads to altered glucose metabolism, dyslipidemia, and hypertension.[4,6] Metabolic syndrome also leads to changes in insulin resistance, increased inflammatory cytokine production, altered leptin production, and vitamin D deficiency.[4,6,9,13] These alterations have negative effects on bone physiology.

Hyperinsulinemia, which is caused by insulin resistance, has a negative impact on osteoblast/osteoclast function and is associated with decreased numbers of osteoclasts and markers of bone resorption, leading to reduced bone turnover and poor bone quality.[14,15] This is due to an imbalance between osteoblast/osteoclast activity from the increased differentiation of mesenchymal stem cells to adipocytes at the expense of osteoblasts, leading to decreased bone formation.[14,16] The hallmark mechanism of bone pathology in these clinical situations is an increased engagement of RANKL with its receptor RANK which increases osteoclastogenesis. The increased signaling may derive from increased production of RANKL by inflammatory and fat cells and/or decreased production of the soluble inhibitor of this system, osteoprotegerin (OPG). Regardless of the specific change that occurs, the result is increased bone resorption.[14,17–19]

Obesity-related bone disease has also been linked to leptin resistance.[20–23] Leptin, produced by adipocytes, is a key regulator of metabolism and satiety and levels change throughout the day most often peaking at night.[24,25] Elevated leptin levels increase bone resorption and decrease bone formation through increased RANK expression and the inhibition of OPG. This triggers the RANK/RANKL pathway, leading to increased bone resorption through increased osteoclast activity,[4,6,12,14,26] resulting in decreased bone mass, decreased trabecular thickness, and increased cortical porosity.[24,25,27] This is evidenced by the decreased radial cortical porosity and tibial trabecular thickness seen in obese children compared with normal-weight children.[14,24,27,28]

Due to the sequestration of vitamin D (a fat-soluble vitamin) in adipose tissue, obesity leads to decreased availability of vitamin D for bone remodeling, which negatively affects bone physiology.[4,11] Based on a sample of children aged 6 to 18 years who have enrolled in the 2003 to 2006 National Health and Nutrition Examination Survey the prevalence of vitamin D deficiency is 21% in normal-weight children, 29% in overweight children, 34% in obese children, and 49% in severely obese children.[4,13]

How Obesity Affects Spine Deformities?

Bracing is usually the first line of treatment of children with adolescent idiopathic scoliosis (AIS) and in many children, bracing can slow the progression of a curve;[29] however, a child's body mass index (BMI) may affect the outcomes of bracing. O'Neill and colleagues evaluated how effective a Boston or custom-molded thoracolumbosacral orthosis was in controlling curve progression in children stratified by BMI.[30] They found that overweight (OW) children with AIS who were treated with a brace had a curve progression of $9.6° \pm 7.3°$ as compared with normal weight (NW) patients, who had a curve progression of $3.6° \pm 9.4°$. Interestingly, 15 years later, Karol and colleagues provided more clarity on the topic by reporting on the effectiveness of brace wear in 175 children with AIS based on the number of hours the brace was worn.[31] They found that underweight (UW) patients had the highest brace wear compliance at 15 hours per day; however, this still resulted in a 60% progression of their curves to a surgical magnitude. When comparing the NW, OW, and obese (OB) BMI groups, brace wear compliance, measured in hours, decreased as the child's BMI increased. In addition, of the NW, OW, and OB children with AIS who were wearing their brace, the obese children had the greatest progression of their curves to a surgical magnitude. The current consensus in the literature is that obesity itself is a risk factor for multiple perioperative complications such as increased operative times, increased blood loss, increased use of intraoperative crystalloids, difficulty with spinal anesthesia administration, and prolonged opioid use postoperatively.[32,33] Hospital readmission rates are also significantly higher for patients with OB and OW compared with their NW and UW peers.[34–36]

McDonald and colleagues[37] recently published the largest, multicenter study on the effects of childhood obesity on idiopathic scoliosis after posterior spinal fusions to correct these deformities. They found a significantly higher rate of superficial surgical site infections (SSIs) based on BMI with an SSI rate of 0.8% for patients with NW, 4.3% patients with OW, and 5.4% patients with OB ($P = .012$). Interestingly they also found that patients with OB and OW also presented with a lower socioeconomic status as measured by the area deprivation index as compared with patients with NW, further highlighting the interplay between obesity and poverty. The presentation of larger curve magnitudes in overweight and obese children is likely related to the difficulty in the early detection of asymmetry of the spine in these children due to their body composition (Fig. 1). Interestingly, a recent study showed that fat and muscle mass correlated with curve severity, especially in overweight patients. Goodbody and colleagues compared curve magnitude at presentation based on BMI-for-age; patients with OW and obese were 14% to 16% more likely to present with curve magnitudes that required surgery ($P = .010$). Additionally, higher BMI patients presented with high average Risser scores

indicating an advanced skeletal maturity compared with their peers ($P = .010$).[38]

There are very little data related to how obesity affects kyphotic deformities in children. Valvodino and colleagues compared the radiographs of 1551 patients with idiopathic scoliosis to those without scoliosis based on BMI. Interestingly, they found that in children with idiopathic scoliosis, their thoracic kyphosis increased significantly as their BMI also increased. This positive correlation was also found in children who didn't have scoliosis, showing the impact overall of obesity on the sagittal alignment of children.[39,40]

How Obesity Affects Lower Extremity Alignment?

Obesity has been linked with increased prevalence of Blount's disease in the pediatric population, and the effect seems to be mechanical in nature.[41,42] Excessive body weight in children can translate to compounding stress on the joints before their full development (Fig. 2). It is postulated that the increased compressive forces present in knee joints in OW and OB children may inhibit growth around the knees.[41] In observing data obtained at Boston Children's Hospital, Dietz and colleagues confirmed a statistically significant correlation of obese children with infantile Blount disease.[43] Most notably, there was a positive correlation between the

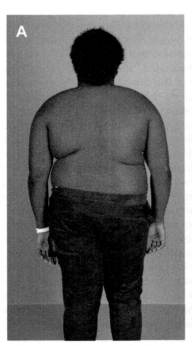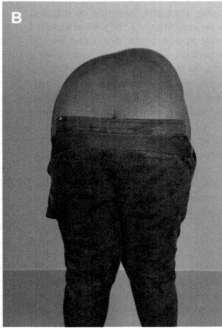

Fig. 1. (A) Clinical photo of an obese child with adolescent idiopathic scoliosis who presented with scoliosis that already surpassed the surgical threshold. On a forward bend test his rib asymmetry is more clearly delineated (B).

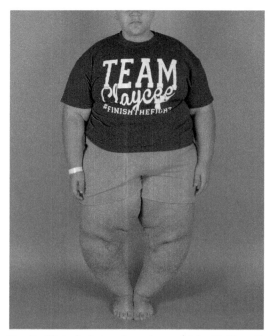

Fig. 2. Clinical photo of an obese child with Blount's disease.

angular magnitude of tibial deformity and the magnitude of the child's BMI.[43] Sabharwal and colleagues observed a direct link of BMI and varus malalignment of the affected extremity in children with early-onset Blount disease (r = 0.74; P<.001) given a BMI ≥ 40 kg/m[2].[41] Thus, proposing that the severity of obesity may often be an indicator of how severe a child's tibial deformity appears. As discussed in the basic science section, obesity leads to increased osteoclast activity and thus, decreased bone density. This decrease in bone density exposes obese children with Blount's disease to intensifying deformities as they continue to gain weight.[44]

Nonoperative treatment of Blount's disease can include braces that extend from the upper thigh to the foot, applying valgus force to the knee.[44] The efficacy of braces to treat Blount's disease is controversial and often questioned due to the high rate of spontaneous correction among patients. Shinohara and colleagues observed 29 patients who all had early-onset Blount's disease and found that all 22 limbs showed signs of Langenskiold stage-I changes, which resolved without treatment.[45] Obesity may also play a role in the outcomes of surgery in this patient population. Lateral tension band hemiepiphysiodesis has been popularized as a method for guided growth; however, high failure rate has been observed with obese patients

when small diameter titanium screws were used.[46] Loder and Johnston observed that an increase in the Langenskiold stage is seen with age; thus, causing high recurrence rates following osteotomy.[47] This is possibly attributed to the fact that the Langenskiold stage progressively worsens as obese patients continually impose greater strains over longer periods of time.

Obesity has been known to alter children's physiology; thus, multiple organ systems. As a result, obesity itself poses a multitude of risks for perioperative complications. Morbidly obese children with Blount disease have been identified to have obstructive sleep apnea which may pose complications during surgery.[48,49] Gordon and colleagues found a 61% incidence of sleep apnea in children with Blount's disease, who were older than 9 years old, that required surgical correction of their deformities. Preoperatively, these patients were treated with noninvasive positive pressure ventilation and had uneventful anesthetic and pulmonary postoperative recoveries.[50] Precocious puberty is also linked to childhood obesity and should be considered when planning for the appropriate time to perform growth modulation to treat tibia vara in Blount's disease.[51]

How Obesity Affects Flat Feet (pes planovalgus)?

The prevalence of pes planovalgus in children is influenced by age, gender, and weight with 54% of 3-year olds having flat feet, while only 24% of 6-year olds had flat feet.[52] More salient to our discussion, Pfeiffer and colleagues also found that the prevalence of flat feet increased significantly between normal weight (42%), overweight (51%) and obese children (62%). The collapse or disappearance of the medial longitudinal arch is what inevitably leads to flatfoot in children[53] (Fig. 3). In obese and overweight children, the excessive loads applied to the foot as their BMI increases have shown a positive correlation in the severity of the pes planovalgus present in children of preschool age.[54] Chen and colleagues evaluated 580 children to determine how obesity affected the presentation of pes planovalgus. They found that obese children are significantly more likely to develop bilateral pes planovalgus as compared with nonobese children (odds ratio (OR): 1.9; 95% confidence interval (CI): 1.2–2.9).[54] In children with baseline developmental delay who also are overweight and obese, the prevalence of pes planovalgus was reported by Chen and colleagues to be nearly 96%, highlighting the synergistic effect

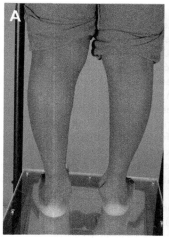 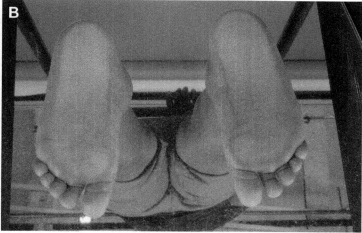

Fig. 3. (A) Clinical photo of an overweight child with pes planovalgus highlighting the loss of the medial arch. The associated pedobarogram confirms that a significant amount of pressure is being placed on the medial column of the foot (B).

of obesity with the ligamentous laxity often seen in children with developmental delay.[55]

The Effect of Obesity on Legg–Calvé–Perthes Disease

When a clinician thinks about the typical child with a slipped capital femoral epiphysis (SCFE), the picture of an obese or overweight male with a limp is easy to imagine. For children with Legg–Calvé–Perthes Disease (LCPD) there is less clarity on how these kids typically present. Additionally, there is a dearth of literature that discusses how childhood obesity affects outcomes, if at all, in children with LCPD. To date, the best paper describing the association between LCPD and BMI was published in 2016 by Neal and colleagues who reported their findings on 150 patients (172 hips) with LCPD.[56] In their cohort, most of the patients with LCPD were categorized as normal weight (51%, N = 76), followed by 32% being obese (N = 48), 16% being overweight (N = 24), and 1% being underweight (N = 1). Compared with an age-matched cohort of children without LCPD, they found that obesity was twice as common in children with LCPD. Sixty-four patients (43%) were treated with some type of operative procedure including hip arthrograms and Petrie casting or femoral/pelvic osteotomies. Interestingly they found that being obese or overweight was actually protective for surgical interventions in patients with LCPD; the odds of requiring surgery for LCPD was 2.4 times lower for obese children versus normal-weight children (P = .02). This finding is likely explained by the fact that obese children with LCPD presented to the clinic at significantly advanced Waldenstrom

stages (3 or 4) as compared with normal weight patients (P = .003). What is not known is whether an advanced Waldenstrom stage combined with obesity results in worse long-term functional outcomes in children with LCPD.

The association between obesity and LCPD was later reaffirmed by Morlin and Hailer, who queried the Swedish National Quality Register for Pediatric Orthopedics for all patients with LCPD over a 3 year period.[57] The purpose of their study was to determine if there was a correlation between LCPD and childhood hypertension. Similar to Neal and colleagues,[56] they found a prevalence of obesity in children with LCPD of 32% at 2 years of follow-up. They also found that 19% of children with LCPD also had hypertension at the time of LCPD diagnosis which decreased to 13% at 2 years of follow-up. The etiology of this association between hypertension and LCPD remains unclear; however, it should remind the clinician to think outside the musculoskeletal system when evaluating children with LCPD.

The etiology of the association between obesity and LCPD was investigated by Lee and colleagues in a cohort of 41 Korean children with LCPD.[58] They measured the serum levels of leptin, soluble leptin receptor (sOB-R), and free leptin index (FLI) in the LCPD cohort and in an age-matched cohort without LCPD. They found that leptin, sOB-R, and FLI levels are all significantly different in the LCPD cohort compared with the normal cohort (P = .002). Interestingly, as the severity of LCPD increased, according to the lateral pillar and Stulberg classification, the serum levels of leptin and sOB-R also increased significantly. With the increased prevalence of obesity in LCPD and the significant association between LCPD and serum leptin levels, it seems that LCPD has more in common with SCFEs than previously thought.

The Effect of Obesity on Slipped Capital Femoral Epiphysis

It is well known that obese and overweight children are more susceptible to the development of SCFEs and recent literature has shed light on just how susceptible they are. Perry and colleagues evaluated a cohort of 615,950 children in Scotland and found that the risk of developing an SCFE increased by a factor of 1.7 for every integer increase in BMI.[59] Perry and colleagues also found that the age of the child at SCFE diagnosis independently affected the risk of developing an SCFE with obese children aged 5 to 6 years old having a 5.9 greater risk of SCFE and obese children aged 11 to 12 years old having a 17 times greater risk of developing an SCFE as compared with children with a normal BMI. While the orthopedic surgeon often focuses on the technical details of reducing and instrumenting the hip in a child with an SCFE, the downstream metabolic effects of obesity in this patient population are truly deleterious. Hailer used a large, Swedish patient registry to identify all patients with an SCFE between 1964 and 2011 and compared these patients to controls without SCFE.[60] In her cohort of 2564 patients with SCFEs there was 2 times all-cause, greater hazard ratio of mortality as compared with controls and 3 times greater hazard ratio of developing hypothyroidism as compared with controls. The relatively high prevalence of obesity in children with SCFEs has also been shown to result in significantly higher serum leptin levels as compared with controls,[20] and significantly higher serum levels of insulin, triglycerides, and low-density lipoproteins as compared with controls.[61] This data compels clinicians treating children with SCFEs to educate the family on the long-term effects of obesity on their child's condition and may support the argument that all overweight and obese children with SCFEs should be under the care of metabolic specialists or referred to a weight loss clinic.

The Effect of Obesity on Children with Traumatic Injuries

Obesity has been found to be a risk fracture for the increased incidence of skeletal fractures in children, with contributors thought to be poor mobility, balance, nutrition, and mechanical disadvantage.[62] Studies have shown that the prevalence of skeletal fractures after high energy traumas in obese children are five times more likely to occur than in nonobese children (OR: 4.54 95% CI: 1.6–13.2, $P = .0053$).[63] These differences between obese and normal-weight children occur both with low mechanism injuries as well as high mechanism injuries. It has been noted by Valerio and colleagues that it was more common for girls to be obese if they had sustained a fracture while the same was only true in the lower extremity for boys.[64] Pomerantz found that obese children were almost two times more likely to sustain lower extremity injuries when compared with normal-weight children (OR: 1.71).[65] Kessler noted that children ages 6 to 11 were more likely to sustain fractures of the foot, ankle, leg, and knee if they were obese or overweight. The risk of lower extremity fracture increased with increasing obesity.[66] Gilbert and colleagues looked into trauma activations at 2 level one trauma centers in patients with lower extremity long bone fractures and found that obese children had a higher Injury Severity Score (ISS) ($P = .0002$), Abbreviated Injury Scale (AIS) >3 to head/neck ($P = .026$), chest ($P = .0008$), abdomen (p+.065) and extremities ($P = .0338$) than normal-weight children. There was also an increase in pelvic and spinal fractures compared with normal-weight children.[67] There are several notable differences in fracture pattern due to location in children who are obese versus normal weight.

In upper extremity injuries, Seeley and colleagues looked at 354 fractures and found that complex supracondylar fractures were more likely to occur in obese and overweight children versus normal-weight children (OR: 9.19 95% CI: 4.25–19.92 $P<.001$ and OR: 2.05 95% CI: 1.11–3.80 $P = .02$, respectively).[68] It was also noted that patients who fell from standing who were obese were more likely to suffer a complex type supracondylar fracture when compared with normal weight patients. Seeley also noted a higher incidence of preoperative nerve injury in obese patients (OR: 2.69 CI: 1.15–6.29 $P = .02$) as well as persistence in postoperative nerve palsies when compared with normal-weight children. Fornari and colleagues looked at the incidence of lateral condyle fractures versus supracondylar fractures and found that the lateral condyle fracture group had a higher BMI ($P = .001$). It was also noted that there was a significant difference in the type of lateral condyle fracture with obesity being a risk fracture for a more complex fracture pattern.[69] In upper extremity injuries Chang and colleagues noted that obese children with a type 3 supracondylar fracture were more likely to develop postoperative loss of reduction and varus alignment.[70] Li and colleagues noted an increased rate of open reduction in obese patients when compared with normal-weight children for the ages of 8 to 12 years old (OR: 4.29 95% CI: 1.17–10.36 P = .001). There was no difference in requirement for open reduction in children under the age of 8 who sustained supracondylar fractures.[71] Multiple reports have been published showing obese patients with diaphyseal both bone forearm fractures are more likely to experience loss of reduction during cast treatment than normal weight patients (44.4% vs 7.2% P = .005; 34% vs 18% P = .04, respectively).[72,73]

When reviewing fracture patterns in lower extremity long bone injuries, Gilbert and colleagues found that obese patients were almost two times more likely to sustain an injury to the epiphysis than normal-weight children (P = .004 for femur, p=<0.007 tibia).[74] It was also noted that obese children were more likely to sustain bilateral lower extremity injuries than normal-weight children (bilateral femur P = .08, bilateral tibia P = .033).[67]

For lower extremity injuries, age-adjusted obese children had more fractures treated operatively (P = .022). This has been postulated to be a combination of factors including a more severe injury pattern as well as more difficult management of fractures due to increased fat distribution and difficulty with cast molding as well as increased caregiver burden.[75] It has also been noted that obese children may be at risk for increased surgical complications including refracture, loss of reduction, infection, compartment syndrome, and malunion.[76,77] In the lower extremity there has been controversy regarding treatment, with several studies showing increased failure rate of using flexible titanium nails in children greater than 49 kg[77–79]; however, this has not been proven with stainless steel nails as far as angulation or union.[80] In regards to the tibia, Goodbody found no significant difference in rate of malunion or time to union between children above and below 50 kg when using flexible titanium nails.[81] Fracture evaluation of the obese child continues to evolve and often requires adaptation by the treating provider to avoid an increase in complications.

The Effect of Obesity on Sports Injuries

Obese children are more likely than their peers to experience musculoskeletal injury.[82,83] Lower extremity injuries predominate, likely as a result of altered biomechanics associated with increased weight. Compared with healthy BMI controls, obese adolescent children have greater knee valgus in standing and greater knee external rotation with jogging[84] with 1.8 times greater patellofemoral contact forces normalized for the patellar area.[85] Slower walking speeds with shorter step length and longer support phases are considered to be compensatory for an underlying instability in gait with obesity.[86] Balance skills have also been shown to be decreased in overweight prepubertal boys,[87] a risk factor which has separately been shown to increase lower extremity sporting injury.[88,89]

In a Dutch database study of children (aged 2–11) and adolescents (aged 12–17) presenting to a primary care provider, overweight and obese patients were more likely to report musculoskeletal injuries, specifically more lower extremity, foot, and ankle problems.[90] Similarly, in children with an average age of 10 years, those with a BMI greater than 95th percentile were more likely to complain of joint pain than those a BMI of less than 80th percentile.[90] Obesity was significantly associated with low back pain, tight quadriceps and knee deformities such as genu valgum and genu recurvatum.

Acute injuries requiring presentation to the emergency room also reveal an increased predominance of lower extremity injuries in obese children.[65] Increasing BMI percentile is significantly associated with ankle injury in an urban pediatric emergency department with patients aged 5 to 19 years old.[91] Notably, obese youth who sustain an ankle injury experience greater morbidity, with persistent ankle instability and symptoms more than 6 months out from ankle sprain.[92]

The effects of obesity in sport-specific activities have been best studied in football, as larger size may confer a competitive advantage to participants. Increased BMI imparts a 2.5 times increased relative risk of adolescent football injury.[93] A study of American high school lineman showed higher body fat percentage and BMI significantly increased lower extremity injuries during a single season.[94] It should be noted, however, that despite a correlation coefficient of 0.8 for percent body fat and BMI in high school football lineman,[94] BMI may not be the most accurate representation of obesity in sports given the propensity for muscular development above normal for their given age and height.[95] Common sports pathology of the lower extremity is expectedly affected by obesity. Increased BMI percentile in children was associated with osteochondritis dissecans of the knee and ankle, but not the elbow.[96] Though not statistically significant, children who were overweight or obese tended toward lower volume and accrual rates of articular cartilage formation during development. Vigorous sporting activity, on the contrary, was protective with increased articular cartilage about the knee.[97]

Anterior cruciate ligament (ACL) injury is also associated with higher BMI, independent of age, sex, and sport.[98] In those who undergo reconstruction, however, BMI did not have a significant effect on rates of rerupture or contralateral injury.[99] Weight gain is also seen as a consequence of surgery and postoperative limitations, with a median increase in BMI of 1.8 percentile points after pediatric ACL reconstruction. While the effect was less pronounced in those who were already obese, this postop elevation in BMI persists out to 2 years from index surgery.[100] Concomitant injury described at the time of ACL reconstruction reveals increasing morbidity in the setting of obesity. Numerous studies have described an association with elevated weight or BMI and concomitant meniscal tears in pediatric patients.[98,99,101–104] This specifically affects the medial meniscus with reported tear rates of 6% to 8% and an increase in concomitant meniscus tears for each integer increase in BMI.[98,103] Pediatric obesity in the setting of ACL reconstructions confers 16 times increased odds of meniscectomy[99] and in all meniscal surgeries is associated with increasing tear complexity.[105] Concomitant chondral injuries are also elevated, with a 12% increased incidence for each point increase in BMI.[98]

SUMMARY

The effects of childhood obesity are widespread, with implications for a multitude of orthopedic pathologies. Some problems such as SCFE and Blount's disease are easily associated with and rather unique to the obese child. Others, such as scoliosis, fractures, and sports injuries, affect all children but have unique considerations and increased complexity related to increased body mass.

Increased rates of musculoskeletal complaints and injuries among obese children will inevitably bring them into the orthopedic clinic for evaluation. Providers should not treat the orthopedic pathology in isolation and instead address the patient holistically. Addressing pain and limitation will permit patients to return to youth activity participation, an important component of combatting obesity. It is essential for orthopedic surgeons to recognize how obesity may affect both operative and nonoperative treatment outcomes and counsel patients and families accordingly.

CLINICS CARE POINTS

- The adolescent growth spurt is a critical time to amass bone density and obesity, through the effect of increased insulin and leptin levels via the RANK pathway, results in decreased bone mass and bone quality.

- In the nonoperative treatment of scoliosis, increased BMI negatively impacts both brace wear compliance and effectiveness. Obese adolescents present more often with a curve of surgical magnitude and are at an increased risk of surgical site infections.

- Obesity has been associated with childhood pathology of the lower extremity including slipped capital femoral epiphysis (SCFE), Legg–Calvé–Perthes (LCP), Blount's, and flatfoot. There is a clearly established association between metabolic syndrome and SCFE, with increased risk up to 17 times greater in obese children compared with those with normal BMI. Obesity is associated with increased prevalence among those with LCPD compared with those without but is also seen to be protective against the need for surgical intervention.

- Acute injury also disproportionately affects the lower extremities in obese children-both with sporting activities and higher mechanism trauma. Increased BMI has been associated with increased complexity of bony and soft tissue injuries.

DISCLOSURE

The authors have nothing to disclose.

REFERENCES

1. de Onis M, Blössner M, Borghi E. Global prevalence and trends of overweight and obesity among preschool children. Am J Clin Nutr 2010; 92(5):1257–64.

2. Ogden CL, Carroll MD, Kit BK, et al. Prevalence of obesity and trends in body mass index among US children and adolescents, 1999-2010. JAMA 2012; 307(5):483–90.

3. Ogden C, Carroll M, for Disease Control C, Prevention, Others. NCHS Health EStat: Prevalence of obesity among children and adolescents: United States, Trends 1963-1965 Through 2007-

2008. 2010. Available at: https://www.cdc.gov/nchs/products/hestats.htm.

4. Nowicki P, Kemppainen J, Maskill L, et al. The Role of Obesity in Pediatric Orthopedics. J Am Acad Orthop Surg Glob Res Rev 2019;3(5):e036.

5. Kelley JC, Crabtree N, Zemel BS. Bone Density in the Obese Child: Clinical Considerations and Diagnostic Challenges. Calcif Tissue Int 2017; 100(5):514–27.

6. da Silva VN, Fiorelli LNM, da Silva CC, et al. Do metabolic syndrome and its components have an impact on bone mineral density in adolescents? Nutr Metab 2017;14:1.

7. Chan G, Chen CT. Musculoskeletal effects of obesity. Curr Opin Pediatr 2009;21(1):65–70.

8. Golden NH, Abrams SA, Committee on Nutrition. Optimizing bone health in children and adolescents. Pediatrics 2014;134(4):e1229–43.

9. Pollock NK. Childhood obesity, bone development, and cardiometabolic risk factors. Mol Cell Endocrinol 2015;410:52–63.

10. Leonard MB, Shults J, Wilson BA, et al. Obesity during childhood and adolescence augments bone mass and bone dimensions. Am J Clin Nutr 2004;80(2):514–23.

11. Bialo SR, Gordon CM. Underweight, overweight, and pediatric bone fragility: impact and management. Curr Osteoporos Rep 2014;12(3):319–28.

12. Lazar-Antman MA, Leet AI. Effects of obesity on pediatric fracture care and management. J Bone Joint Surg Am 2012;94(9):855–61.

13. Turer CB, Lin H, Flores G. Prevalence of vitamin D deficiency among overweight and obese US children. Pediatrics 2013;131(1):e152–61.

14. Fintini D, Cianfarani S, Cofini M, et al. The Bones of Children With Obesity. Front Endocrinol 2020; 11:200.

15. Huang S, Kaw M, Harris MT, et al. Decreased osteoclastogenesis and high bone mass in mice with impaired insulin clearance due to liver-specific inactivation to CEACAM1. Bone 2010; 46(4):1138–45.

16. da Silva SV, Renovato-Martins M, Ribeiro-Pereira C, et al. Obesity modifies bone marrow microenvironment and directs bone marrow mesenchymal cells to adipogenesis. Obes 2016; 24(12):2522–32.

17. Roy B, Curtis ME, Fears LS, et al. Molecular Mechanisms of Obesity-Induced Osteoporosis and Muscle Atrophy. Front Physiol 2016;7:439.

18. Riches PL, McRorie E, Fraser WD, et al. Osteoporosis associated with neutralizing autoantibodies against osteoprotegerin. N Engl J Med 2009; 361(15):1459–65.

19. Souza PPC, Lerner UH. The role of cytokines in inflammatory bone loss. Immunol Invest 2013;42(7): 555–622.

20. Halverson SJ, Warhoover T, Mencio GA, et al. Leptin Elevation as a Risk Factor for Slipped Capital Femoral Epiphysis Independent of Obesity Status. J Bone Joint Surg Am 2017; 99(10):865–72.

21. Friedman JM, Halaas JL. Leptin and the regulation of body weight in mammals. Nature 1998; 395(6704):763–70.

22. Maor G, Rochwerger M, Segev Y, et al. Leptin acts as a growth factor on the chondrocytes of skeletal growth centers. J Bone Miner Res 2002;17(6): 1034–43.

23. Myers MG Jr, Leibel RL, Seeley RJ, et al. Obesity and leptin resistance: distinguishing cause from effect. Trends Endocrinol Metab 2010;21(11): 643–51.

24. Beck JJ, Mahan ST, Nowicki P, et al. What Is New in Pediatric Bone Health. J Pediatr Orthop 2021; 41(8):e594–9.

25. Farr JN, Dimitri P. The Impact of Fat and Obesity on Bone Microarchitecture and Strength in Children. Calcif Tissue Int 2017;100(5):500–13.

26. Lamghari M, Tavares L, Camboa N, et al. Leptin effect on RANKL and OPG expression in MC3T3-E1 osteoblasts. J Cell Biochem 2006; 98(5):1123–9.

27. Dimitri P, Jacques RM, Paggiosi M, et al. Leptin may play a role in bone microstructural alterations in obese children. J Clin Endocrinol Metab 2015; 100(2):594–602.

28. Fujita Y, Watanabe K, Maki K. Serum leptin levels negatively correlate with trabecular bone mineral density in high-fat diet-induced obesity mice. J Musculoskelet Neuronal Interact 2012;12(2): 84–94. Available at: https://www.ncbi.nlm.nih.gov/pubmed/22647282.

29. Tsaknakis K, Braunschweig L, Lorenz HM, et al. [Claims and realities of brace treatment : Primary correction of scoliosis in children and adolescents]. Orthopade 2020;49(1):59–65.

30. O'Neill PJ, Karol LA, Shindle MK, et al. Decreased orthotic effectiveness in overweight patients with adolescent idiopathic scoliosis. J Bone Joint Surg Am 2005;87(5):1069–74.

31. Karol LA, Wingfield JJ, Virostek D, et al. The Influence of Body Habitus on Documented Brace Wear and Progression in Adolescents With Idiopathic Scoliosis. J Pediatr Orthop 2020;40(3): e171–5.

32. Hardesty CK, Poe-Kochert C, Son-Hing JP, et al. Obesity negatively affects spinal surgery in idiopathic scoliosis. Clin Orthop Relat Res 2013; 471(4):1230–5.

33. Kendall MC, Castro Alves LJ. Risk Factors for Prolonged Postoperative Opioid Use After Spinal Fusion for Adolescent Idiopathic Scoliosis. J Pediatr Orthop 2019;39(9):e729.

34. Lee NJ, Fields MW, Boddapati V, et al. The risks, reasons, and costs for 30- and 90-day readmissions after fusion surgery for adolescent idiopathic scoliosis. J Neurosurg Spine 2020;1–9. https://doi.org/10.3171/2020.6.SPINE20197.

35. Minhas SV, Chow I, Feldman DS, et al. A Predictive Risk Index for 30-day Readmissions Following Surgical Treatment of Pediatric Scoliosis. J Pediatr Orthop 2016;36(2):187–92.

36. De la Garza Ramos R, Nakhla J, Nasser R, et al. Effect of body mass index on surgical outcomes after posterior spinal fusion for adolescent idiopathic scoliosis. Neurosurg Focus 2017;43(4):E5.

37. McDonald TC, Heffernan MJ, Ramo B, et al. Surgical Outcomes of Obese Patients With Adolescent Idiopathic Scoliosis From Endemic Areas of Obesity in the United States. J Pediatr Orthop 2021;41(10):e865–70.

38. Goodbody CM, Sankar WN, Flynn JM. Presentation of Adolescent Idiopathic Scoliosis: The Bigger the Kid, the Bigger the Curve. J Pediatr Orthop 2017;37(1):41–6.

39. Lonner BS, Toombs CS, Husain QM, et al. Body Mass Index in Adolescent Spinal Deformity: Comparison of Scheuermann's Kyphosis, Adolescent Idiopathic Scoliosis, and Normal Controls. Spine Deform 2015;3(4):318–26.

40. Valdovino AG, Bastrom TP, Reighard FG, et al. Obesity Is Associated With Increased Thoracic Kyphosis in Adolescent Idiopathic Scoliosis Patients and Nonscoliotic Adolescents. Spine Deform 2019;7(6):865–9.

41. Sabharwal S. Blount disease. J Bone Joint Surg Am 2009;91(7):1758–76.

42. Wills M. Orthopedic complications of childhood obesity. Pediatr Phys Ther 2004;16(4):230–5.

43. Dietz WH Jr, Gross WL, Kirkpatrick JA Jr. Blount disease (tibia vara): another skeletal disorder associated with childhood obesity. J Pediatr 1982;101(5):735–7.

44. Janoyer M. Blount disease. Orthop Traumatol Surg Res 2019;105(1S):S111–21.

45. Shinohara Y, Kamegaya M, Kuniyoshi K, et al. Natural history of infantile tibia vara. J Bone Joint Surg Br 2002;84(2):263–8.

46. Robbins CA. Deformity Reconstruction Surgery for Blount's Disease. Children 2021;8(7). https://doi.org/10.3390/children8070566.

47. Loder RT, Johnston CE 2nd. Infantile tibia vara. J Pediatr Orthop 1987;7(6):639–46.https://www.ncbi.nlm.nih.gov/pubmed/3429646.

48. Jardaly A, McGwin G Jr, Gilbert SR. Blount Disease and Obstructive Sleep Apnea: An Underrecognized Association? J Pediatr Orthop 2020;40(10):604–7.

49. Sabharwal S. Blount disease: an update. Orthop Clin North Am 2015;46(1):37–47.

50. Gordon JE, Hughes MS, Shepherd K, et al. Obstructive sleep apnoea syndrome in morbidly obese children with tibia vara. J Bone Joint Surg Br 2006;88(1):100–3.

51. Sabharwal S, Sakamoto SM, Zhao C. Advanced bone age in children with Blount disease: a case-control study. J Pediatr Orthop 2013;33(5):551–7.

52. Pfeiffer M, Kotz R, Ledl T, et al. Prevalence of flat foot in preschool-aged children. Pediatrics 2006;118(2):634–9.

53. Staheli LT, Chew DE, Corbett M. The longitudinal arch. A survey of eight hundred and eighty-two feet in normal children and adults. J Bone Joint Surg Am 1987;69(3):426–8. Available at: https://www.ncbi.nlm.nih.gov/pubmed/3818704.

54. Malden S, Gillespie J, Hughes A, et al. Obesity in young children and its relationship with diagnosis of asthma, vitamin D deficiency, iron deficiency, specific allergies and flat-footedness: A systematic review and meta-analysis. Obes Rev 2021;22(3):e13129.

55. Chen KC, Tung LC, Tung CH, et al. An investigation of the factors affecting flatfoot in children with delayed motor development. Res Dev Disabil 2014;35(3):639–45.

56. Neal DC, Alford TH, Moualeu A, et al. Prevalence of Obesity in Patients With Legg-Calvé-Perthes Disease. J Am Acad Orthop Surg 2016;24(9):660–5.

57. Mörlin GB, Hailer YD. High blood pressure and overweight in children with Legg-Calvé-Perthes disease: a nationwide population-based cohort study. BMC Musculoskelet Disord 2021;22(1):32.

58. Lee JH, Zhou L, Kwon KS, et al. Role of leptin in Legg-Calvé-Perthes disease. J Orthop Res 2013;31(10):1605–10.

59. Perry DC, Metcalfe D, Lane S, et al. Childhood Obesity and Slipped Capital Femoral Epiphysis. Pediatrics 2018;142(5). https://doi.org/10.1542/peds.2018-1067.

60. Hailer YD. Fate of patients with slipped capital femoral epiphysis (SCFE) in later life: risk of obesity, hypothyroidism, and death in 2,564 patients with SCFE compared with 25,638 controls. Acta Orthop 2020;91(4):457–63.

61. Montañez-Alvarez M, Flores-Navarro HH, Cuevas-De Alba C, et al. The Role of Hyperinsulinemia in Slipped Capital Femoral Epiphysis. J Pediatr Orthop 2020;40(8):413–7.

62. Lee RJ, Hsu NN, Lenz CM, et al. Does obesity affect fracture healing in children? Clin Orthop Relat Res 2013;471(4):1208–13.

63. Taylor ED, Theim KR, Mirch MC, et al. Orthopedic complications of overweight in children and adolescents. Pediatrics 2006;117(6):2167–74.

64. Valerio G, Gallè F, Mancusi C, et al. Prevalence of overweight in children with bone fractures: a case control study. BMC Pediatr 2012; 12:166.

65. Pomerantz WJ, Timm NL, Gittelman MA. Injury patterns in obese versus nonobese children presenting to a pediatric emergency department. Pediatrics 2010;125(4):681–5.

66. Kessler J, Koebnick C, Smith N, et al. Childhood obesity is associated with increased risk of most lower extremity fractures. Clin Orthop Relat Res 2013;471(4):1199–207.

67. Backstrom IC, MacLennan PA, Sawyer JR, et al. Pediatric obesity and traumatic lower-extremity long-bone fracture outcomes. J Trauma Acute Care Surg 2012;73(4):966–71.

68. Seeley MA, Gagnier JJ, Srinivasan RC, et al. Obesity and its effects on pediatric supracondylar humeral fractures. J Bone Joint Surg Am 2014; 96(3):e18.

69. Fornari ED, Suszter M, Roocroft J, et al. Childhood obesity as a risk factor for lateral condyle fractures over supracondylar humerus fractures. Clin Orthop Relat Res 2013;471(4):1193–8.

70. Chang CH, Kao HK, Lee WC, et al. Influence of obesity on surgical outcomes in type III paediatric supracondylar humeral fractures. Injury 2015; 46(11):2181–4.

71. Li NY, Bruce WJ, Joyce C, et al. Obesity's Influence on Operative Management of Pediatric Supracondylar Humerus Fractures. J Pediatr Orthop 2018;38(3):e118–21.

72. DeFrancesco CJ, Rogers BH, Shah AS. Obesity Increases Risk of Loss of Reduction After Casting for Diaphyseal Fractures of the Radius and Ulna in Children: An Observational Cohort Study. J Orthop Trauma 2018;32(2):e46–51.

73. Okoroafor UC, Cannada LK, McGinty JL. Obesity and Failure of Nonsurgical Management of Pediatric Both-Bone Forearm Fractures. J Hand Surg Am 2017;42(9):711–6.

74. Gilbert SR, MacLennan PA, Backstrom I, et al. Altered lower extremity fracture characteristics in obese pediatric trauma patients. J Orthop Trauma 2015;29(1):e12–7.

75. Gettys FK, Jackson JB, Frick SL. Obesity in pediatric orthopaedics. Orthop Clin North Am 2011; 42(1):95–105, vii.

76. Leet AI, Pichard CP, Ain MC. Surgical treatment of femoral fractures in obese children: does excessive body weight increase the rate of complications? J Bone Joint Surg Am 2005;87(12): 2609–13.

77. Weiss JM, Choi P, Ghatan C, et al. Complications with flexible nailing of femur fractures more than double with child obesity and weight >50 kg. J Child Orthop 2009;3(1):53–8.

78. Li Y, Stabile KJ, Shilt JS. Biomechanical analysis of titanium elastic nail fixation in a pediatric femur fracture model. J Pediatr Orthop 2008;28(8):874–8.

79. Moroz LA, Launay F, Kocher MS, et al. Titanium elastic nailing of fractures of the femur in children. Predictors of complications and poor outcome. J Bone Joint Surg Br 2006;88(10):1361–6.

80. Basques BA, Lukasiewicz AM, Samuel AM, et al. Which Pediatric Orthopaedic Procedures Have the Greatest Risk of Adverse Outcomes? J Pediatr Orthop 2017;37(6):429–34.

81. Goodbody CM, Lee RJ, Flynn JM, et al. Titanium Elastic Nailing for Pediatric Tibia Fractures: Do Older, Heavier Kids Do Worse? J Pediatr Orthop 2016;36(5):472–7.

82. Confroy K, Miles C, Kaplan S, et al. Pediatric Obesity and Sports Medicine: A Narrative Review and Clinical Recommendations. Clin J Sport Med 2021;31(6):e484–98.

83. Bazelmans C, Coppieters Y, Godin I, et al. Is obesity associated with injuries among young people? Eur J Epidemiol 2004;19(11):1037–42.

84. Briggs MS, Bout-Tabaku S, McNally MP, et al. Relationships Between Standing Frontal-Plane Knee Alignment and Dynamic Knee Joint Loading During Walking and Jogging in Youth Who Are Obese. Phys Ther 2017;97(5):571–80.

85. Kim N, Browning RC, Lerner ZF. The effects of pediatric obesity on patellofemoral joint contact force during walking. Gait Posture 2019;73: 209–14.

86. McGraw B, McClenaghan BA, Williams HG, et al. Gait and postural stability in obese and nonobese prepubertal boys. Arch Phys Med Rehabil 2000; 81(4):484–9.

87. Deforche BI, Hills AP, Worringham CJ, et al. Balance and postural skills in normal-weight and overweight prepubertal boys. Int J Pediatr Obes 2009;4(3):175–82.

88. Tropp H, Ekstrand J, Gillquist J. Stabilometry in functional instability of the ankle and its value in predicting injury. Med Sci Sports Exerc 1984; 16(1):64–6. Available at: https://www.ncbi.nlm. nih.gov/pubmed/6708781.

89. McGuine TA, Greene JJ, Best T, et al. Balance as a predictor of ankle injuries in high school basketball players. Clin J Sport Med 2000;10(4):239–44.

90. Krul M, van der Wouden JC, Schellevis FG, et al. Musculoskeletal problems in overweight and obese children. Ann Fam Med 2009;7(4):352–6.

91. Zonfrillo MR, Seiden JA, House EM, et al. The association of overweight and ankle injuries in children. Ambul Pediatr 2008;8(1):66–9.

92. Timm NL, Grupp-Phelan J, Ho ML. Chronic ankle morbidity in obese children following an acute ankle injury. Arch Pediatr Adolesc Med 2005; 159(1):33–6.

93. Kaplan TA, Digel SL, Scavo VA, et al. Effect of obesity on injury risk in high school football players. Clin J Sport Med 1995;5(1):43–7.

94. Gómez JE, Ross SK, Calmbach WL, et al. Body fatness and increased injury rates in high school football linemen. Clin J Sport Med 1998;8(2):115–20.

95. McHugh MP. Oversized young athletes: a weighty concern. Br J Sports Med 2010;44(1):45–9.

96. Kessler JI, Jacobs JC Jr, Cannamela PC, et al. Childhood Obesity is Associated With Osteochondritis Dissecans of the Knee, Ankle, and Elbow in Children and Adolescents. J Pediatr Orthop 2018;38(5):e296–9.

97. Jones G, Ding C, Glisson M, et al. Knee articular cartilage development in children: a longitudinal study of the effect of sex, growth, body composition, and physical activity. Pediatr Res 2003;54(2):230–6.

98. Vavken P, Tepolt FA, Kocher MS. Concurrent Meniscal and Chondral Injuries in Pediatric and Adolescent Patients Undergoing ACL Reconstruction. J Pediatr Orthop 2018;38(2):105–9.

99. Patel NM, Talathi NS, Bram JT, et al. How Does Obesity Impact Pediatric Anterior Cruciate Ligament Reconstruction? Arthroscopy 2019;35(1):130–5.

100. MacAlpine EM, Talwar D, Storey EP, et al. Weight Gain After ACL Reconstruction in Pediatric and Adolescent Patients. Sports Health 2020;12(1):29–35.

101. Newman JT, Carry PM, Terhune EB, et al. Factors predictive of concomitant injuries among children and adolescents undergoing anterior cruciate ligament surgery. Am J Sports Med 2015;43(2):282–8.

102. Dumont GD, Hogue GD, Padalecki JR, et al. Meniscal and chondral injuries associated with pediatric anterior cruciate ligament tears: relationship of treatment time and patient-specific factors. Am J Sports Med 2012;40(9):2128–33.

103. Perkins CA, Christino MA, Busch MT, et al. Rates of Concomitant Meniscal Tears in Pediatric Patients With Anterior Cruciate Ligament Injuries Increase With Age and Body Mass Index. Orthop J Sports Med 2021;9(3). 2325967120986565.

104. Raad M, Thevenin Lemoine C, Bérard E, et al. Delayed reconstruction and high BMI z score increase the risk of meniscal tear in paediatric and adolescent anterior cruciate ligament injury. Knee Surg Sports Traumatol Arthrosc 2019;27(3):905–11.

105. Shieh A, Bastrom T, Roocroft J, et al. Meniscus tear patterns in relation to skeletal immaturity: children versus adolescents. Am J Sports Med 2013;41(12):2779–83.

Shoulder and Elbow

Management of Failed Rotator Cuff Repairs: A Review

Ian J. Wellington, MD[a],*, Annabelle P. Davey, MD[a],
Michael R. Mancini, MD[a], Benajmin C. Hawthorne, BS[a],
Maxwell T. Trudeau, BS[a], Colin L. Uyeki, BA[b],
Augustus D. Mazzocca, MS, MD[c]

KEYWORDS

• Rotator cuff repair • Revision • Augmentation • Biologics • Reverse shoulder arthroplasty

KEY POINTS

• Recurrent rotator cuff tears are a complex pathology.
• Revision rotator cuff repair can be augmented with autografts, allografts, or biologics.
• Superior capsule reconstruction, balloon arthroplasty, and bursal acromial reconstruction are each methods for preventing humeral head migration and subsequent arthropathy.
• Reverse total shoulder arthroplasty is an effective solution for older patients with recurrent or massive rotator cuff tears.

INTRODUCTION

Rotator cuff tears are one of the most common sources of shoulder disability treated by orthopedic surgeons, with an incidence of greater than 54% in patients 60 years or older of which 34.7% are symptomatic.[1,2] With our aging population, the incidence of rotator cuff tears and subsequent repairs will only increase over the coming decades. Unfortunately, current literature demonstrates high retear rates ranging between 13% and 80%.[3,4] Surgical technique, initial tear size, tendon retraction, fatty infiltration, and muscle atrophy are all thought to contribute to these unsatisfactory rates.[4]

Revision surgery presents surgeons with the unique challenge of managing intrinsic and extrinsic factors that may have led to a recurrent tear and influence the likelihood of a successful reoperation.[5–8] Intrinsic factors include poor tissue quality, postoperative complications, and retained hardware.[7,9] Often not considered in the same light, but just as essential to management are the extrinsic patient factors such as demographics, comorbidities, work/lifestyle requirements, and expectations.[10–12]

PATIENT EVALUATION

The evaluation of patients with a potential failure of their rotator cuff repair should begin with a thorough history and examination. Patients with failure of repair often present with continued shoulder pain and weakness.[13] The patient should be asked if there was a period of symptomatic improvement following the initial repair.[13] Timing of symptom onset following their repair, or a traumatic event, may suggest a failure of repair rather than another pathologic condition. Other causes of shoulder pain such as cervical spine pathology and adhesive capsulitis must be ruled out. Active

[a] University of Connecticut, 120 Dowling Way, Farmington, CT 06032, USA; [b] Frank H. Netter School of Medicine, Quinnipiac University, 370 Bassett Rd, North Haven, CT 06473, USA; [c] Massachusetts General Hospital, 55 Fruit St, Boston, MA 02114, USA
* Corresponding author.
E-mail address: iwellington@uchc.edu

Orthop Clin N Am 53 (2022) 473–482
https://doi.org/10.1016/j.ocl.2022.05.002
0030-5898/22/© 2022 Elsevier Inc. All rights reserved.

and passive range of motion should be evaluated; a decrease in passive range of motion may suggest adhesive capsulitis. A patient's rotator cuff strength should also be assessed: a positive Jobe sign may suggest recurrent supraspinatus tear or a positive liftoff or the belly-press test may point to a subscapularis tear. Evaluation of the biceps tendon in patients not treated with prior biceps tenotomy or tenodesis should be performed as Chen and colleagues found that 96% of patients with massive rotator cuff tears had concomitant biceps tendon pathology.[14]

Initial imaging should consist of standard radiographs of the shoulder, including a Grashey, lateral, scapular Y, and axillary views. The presence of joint degeneration should be evaluated, as well as any presence of static proximal humeral head migration. Magnetic resonance imaging (MRI) should be obtained; Motamedi and colleagues described a high sensitivity (91%) but low specificity (25%) of MRI in diagnosing a recurrent rotator cuff tear.[15] The MRI can be used to assess for non-rotator cuff pathologies, such as biceps tenosynovitis or a concurrent superior labrum from anterior to posterior tear (SLAP) tear. For recurrent rotator cuff tearing, MRI can be used to determine the extent of fatty infiltration of the involved muscles, number of tendons torn, and amount of retraction. MRI arthrogram can be helpful to detect a recurrent rotator cuff as it is difficult to determine between postoperative changes and intact tendon. Optionally, an ultrasound can be obtained with studies showing that ultrasound by an experienced sonographer has a sensitivity of 91% and specificity of 86% for diagnosis of rotator cuff tear.[16]

BIOLOGIC AUGMENTATION OF REVISION REPAIR

Revision arthroscopic rotator cuff repairs have had mixed success; good or excellent outcomes are seen in only 64% of patients with the remainder having fair or poor outcomes.[17] As such, graft and biologic augmentations have been investigated to optimize successful outcomes in patients undergoing revision repair. Biological modalities such as platelet-rich plasma (PRP), connective tissue progenitor (CTP) cells, and extracellular matrices (ECMs) have been studied for their potential role in reducing retear rates and improving healing of torn rotator cuffs. PRP has been shown to have proliferative effects on tenocytes via several growth factors, which promote cell growth and inhibit inflammation.

ALLOGRAFTS

Sears and colleagues published a case series following patients who underwent revision rotator cuff repair augmented with ECM patches for a minimum of 50 months and showed a 50% (8/16) retear rate. Subgroup analysis showed that patients with healed cuffs had significantly higher single assessment numeric evaluation (SANE) and American Shoulder and Elbow Surgeons (ASES) scores when compared with patients who suffered repair failure. Type of ECM patch had no effect on overall outcome. Although smokers and worker's compensation patients trended toward worse outcomes, there was no significant difference. Furthermore, there was no significant difference observed when comparing the number of tendons involved, age, previous infection, or deltoid dehiscence.[18]

Namdari and colleagues followed 23 revision rotator cuff tears using dermal allograft augmentation. At final follow-up, MRIs showed repeat tearing in 57% (8/14) of cases. A comparison of clinical outcomes in the healed versus unhealed patients revealed significantly more favorable ASES and SANE scores for healed patients ($P = .04$ and $P = .02$). The investigators concluded that although the patch provided significant benefit in patients without retear, the benefits and drawbacks of this augmentation need further investigation due to the complexity and cost of the augmented procedure.[19]

SYNTHETIC GRAFTS

Synthetic patches are available in various formulations and aim to improve the mechanical integrity of the repair and can be imbibed with adjuvants to promote cellular infiltration, however, these grafts have mixed success in reducing retear rates.[20] In the only study to date including revision repair, Lenart and colleagues followed 13 patients who underwent revision rotator cuff repair or rotator cuff repair following massive irreparable rotator cuff tears, augmented with a poly-L-lactide graft (X-Repair; Synthasome) and PRP. After a mean follow-up of 1.5 years, 5 of the 13 patients (38.4%) had an intact repair confirmed by MRI, whereas the remaining eight (61%) patients had full thickness recurrent tears.[21]

PLATELET-RICH PLASMA AND BONE MARROW

PRP and concentrated bone marrow aspirate (cBMA) have been commonly used as biologic adjuvants for rotator cuff repairs (Fig. 1). PRP

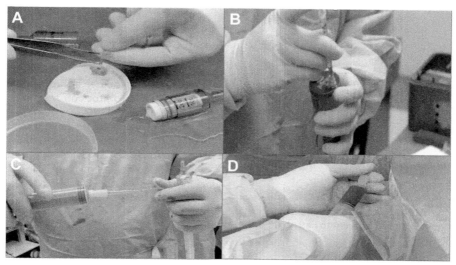

Fig. 1. Preparation of biologically augmented bursal tissue. (A) Preparation of bursal tissue collected with arthroscopic shaver using a tissue collector system (GraftNet; Arthrex, Naples, FL). (B) Combination of PRP with collected bursal tissue. (C) A pediatric chest tube is placed on a syringe. (D) Augmented bursal tissue is injected into the repair using pediatric chest tube.

has a high concentration of growth factors which have been shown to induce both inflammation and proliferation of new cells.[22,23] cBMA has been used as a common source of mesenchymal stem cells and has been shown to have potential to impact retear rates after rotator cuff repairs.[24,25]

Muench and colleagues followed 23 patients who underwent revision rotator cuff repair (RCR) augmented with an acellular dermal allograft that had been soaked and injected with intraoperatively extracted PRP and cBMA.[26] Patients were assessed after a mean two-and-a-half years for clinical improvement. Eight (36%) patients suffered clinical failure, and five (22.7%) patients required reoperation. A secondary analysis of cell cultures grown in the cBMA extracted from patients comparing failures to non-failures was also done. This analysis showed significantly more cells in the non-failure group on the 21st day of culture ($P = .02$) but no difference in CTP cell prevalence ($P = .81$) or concentration ($P = .73$).

SUPERIOR CAPSULAR RECONSTRUCTION

Superior capsular reconstruction (SCR) is an emerging option for younger, higher demand patients with recurrent rotator cuff tears (RCTs). The superior capsule of the glenohumeral joint and the rotator cuff work in conjunction to resist superior translation of the humeral head, with the superior capsule providing static stability and the rotator cuff providing dynamic

stability.[27] Reconstruction of the superior capsule is an option to maintain coronal stability of the glenohumeral joint in the rotator cuff deficient shoulder and to prevent progression to rotator cuff arthropathy.

SCR is often indicated in the setting of a retear because of the poor tissue quality in these patients limiting the feasibility of revision primary repair. SCR is an attractive option for patients with recurrent irreparable RCTs who are not candidates for reverse total shoulder arthroplasty (rTSA) due to younger age or higher demand.

SCR is performed arthroscopically by anchoring the graft from the greater tuberosity to the superior glenoid (Fig. 2).[28] Graft types that have been described include acellular dermal allograft, long head of the biceps tendon autograft, and fascia lata autograft or allograft.[29–31] If a subscapularis tear is present, it should be repaired at the time of surgery. The supraspinatus and infraspinatus may also be addressed concomitantly with either a partial rotator cuff repair or an "over-the-top" repair, which incorporates native rotator cuff tissue when fixing the graft to the greater tuberosity.[32]

Long-term clinical outcomes of SCR are limited, mainly due to the novelty of the procedure. Mihata and colleagues reported on a case series of 30 patients with 5-year follow-up.[33] They found a graft tear rate of 10% at 5 years, with overall statistically significant improvements in postoperative ASES scores, improvements in postoperative ROM, and increased acromiohumeral distance.[33] The

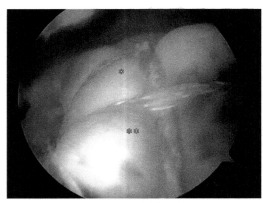

Fig. 2. Arthroscopic view of SCR demonstrating the dermal allograft (*asterisk*) adjacent to native cuff tissue (*double asterisk*).

failure and/or retear rate ranges from 3.4% to 36.1%.[29] There is a lack of data regarding SCR after recurrent rotator cuff tear. In one case-control study examining risk factors for SCR failure, Lee and colleagues found no significant correlation of SCR failure with prior failed rotator cuff repair.[34] This is a promising finding supporting the use of SCR in patients with recurrent rotator cuff tears, but further research is needed to fully understand the risk factors for poor outcome after SCR.

SUBACROMIAL BALLOON SPACERS

Subacromial balloon spacers are a novel advancement in managing irreparable rotator cuff tears. Although available in the European market since 2010, the first subacromial balloon spacer was recently granted clearance by the US Food and Drug Administration (FDA) in July 2021. Balloon spacers are made from a pre-shaped biodegradable copolymer which gets implanted in the subacromial space and filled with sterile saline. Over 12 months, the balloon progressively compresses and eventually degrades into a thick layer of fibrosis by 24 months.[35] Spacers aim to restore native glenohumeral biomechanics by providing a physical barrier to depress the humeral head and reduce subacromial friction.[36] A recent study by Lobao and colleagues found that spacers restored intact-state glenohumeral contact pressures at most abduction angles, lowered the humeral head, and increased the deltoid load.[37] By lowering the humeral head to a more native position in the glenoid and increasing tension on the deltoid, improved muscle contraction may be obtained, similar to the effects of reverse shoulder arthroplasty.

Subacromial balloon spacers are indicated to treat massive irreparable rotator cuff tears and failed rotator cuff repairs but can also be used in primary procedures with complex pathology. Balloon spacers can be used preemptively before reverse shoulder arthroplasty in patients with irreparable rotator cuff tears who lack glenohumeral arthritis.

Very few complications have been attributed to balloon implantation. A systematic review of 375 patients by Osti and colleagues determined an overall complication rate of 6.7%, which included 18 persistent shoulder pain, 3 balloon migrations, and 1 deep infection.[38]

BURSAL ACROMIAL RECONSTRUCTION

Bursal acromial reconstruction (BAR) is another novel technique developed for the management of irreparable rotator cuff tears. The BAR technique uses an acellular dermal allograft to recreate the normal subacromial bursa layer and provide interposition between the humeral head and acromion (Fig. 3).[39] Like the subacromial balloon spacers, the purpose of BAR is to reduce abnormal acromiohumeral articulation and minimize pain; however, unlike spacers, it serves as a permanent solution that does not biodegrade with time. BAR is indicated for elderly patients with irreparable rotator cuff tears and minimal glenohumeral arthritis.

The effect of BAR with an acellular dermal allograft on glenohumeral joint kinematics was recently analyzed in a biomechanical cadaveric study by Berthold and colleagues.[40] The investigators found that BAR improves glenohumeral joint kinematics compared with irreparable rotator cuff tear. There is limited literature assessing clinical outcomes following the BAR technique, which warrants further investigation.

TENDON TRANSFER

Originally described by Gerber and colleagues transfer of the latissimus dorsi tendon from its insertion on the humeral shaft to the superolateral humeral head serves as a treatment option for large irreparable posterosuperior cuff defects but can also be used for the treatment of failed primary rotator cuff repairs.[41] This treatment modality is generally used to treat younger patients with large rotator cuff defects without glenohumeral arthritis.[42]

Biomechanically, latissimus dorsi transfer alters the function of the latissimus dorsi muscle from an internal rotator that also imparts retroversion and abduction to the shoulder and

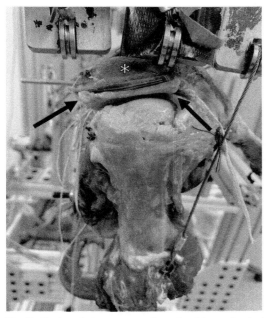

Fig. 3. Cadaveric humerus undergoing biomechanical testing following BAR. Dermal allograft (*arrows*) attached to the undersurface of the acromion (*asterisk*).

converts it into an external rotator.[42,43] Currently, it is unclear if this tendon transfer functions primarily via a tenodesis effect or by acting as a functional tendon.[44–46] Burkhart and colleagues showed that the balance of forces acting on the glenohumeral joint provided by latissimus dorsi transfer may allow the deltoid to function more effectively.[47] In addition to this mechanical function, this transfer serves as a large, vascularized flap for coverage of substantial cuff defects.[41]

Latissimus dorsi tendon transfer has shown promising outcomes in appropriately selected patients. A meta-analysis of 10 studies showed the significant improvement of Constant scores, reduction in pain scores, and improvement of subjective shoulder value scores in patients treated with latissimus dorsi transfer.[42] In addition, these patients showed a significant improvement in active forward elevation and external rotation. The preoperative status of the teres minor and subscapularis tendons have been shown to affect the outcomes following tendon transfer.[45,48,49] Iannotti and colleagues found that female gender, poor preoperative shoulder function, and generalized muscular weakness were all associated with poor clinical outcomes following latissimus transfer.[46] Finally, patients treated primarily with

latissimus transfer have been shown to have greater postoperative improvements of Constant scores and lower risk of latissimus tendon rupture when compared with those treated with transfer as a revision procedure.[50]

Latissimus tendon transfer has a total reported complication rate of 9.5% to 27%, with the most common complications being tears of the transferred tendon (3.4%), neuropraxia (2.7%), wound dehiscence (1.5%), failure of deltoid repair (0.7%), hematoma (0.7%), and infection (0.4%).[42,51] In addition, Muench and colleagues reported a clinical failure rate of 41% after latissimus transfer.[51]

Historically used for brachial plexus pathologies with a paralytic shoulder, transfer of the lower trapezius tendon has gained traction in the management of massive irreparable rotator cuff tears.[52] Lower trapezius transfer can be performed either open or with arthroscopic assistance. A study by Elhassan and colleagues followed 33 patients who underwent lower trapezius transfer with Achilles tendon allograft and found that 97% showed a significant improvement of shoulder flexion and abduction.[53] Omid and colleagues evaluated eight cadaveric shoulders treated with lower trapezius transfers or latissimus transfers and found that the lower trapezius transfers corrected shoulder kinematics throughout abduction range of motion, although the latissimus transfer only restored normal kinematics at 0° of abduction.[54] This is thought to be due to the more cranial origin of the lower trapezius relative to the latissimus, which closely mimics the line of pull of the infraspinatus. Although early results with lower trapezius transfers are promising, further study is warranted for this technique.

REVERSE TOTAL SHOULDER ARTHROPLASTY

An rTSA is typically the final option for patients with irreparable rotator cuff repairs (Fig. 4). First designed in France in 1985 by Paul Grammont for the treatment of arthritic shoulders with cuff insufficiency, the US FDA approved rTSA for treatment of cuff tear arthropathy (CTA) in 2004.[55,56] Since that time, the indications for rTSA have expanded to include primary osteoarthritis, rheumatoid arthritis, revision arthroplasty, and proximal humerus fractures, among others.[57]

The primary indication for rTSA following failed RCR remains CTA (typically reserved for Hamada grade 3 or greater). Advanced cuff tears may ultimately progress to CTA without

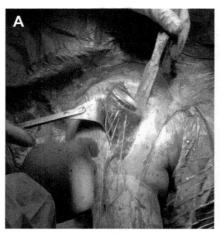 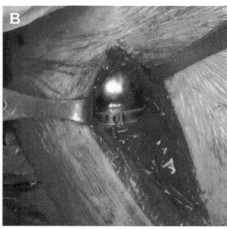

Fig. 4. Reverse total shoulder arthroplasty. (A) Humerus with trial components and (B) implants in position with trial liner between humeral implant and glenosphere.

appropriate diagnosis and management of patients with failed RCRs. With its biomechanical advantage in rotator cuff-deficient shoulders, rTSA has also gained favor in treating massive irreparable cuff tears in the absence of arthritis. However, for both indications, rTSA is typically reserved for patients older than 70 years due to concerns for implant survivorship in young, active patients.[58,59] rTSA for CTA has demonstrated success in providing reliable pain relief and improved function in an older population.[60] In addition, sufficient deltoid muscle integrity is required to elevate the arm and stabilize the joint without a functional rotator cuff. Along this line, permanent axillary nerve dysfunction is a contraindication for rTSA.

When evaluating a patient for potential rTSA, it is important to assess for pseudoparalysis (intact passive motion with an inability to elevate the arm beyond 90° actively) during physical examination. Computed tomography scans can assess bone stock, classify the glenoid morphology, and are used by commercially available preoperative planning software. Finally, MRI can evaluate the rotator cuff muscles by the Goutallier classification and the surrounding dynamic stabilizers such as the deltoid. In younger patients (less than 70) without glenohumeral arthritis or pseudoparalysis, joint-preserving interventions should be considered before rTSA.[61]

Dislocation is the most common complication following rTSA, with rates ranging from 1.5% to 31%.[62–65] Factors associated with dislocation are body mass index greater than 30, males, subscapularis deficiency, previous surgery, surgical approach, bone deficiency, and previous

trauma.[62–67] Other significant complications include acromial stress fractures, scapular notching, and glenoid baseplate failure. Fortunately, complication rates have declined with time, as one study demonstrated the overall complication rate decreased from 19% to 10.8%, and the revision rate decreased from 7.5% to 5%.[68] The lateralized rTSA designs demonstrate a 3% revision rate at a minimum 2-year follow-up.[69,70]

EVALUATION OF OUTCOME/LONG-TERM RECOMMENDATIONS

Following revision RCR, early therapy has focused on regaining preoperative motion and minimizing development of adhesive capsulitis.[71,72] However, following revision RCR, it is important to avoid over-tensioning the repair in the postoperative period.[73] Rehabilitation should be tailored to tendon integrity, which is influenced by clinical features of the patient, smoking, diabetes, and age.[74–76] During the initial period of immobilization, the goal is to achieve tendon healing while avoiding excessive stress on the repair. Several randomized controlled trials and meta-analyses have evaluated the efficacy between early versus delayed motion after RCR.[77,78] These studies demonstrated that early motion improves range of motion, but may increase the risk of rotator cuff retear. However, these studies did not specifically focus on patients with recurrent tears, which may limit generalizability. In addition, ideal form of rehabilitation after rotator cuff repair remains controversial.

As outlined by the American Society of Shoulder and Elbow Therapist, for small- to medium-sized tears, it is recommended to have 2 weeks of strict immobilization followed by staged introduction of protected range of motion.[74,76] At 6 weeks, the patient should progress to active range of motion, and at 12-week gradual strengthening exercises.[76] Protocols that focus on gradual strengthening targeting the deltoid, such as the Reading anterior deltoid program, can be helpful.[79] Return to work and sports is typically recommended 4 to 5 months after surgery.[73] For patients with poor tendon integrity and other risk factors for nonhealing, a more conservative approach featuring 6 weeks of strict immobilization should be pursued.[74]

NEW DEVELOPMENTS

Although novel treatments such as bone marrow stimulation or the use of xenografts have been investigated, they have shown the mixed results.[80–83] Given how new the techniques describe above are for the treatment of failed rotator cuff repairs, most of the current research is focused on refining these techniques.

DISCUSSION

Although recurrent rotator cuff tears present a complex challenge for treating surgeons, many management options exist. The decision of which of these modalities to pursue should be made between the surgeon and the patient, with careful consideration for patient selection and disease pathology. Although these different options have shown varying degrees of success, reverse shoulder arthroplasty provides a highly successful bailout solution in patients with a functioning deltoid muscle, although it is preferable to avoid its use in younger patients. New and improved solutions for this pathology continue to be developed as novel surgical techniques and biologic augmentation modalities are further investigated.

SUMMARY

Recurrent rotator cuff tears are a challenging pathology. After a thorough history and physical examination to confirm failure of a primary rotator cuff repair many revision surgical options exist. A repeat rotator cuff repair can be attempted with or without biologic or graft augmentation. The SCR, balloon arthroplasty, and BAR all can be used in large tears to prevent humeral head migration and reduce the risk of the development of arthropathy. Latissimus dorsi transfer provides a functional augmentation to a massive tear. Finally, if other methodologies prove unsuccessful, or the patient has developed CTA, reverse shoulder arthroplasty serves as a salvage procedure.

CLINICS CARE POINTS

- Recurrent rotator cuff tears are a complex pathology with many available treatment options.
- Diagnosis of recurrent tears should involve both physical examination and magnetic resonance imaging).
- Revision rotator cuff repair can be augmented with autografts, allografts, or biologics such as platelet-rich plasma or concentrated bone marrow aspirate.
- Superior capsule reconstruction, balloon arthroplasty, and bursal acromial reconstruction are each methods for preventing humeral head migration and subsequent arthropathy following massive rotator cuff tears.
- Reverse total shoulder arthroplasty is an effective solution for older patients with recurrent or massive rotator cuff tears.

REFERENCES

1. Bartolozzi A, Andreychik D, Ahmad S. Determinants of outcome in the treatment of rotator cuff disease. Clin Orthop Relat Res 1994;308(308):90–7.
2. Minagawa H, Yamamoto N, Abe H, et al. Prevalence of symptomatic and asymptomatic rotator cuff tears in the general population: From mass-screening in one village. J Orthop 2013;10(1):8–12.
3. Henry P, Wasserstein D, Park S, et al. Arthroscopic Repair for Chronic Massive Rotator Cuff Tears: A Systematic Review. Arthroscopy 2015;31(12):2472–80.
4. Kim I-B, Kim M-W. Risk factors for retear after arthroscopic repair of full-thickness rotator cuff tears using the suture bridge technique: classification system. Arthroscopy 2016;32(11):2191–200.
5. Denard PJ, Burkhart SS. Arthroscopic revision rotator cuff repair. J Am Acad Orthop Surg 2011;19(11):657–66.
6. Hartzler RU, Sperling JW, Schleck CD, et al. Clinical and radiographic factors influencing the results of revision rotator cuff repair. Int J Shoulder Surg 2013;7(2):41.
7. Keener JD, Wei AS, Kim HM, et al. Revision arthroscopic rotator cuff repair: repair integrity and clinical outcome. J Bone Joint Surg Am 2010;92(3):590–8.

8. Mora MV, Barrenechea DM, Ríos MDM, et al. Clinical outcome and prognostic factors of revision arthroscopic rotator cuff tear repair. Knee Surg Sports Traumatol Arthrosc 2017;25(7):2157–63.

9. Cho NS, Yi JW, Lee BG, et al. Retear patterns after arthroscopic rotator cuff repair: single-row versus suture bridge technique. Am J Sports Med 2010; 38(4):664–71.

10. Chen AL, Shapiro JA, Ahn AK, et al. Rotator cuff repair in patients with type I diabetes mellitus. J Shoulder Elb Surg 2003;12(5):416–21.

11. Clement ND, Hallett A, MacDonald D, et al. Does diabetes affect outcome after arthroscopic repair of the rotator cuff? J Bone Joint Surg Br 2010; 92(8):1112–7.

12. Mallon WJ, Misamore G, Snead DS, et al. The impact of preoperative smoking habits on the results of rotator cuff repair. J Shoulder Elb Surg 2004;13(2):129–32.

13. Strauss EJ, McCormack RA, Onyekwelu I, et al. Management of failed arthroscopic rotator cuff repair. J Am Acad Orthop Surg 2012;20(5):301–9.

14. Chen CH, Hsu KY, Chen WJ, et al. Incidence and severity of biceps long head tendon lesion in patients with complete rotator cuff tears. J Trauma 2005;58(6):1189–93.

15. Motamedi AR, Urrea LH, Hancock RE, et al. Accuracy of magnetic resonance imaging in determining the presence and size of recurrent rotator cuff tears. J Shoulder Elb Surg 2002;11(1):6–10.

16. Prickett WD, Teefey SA, Galatz LM, et al. Accuracy of ultrasound imaging of the rotator cuff in shoulders that are painful postoperatively. J Bone Joint Surg Am 2003;85(6):1084–9.

17. Lo IKY, Burkhart SS. Arthroscopic revision of failed rotator cuff repairs: technique and results. Arthroscopy 2004;20(3):250–67.

18. Sears BW, Choo A, Yu A, et al. Clinical outcomes in patients undergoing revision rotator cuff repair with extracellular matrix augmentation. Orthopedics 2015;38(4):e292–6.

19. Namdari S, Nicholson T, Brolin TJ, et al. Healing and Functional Results of Dermal Allograft Augmentation of Complex and Revision Rotator Cuff Repairs. Am J Sports Med 2021;49(8):2042–7.

20. Karuppaiah K, Sinha J. Scaffolds in the management of massive rotator cuff tears: current concepts and literature review. EFORT Open Rev 2019;4(9): 557–66.

21. Lenart BA, Martens KA, Kearns KA, et al. Treatment of massive and recurrent rotator cuff tears augmented with a poly-l-lactide graft, a preliminary study. J Shoulder Elb Surg 2015;24(6):915–21.

22. Foster TE, Puskas BL, Mandelbaum BR, et al. Platelet-rich plasma: from basic science to clinical applications. Am J Sports Med 2009;37(11):2259–72.

23. Jo CH, Kim JE, Yoon KS, et al. Platelet-rich plasma stimulates cell proliferation and enhances matrix gene expression and synthesis in tenocytes from human rotator cuff tendons with degenerative tears. Am J Sports Med 2012;40(5):1035–45.

24. Hernigou P, Flouzat Lachaniette CH, Delambre J, et al. Biologic augmentation of rotator cuff repair with mesenchymal stem cells during arthroscopy improves healing and prevents further tears: a case-controlled study. Int Orthop 2014;38(9): 1811–8.

25. Imam MA, Holton J, Horriat S, et al. A systematic review of the concept and clinical applications of bone marrow aspirate concentrate in tendon pathology. SICOT-J 2017;3:58.

26. Muench LN, Kia C, Jerliu A, et al. Clinical outcomes following biologically enhanced patch augmentation repair as a salvage procedure for revision massive rotator cuff tears. Arthroscopy 2020;36(6): 1542–51.

27. Adams CR, DeMartino AM, Rego G, et al. The rotator cuff and the superior capsule: Why we need both. Arthroscopy 2016;32(12):2628–37.

28. Mihata T, Lee TQ, Watanabe C, et al. Clinical results of arthroscopic superior capsule reconstruction for irreparable rotator cuff tears. Arthroscopy 2013;29(3):459–70.

29. Catapano M, Ekhtiari S, Lin A, et al. Arthroscopic superior capsular reconstruction for massive, irreparable rotator cuff tears: A systematic review of modern literature. Arthroscopy 2019;35(4):1243–53.

30. Galvin JW, Kenney R, Curry EJ, et al. Superior capsular reconstruction for massive rotator cuff tears: A critical analysis review. JBJS Rev 2019; 7(6):e1.

31. Gao I, Sochacki KR, Freehill MT, et al. Superior capsular reconstruction: A systematic review of surgical techniques and clinical outcomes. Arthroscopy 2021;37(2):720–46.

32. Frank RM, Cvetanovich G, Savin D, et al. Superior capsular reconstruction: indications, techniques, and clinical outcomes. JBJS Rev 2018;6(7):e10.

33. Mihata T, Lee TQ, Hasegawa A, et al. Five-year Follow-up of Arthroscopic Superior Capsule Reconstruction for Irreparable Rotator Cuff Tears. J Bone Joint Surg Am 2019;7(3_suppl2). 2325967119S0019.

34. Lee S-J, Kang S-W, Chung I, et al. Which factors influence clinical outcomes after superior capsular reconstruction surgery? Orthop J Sport Med 2020; 8(12). 2325967120966410.

35. Ricci M, Vecchini E, Micheloni GM, et al. A clinical and radiological study of biodegradable subacromial spacer in the treatment of massive irreparable rotator cuff tears. Acta Bio Med Atenei Parm 2017; 88(Suppl 4):75.

36. Chevalier Y, Pietschmann MF, Thorwächter C, et al. Biodegradable spacer reduces the subacromial

pressure: A biomechanical cadaver study. Clin Biomech 2018;52:41–8.

37. Lobao MH, Canham RB, Melvani RT, et al. Biomechanics of Biodegradable Subacromial Balloon Spacer for Irreparable Superior Rotator Cuff Tears: Study of a Cadaveric Model. J Bone Joint Surg Am 2019;101(11). https://doi.org/10.2106/JBJS.18.00850.

38. Osti L, Milani L, Maggiore O, et al. Subacromial spacer implantation: an alternative to arthroscopic superior capsular reconstruction. A systematic review. Br Med Bull 2021. https://doi.org/10.1093/bmb/ldab014.

39. Ravenscroft M, Barnes MW, Muench LN, et al. Bursal Acromial Reconstruction (BAR) Using an Acellular Dermal Allograft as a Surgical Solution for the Treatment of Massive Irreparable Rotator Cuff Tears. Arthrosc Tech 2021;10(3):e877–85.

40. Berthold DP, Ravenscroft M, Bell R, et al. Bursal Acromial Reconstruction (BAR) Using an Acellular Dermal Allograft for Massive, Irreparable Posterosuperior Rotator Cuff Tears: A Dynamic Biomechanical Investigation. Arthroscopy 2021. https://doi.org/10.1016/J.ARTHRO.2021.07.021.

41. Gerber C, Vinh TS, Hertel R, et al. Latissimus dorsi transfer for the treatment of massive tears of the rotator cuff. A preliminary report. Clin Orthop Relat Res 1988;232:51–61.

42. Namdari S, Voleti P, Baldwin K, et al. Latissimus dorsi tendon transfer for irreparable rotator cuff tears: A systematic review. J Bone Joint Surg Am 2012;94(10):891–8.

43. Magermans DJ, Chadwick EKJ, Veeger HEJ, et al. Effectiveness of tendon transfers for massive rotator cuff tears: a simulation study. Clin Biomech 2004;19(2):116–22.

44. Aoki M, Okamura K, Fukushima S, et al. Transfer of latissimus dorsi for irreparable rotator-cuff tears. J Bone Joint Surg Br 1996;78(5):761–6.

45. Gerber C, Maquieira G, Espinosa N. Latissimus dorsi transfer for the treatment of irreparable rotator cuff tears. J Bone Joint Surg Am 2006;88(1):113–20.

46. Iannotti JP, Hennigan S, Herzog R, et al. Latissimus dorsi tendon transfer for irreparable posterosuperior rotator cuff tears: Factors affecting outcome. J Bone Joint Surg Am 2006;88(2):342–8.

47. Burkhart SS. Arthroscopic treatment of massive rotator cuff tears: Clinical results and biomechanical rationale. Clin Orthop Relat Res 1991;45–56. https://doi.org/10.1097/00003086-199106000-00006.

48. Costouros JG, Espinosa N, Schmid MR, et al. Teres minor integrity predicts outcome of latissimus dorsi tendon transfer for irreparable rotator cuff tears. J Shoulder Elb Surg 2007;16(6):727–34.

49. Gerber C, Rahm SA, Catanzaro S, et al. Latissimus dorsi tendon transfer for treatment of irreparable posterosuperior rotator cuff tears: long-term results at a minimum follow-up of ten years. J Bone Joint Surg Am 2013;95(21):1920–6.

50. Warner JJP, Parsons IM. Latissimus dorsi tendon transfer: A comparative analysis of primary and salvage reconstruction of massive, irreparable rotator cuff tears. J Shoulder Elb Surg 2001;10(6):514–21.

51. Muench LN, Kia C, Williams AA, et al. High Clinical Failure Rate After Latissimus Dorsi Transfer for Revision Massive Rotator Cuff Tears. Arthroscopy 2020;36(1):88–94.

52. Clouette J, Leroux T, Shanmugaraj A, et al. The lower trapezius transfer: a systematic review of biomechanical data, techniques, and clinical outcomes. J Shoulder Elb Surg 2020;29(7):1505–12.

53. Elhassan BT, Wagner ER, Werthel JD. Outcome of lower trapezius transfer to reconstruct massive irreparable posterior-superior rotator cuff tear. J Shoulder Elb Surg 2016;25(8):1346–53.

54. Omid R, Heckmann N, Wang L, et al. Biomechanical comparison between the trapezius transfer and latissimus transfer for irreparable posterosuperior rotator cuff tears. J Shoulder Elb Surg 2015;24(10):1635–43.

55. Grammont P, Trouilloud P, Laffay JP, et al. Etude et réalisation d'une nouvelle prothèse d'épaule. Rhumatol 1987;39(10):407–18.

56. Grammont PM, Baulot E. Delta shoulder prosthesis for rotator cuff rupture. Orthopedics 1993;16(1):65–8.

57. Erickson BJ, Bohl DD, Cole BJ, et al. Reverse total shoulder arthroplasty: indications and techniques across the world. Am J Orthop (Belle Mead Nj) 2018;47(9). https://doi.org/10.12788/ajo.2018.0079.

58. Ek ETH, Neukom L, Catanzaro S, Gerber C. Reverse total shoulder arthroplasty for massive irreparable rotator cuff tears in patients younger than 65 years old: results after five to fifteen years. J Shoulder Elb Surg 2013;22(9):1199–208.

59. Guery J, Favard L, Sirveaux F, et al. Reverse total shoulder arthroplasty: survivorship analysis of eighty replacements followed for five to ten years. J Bone Joint Surg Am 2006;88(8):1742–7.

60. Bacle G, Nové-Josserand L, Garaud P, et al. Long-term outcomes of reverse total shoulder arthroplasty: a follow-up of a previous study. J Bone Joint Surg Am 2017;99(6):454–61.

61. Goutallier D, Postel J, Bernageau J, et al. Fatty muscle degeneration in cuff ruptures. Pre- and postoperative evaluation by CT scan. Clin Orthop Relat Res 1994;304:78–83. Available at: https://europepmc.org/article/med/8020238. Accessed October 21, 2021.

62. Chalmers PN, Rahman Z, Romeo AA, et al. Early dislocation after reverse total shoulder arthroplasty. J Shoulder Elb Surg 2014;23(5):737–44.

63. Cheung E, Willis M, Walker M, et al. Complications in reverse total shoulder arthroplasty. J Am Acad Orthop Surg 2011;19(7):439–49.

64. Gallo RA, Gamradt SC, Mattern CJ, et al. Instability after reverse total shoulder replacement. J Shoulder Elb Surg 2011;20(4):584–90.

65. Zumstein MA, Pinedo M, Old J, et al. Problems, complications, reoperations, and revisions in reverse total shoulder arthroplasty: a systematic review. J Shoulder Elb Surg 2011;20(1):146–57.

66. Edwards TB, Williams MD, Labriola JE, et al. Subscapularis insufficiency and the risk of shoulder dislocation after reverse shoulder arthroplasty. J Shoulder Elb Surg 2009;18(6):892–6.

67. Trappey GJ, O'Connor DP, Edwards TB. What are the instability and infection rates after reverse shoulder arthroplasty? Clin Orthop Relat Res 2011;469(9):2505–11.

68. Walch G, Bacle G, Lädermann A, et al. Do the indications, results, and complications of reverse shoulder arthroplasty change with surgeon's experience? J Shoulder Elb Surg 2012;21(11):1470–7.

69. Cuff DJ, Virani NA, Levy J, et al. The treatment of deep shoulder infection and glenohumeral instability with debridement, reverse shoulder arthroplasty and postoperative antibiotics. J Bone Joint Surg Br 2008;90(3):336–42.

70. Frankle M, Siegal S, Pupello D, et al. The reverse shoulder prosthesis for glenohumeral arthritis associated with severe rotator cuff deficiency: a minimum two-year follow-up study of sixty patients. J Bone Joint Surg Am 2005;87(8):1697–705.

71. Mansat P, Cofield RH, Kersten TE, et al. Complications of rotator cuff repair. Orthop Clin 1997;28(2):205–13.

72. Schmidt CC, Jarrett CD, Brown BT. Management of rotator cuff tears. J Hand Surg Am 2015;40(2):399–408.

73. Rossi LA, Chahla J, Verma NN, et al. Rotator cuff retears. JBJS Rev 2020;8(1):e0039.

74. Jung C, Tepohl L, Tholen R, et al. Rehabilitation following rotator cuff repair. Obere Extrem 2018;13(1):45–61.

75. Longo UG, Carnevale A, Piergentili I, et al. Retear rates after rotator cuff surgery: a systematic review and meta-analysis. BMC Musculoskelet Disord 2021;22(1):1–14.

76. Thigpen CA, Shaffer MA, Gaunt BW, et al. The American Society of Shoulder and Elbow Therapists' consensus statement on rehabilitation following arthroscopic rotator cuff repair. J Shoulder Elb Surg 2016;25(4):521–35.

77. Houck DA, Kraeutler MJ, Schuette HB, et al. Early versus delayed motion after rotator cuff repair: a systematic review of overlapping meta-analyses. Am J Sports Med 2017;45(12):2911–5.

78. Li S, Sun H, Luo X, et al. The clinical effect of rehabilitation following arthroscopic rotator cuff repair: A meta-analysis of early versus delayed passive motion. Medicine (Baltimore) 2018;97(2):e9625.

79. NHS. Reading Orthopaedic Centre. 2010. Available at: https://www.shouldersurgery.com.au/pdf/reading-anterior-deltoid-program.pdf. Accessed January 18, 2022.

80. Bryant D, Holtby R, Willits K, et al. A randomized clinical trial to compare the effectiveness of rotator cuff repair with or without augmentation using porcine small intestine submucosa for patients with moderate to large rotator cuff tears: a pilot study. J Shoulder Elb Surg 2016;25(10):1623–33.

81. Ciampi P, Scotti C, Nonis A, et al. The benefit of synthetic versus biological patch augmentation in the repair of posterosuperior massive rotator cuff tears: a 3-year follow-up study. Am J Sports Med 2014;42(5):1169–75.

82. Milano G, Saccomanno MF, Careri S, et al. Efficacy of marrow-stimulating technique in arthroscopic rotator cuff repair: a prospective randomized study. Arthroscopy 2013;29(5):802–10.

83. Osti L, Buono A Del, Maffulli N. Pulsed electromagnetic fields after rotator cuff repair: a randomized, controlled study. Orthopedics 2015;38(3):e223–8.

Perioperative Management in Shoulder Arthroplasty
A Review of Current Practice

Christine Park, BA, Kier M. Blevins, MD, MBS*,
Alexandra V. Paul, MD, Jason S. Long, MD, MBA,
Lucy E. Meyer, MD, Oke A. Anakwenze, MD, MBA

KEYWORDS

- Shoulder arthroplasty • Perioperative management • Patient's education • Infection • Pain
- Hemostasis

KEY POINTS

- Perioperative management of patients undergoing shoulder arthroplasty may reduce complications and improve postoperative patient outcomes.
- Important components of perioperative management for shoulder arthroplasty include risk assessment, patient education, infection prevention, hemostasis, and pain control.
- Optimization of patients during the perioperative period may allow shoulder arthroplasty surgeons to maximize the benefit of surgery for patients.

INTRODUCTION

The prevalence of shoulder arthroplasty is projected to increase as the indication for surgery has expanded over the years to include a larger patient demographic.[1–3] Perioperative care is a key facet in mitigating risk for complications and optimizing surgical outcomes.[4] Specifically, attention has been focused on patient factors and selection with the preoperative evaluation of age, social support, and comorbidities.[5,6] In addition, increasing efforts have been made to reduce complications and more effectively manage postoperative pain without the need for inpatient hospital stays. With more studies reporting the advantages of ambulatory procedures in terms of cost-effectiveness and patient satisfaction in hip and knee arthroplasty,[7–9] efforts have been concentrated on improving perioperative practice and facilitating a transition of shoulder arthroplasty to outpatient surgery.[10] This review summarizes the current practice guidelines of perioperative management in shoulder arthroplasty.

DISCUSSION
Patient Baseline Characteristics and Outcomes

Outcome expectation significantly influences overall perception and improvement for patients undergoing shoulder arthroplasty, with positive outcome expectations positively correlated with greater satisfaction and postoperative outcome scores.[11,12] By contrast, psychological instability (ie, depression and anxiety) negatively impacts postoperative improvement in pain and increases the risk for a greater analgesic requirement postoperatively.[13,14] Furthermore, patients with a greater comorbidity burden and a history of substance abuse or narcotic dependence are likely to have a poor preoperative presentation and worse postoperative condition.[15–17] Hence, preoperative risk assessment is essential to identify the patient population that will most likely

---

Department of Orthopaedic Surgery, Duke University Medical Center, 311 Trent Drive, Suite 2214, Box 104002, Durham, NC 27710, USA
* Corresponding author.
E-mail address: kier.blevins@duke.edu

Orthop Clin N Am 53 (2022) 483–490
https://doi.org/10.1016/j.ocl.2022.05.003

benefit from shoulder arthroplasty and to accordingly optimize the treatment plan for this population.

Infection Prevention

As with any arthroplasty surgery, the prevention of periprosthetic joint infection (PJI) is of the utmost importance. There is no single defining patient characteristic regarding the development of PJI; therefore, a variety of factors need to be considered. Similar to hip and knee arthroplasty, *Staphylococcus aureus* and *Staphylococcus epidermidis* are some of the most common pathogens in shoulder arthroplasty. *Cutibacterium acnes* is unique to shoulder arthroplasty with colonization rates between 42% and 73% before skin preparation.[18–20] Even after sterile skin preparation, cultures have demonstrated continued colonization in up to 20% of patients with C acnes.[18]

Preoperative antibiotics, given within 1 hour of incision, are the standard of care for the shoulder arthroplasty surgeons. The antibiotic of choice is cefazolin in patients who do not have a true allergy.[21,22] Cefazolin has good coverage of typical skin flora, including Gram-positive and Gram-negative aerobic bacteria.[23,24] In addition, cefazolin has been shown to have particularly good coverage of C acnes. Some studies have shown that patients who receive antibiotics other than cefazolin, including vancomycin and clindamycin, have a higher rate of PJI postoperatively.[24–26] The addition of a second antibiotic in combination with cefazolin, such as doxycycline, has not been shown to affect postoperative infection rates.[27] In patients who have documented penicillin or cephalosporin allergy but no history of severe reaction to these medications, it may be beneficial to administer a test dose of cefazolin to determine whether the patient can tolerate cefazolin.

In addition, intraoperative topical vancomycin powder is widely used in shoulder arthroplasty. Although data exist refuting the utility of topical vancomycin, there is also contrasting literature supporting its use and reduction in postoperative infections in spine surgery as well as in hip and knee arthroplasty.[28–31] There is limited evidence specific to shoulder arthroplasty, but recent studies suggest that the addition of vancomycin powder is safe and cost-effective and may reduce the bacterial burden within the surgical wound.[32,33] Given the low risk for complication and demonstrated efficacy in other orthopedic subspecialties, it is reasonable to continue the use of intraoperative vancomycin powder in shoulder arthroplasty.

Skin preparation before entering the operating room and immediately before the incision is an important step in reducing the bacterial burden on patients. Standard practice for patients' undergoing shoulder arthroplasty includes a preoperative chlorohexidine-based scrub at home before coming to the hospital. This has been shown to lower the bacterial burden on the skin, although it does not specifically reduce the amount of C acnes.[34] Recently, there has been increasing investigation as to whether the addition of benzoyl peroxide or hydrogen peroxide may reduce the risk of C acnes infection. Randomized controlled trials have not demonstrated that the addition of benzoyl or hydrogen peroxide at home or immediately preoperatively decreases the rate of positive cultures taken before surgery from the skin of shoulder arthroplasty patients.[35–37] Nevertheless, there are prospective data suggesting a lower rate of positive cultures from within the joint following skin preparation with hydrogen peroxide and chlorohexidine.[38] Likewise, topical application of chlorohexidine with benzoyl peroxide and topical clindamycin has shown to reduce rates of positive skin cultures during shoulder surgery.[39] In addition, cultures taken from the end of the procedure compared with the time of incision demonstrate a higher positivity rate.[32] Overall, it is clear that skin preparation before surgery and immediately before the incision is an important step in reducing bacterial burden. Although there are conflicting data as to the efficacy of peroxide solutions in reducing postoperative infections, the risk and costs associated with adding peroxide to the standard preparation of chlorohexidine are low. Further research is needed to determine whether topical antibiotics before incision have clinically significant effects.

Perioperative Pain Management
Preoperative period: patient education and expectations

Pain control is a significant contributor to patient recovery following shoulder arthroplasty.[40,41] In the preoperative setting, it is important to identify patients with a low postsurgical pain threshold secondary to opioid dependence or those who are at risk for increased pain to set proper expectations for effective pain management. Because acute and chronic joint pain is prevalent in shoulder arthroplasty candidates, surgeons should carefully investigate any preoperative opioid use in this patient population. Despite the well-known adverse effects of opioids (including gastrointestinal, hormonal complications, and short-term and long-term dependence), there is limited evidence that opioid therapy is truly more effective for pain control than nonopioid alternatives.[42–44] Despite many significant adverse effects, it remains an unfortunate consequence that the rate of opioid prescriptions and use continues to grow.[45]

Studies have also emphasized the relationship between preoperative opioid use and increased postoperative consumption that correlates with poorer patient-reported outcomes in the shoulder arthroplasty population.[17,46] Cheah and *colleagues* reported that patients consuming opiates for more than 3 months before undergoing shoulder surgery are up to 11 times more likely to require pain medications for a longer period of time postoperatively.[17] The literature also shows that shoulder arthroplasty patients who took opioids preoperatively did not achieve the same functional recovery as those who did not.[47,48] Although the negative effect of opioid use on postoperative outcomes is not fully reversible, patient education has been shown to be an effective method in establishing postoperative expectations and improving pain control and patient satisfaction following shoulder arthroplasty.[49,50]

Intraoperative pain management: general and regional anesthesia

Shoulder arthroplasty has evolved significantly in intraoperative pain control options. Although general anesthesia (GA) has typically been the primary modality of analgesia used in the intraoperative setting, GA alone is not effective in providing local pain control in the immediate postoperative period. This mainstay anesthesia trend likely contributes to the high opioid prescription rates in patients undergoing elective shoulder arthroplasty.[51] Recently, regional anesthesia (RA) has been growing in popularity. In shoulder arthroplasty, RA involves anesthetizing the upper extremity through nerve blocks at the brachial plexus from either the interscalene, supraclavicular or infraclavicular approaches. In addition to providing intraoperative pain control, RA also demonstrates improved postoperative pain control, reduced postoperative opioid use, faster recovery time, and shorter hospital stay compared with GA.[52,53] Although GA is associated with its own risks, RA is prone to nerve injury if improper technique is used. For example, interscalene nerve blocks, which are the most studied and considered the gold standard mode of RA,[54] can result in short-term postoperative nerve injuries in as high as 14% of patients undergoing shoulder arthroplasty.[55]

But the prevalence of nerve injury decreases to less than 1% in the long term (>6 months after surgery).[56,57] Also, for interscalene nerve blocks, the high possibility of concomitant phrenic nerve block during the administration of interscalene nerve block because the phrenic nerve runs near the brachial plexus at the level of C5–6 on the superficial surface of the anterior scalene muscle. The risk of simultaneous phrenic nerve block can be as high as 100% using the traditional landmark-based approach with a high anesthetic dose (usually >20 mL), with dose reduction decreasing the risk to only about 25% to 50%.[58,59] Although this transient phrenic nerve block does not usually cause any significant symptoms and complications that require treatment, patients with pulmonary disease or respiratory restrictions are the exceptions because of their high likelihood of developing symptomatic phrenic nerve palsy associated with their underlying disease.[58] In addition to nerve injuries, RA is prone to rebound pain or a sharp increase in pain once effects decline.[60,61] Given these findings, it is ultimately up to the surgeon to select the appropriate method of anesthesia that is most likely to benefit the patient.

Postoperative pain management: multimodal medication and regional/local anesthesia

As an alternative to opioids, multimodal analgesia therapy is getting increasing attention for early postoperative pain control.[62,63] This combined approach has evolved to help decrease the postoperative opioid requirements and relies on the synergistic effects among analgesics of different mechanisms.[50,64,65] The combined regimen often consists of acetaminophen, nonsteroidal anti-inflammatory medications, opioid analgesic, and gabapentinoids.[40] The several studies have shown excellent results in pain control in patients undergoing various total joint arthroplasty operations with little to no opioid use and fewer complications. In addition to multimodal nonopioid pharmacotherapy, several studies have investigated the efficacy of RA and local anesthesia (LA) in providing comparable pain relief in patients undergoing shoulder arthroplasty.[66] The methods of RA include single-injection interscalene nerve block, continuous interscalene nerve block, and suprascapular (with or without circumflex) nerve block. LA is usually delivered in a peri/intra-articular manner with different anesthetic cocktails. The selection of injection type should depend on treatment goals and the patient's complication profile.

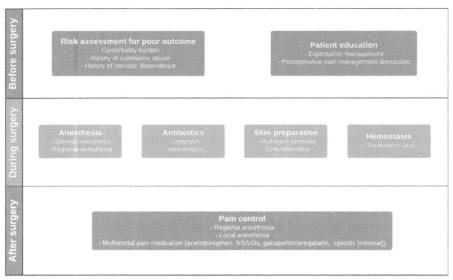

Fig. 1. Flowchart outlining the preoperative, intraoperative, and postoperative management practice for shoulder arthroplasty.

Perioperative Hemostasis

Total joint replacement surgeries are prone to high volume blood loss requiring transfusion.[67–69] Blood transfusions are not without risks that include disease transmission, cardiovascular dysfunction, allergic reactions, and infection.[70,71] Several studies have reported transfusion rates up to 43% after shoulder arthroplasty.[54,72,73] Also, many factors have been reported to be associated with an increased risk of transfusion, including advanced age, female gender, low preoperative hemoglobin levels, low body mass index, and increasing comorbidities.[54,72,73]

Tranexamic acid (TXA) is a synthetic antifibrinolytic agent that mimics the amino acid lysine and stabilizes blood clots by competitively inhibiting the lysine receptor found on plasminogen.[74] The binding of TXA prevents the conversion of plasminogen to its active form plasmin that prevents fibrin matrix degradation. Previous studies have shown that the use of TXA can achieve reduced blood loss and subsequently fewer perioperative blood transfusions in total joint surgery without increasing the risk of thromboembolic events.[73] This finding has been demonstrated in shoulder arthroplasty literature as well,[70,75,76] including recent randomized clinical trials.[77–79] In addition to reducing blood loss and blood transfusion, TXA may also aid in decreasing costs associated with inpatient length of stay and other fiscal measures. In a study done by Anthony and

colleagues, TXA was associated with a 35% reduction in postoperative complications and a 6.2% shorter hospital stay in patients undergoing shoulder arthroplasty.[80]

The present literature does not provide the optimal administration route, timing, and dose of TXA specific to shoulder arthroplasty. In total hip and knee arthroplasty, there was no significant difference in blood loss and postoperative complications between groups that received intravenous (IV) or topical administration of TXA.[81] However, subsequent studies reported that IV and topical TXA delivered in combination was associated with lower total blood loss and transfusion requirements compared with either IV or topical administration alone.[82–84] By contrast, there have also been studies demonstrating an equivalent reduction in blood loss when comparing administration of topical TXA, IV TXA, and in combination.[85] In shoulder arthroplasty, a comparative study done by Belay and colleagues found that IV and topical TXA resulted in similar transfusion rates.[86] Another study done by Budge and colleagues found similar blood loss in patients who received IV or topical TXA during shoulder arthroplasty.[87] In terms of timing of TXA administration, studies report varying points of intervention ranging from 30 to 60 minutes before the incision, immediately after the following anesthesia, or at the incision, or during closure.[88] Regarding the optimal dosage of TXA, findings have been inconclusive throughout total joint arthroplasty literature. Some total hip and knee arthroplasty studies suggest additive benefits of multiple doses of TXA,[89,90] whereas others demonstrate similar effects in minimizing blood loss and the associated complications.[91–93] The literature on shoulder arthroplasty is limited, but a recent meta-analysis of level 1 randomized clinical trials conducted by Fan and *colleagues* showed that multiple doses resulted in similar blood loss compared with a single dose.[73] Further research is needed to clarify the optimal method of use of TXA, but there is nonetheless strong evidence that the use of some form of TXA can reduce intraoperative blood and the need for postoperative blood transfusions.

SUMMARY

This review summarizes the important preoperative factors that influence outcomes in patients undergoing shoulder arthroplasty. The current practice recommends surgeons to consider patient baseline characteristics, infection prevention, pain management, and hemostasis when finalizing the plan for shoulder arthroplasty (Fig. 1).

CLINICS CARE POINTS

- Before shoulder arthroplasty, consider assessing patient risk factors for poor outcomes and providing patient education to manage expectations.
- During surgery, consider the choice of antibiotics for infection, general or regional anesthesia for pain, and tranexamic acid for hemostasis.
- After surgery, consider regional anesthesia or local anesthesia and multimodal pain medication for pain management.

DISCLOSURE

The authors have nothing to disclose.

REFERENCES

1. Farley KX, Wilson JM, Kumar A, et al. Prevalence of Shoulder Arthroplasty in the United States and the Increasing Burden of Revision Shoulder Arthroplasty. JB JS Open Access 2021;6(3). https://doi.org/10.2106/jbjs.Oa.20.00156.
2. Jain NB, Yamaguchi K. The contribution of reverse shoulder arthroplasty to utilization of primary shoulder arthroplasty. J Shoulder Elbow Surg 2014;23(12):1905–12.
3. Kim SH, Wise BL, Zhang Y, et al. Increasing Incidence of Shoulder Arthroplasty in the United States. JBJS 2011;93(24):2249–54.
4. Godlewski M, Knudsen ML, Braman JP, et al. Perioperative Management in Reverse Total Shoulder Arthroplasty. Curr Rev Musculoskelet Med 2021;14(4):282–90.
5. Hijazi A, Padela MT, Sayeed Z, et al. Review article: Patient characteristics that act as risk factors for intraoperative complications in hip, knee, and shoulder arthroplasties. J Orthop 2019;17:193–7.
6. Bernstein DN, Keswani A, Ring D. Perioperative Risk Adjustment for Total Shoulder Arthroplasty: Are Simple Clinically Driven Models Sufficient? Clin Orthop Relat Res 2017;475(12):2867–74.
7. Crawford DC, Li CS, Sprague S, et al. Clinical and Cost Implications of Inpatient Versus Outpatient Orthopedic Surgeries: A Systematic Review of the Published Literature. Orthop Rev (Pavia) 2015;7(4):6177.
8. Kelly MP, Calkins TE, Culvern C, et al. Inpatient Versus Outpatient Hip and Knee Arthroplasty: Which Has Higher Patient Satisfaction? J Arthroplasty 2018;33(11):3402–6.
9. Huang A, Ryu J-J, Dervin G. Cost savings of outpatient versus standard inpatient total knee arthroplasty. Can J Surg 2017;60(1):57–62.
10. Allahabadi S, Cheung EC, Hodax JD, et al. Outpatient Shoulder Arthroplasty—A Systematic Review. J Shoulder Elbow Arthroplasty 2021;5. 24715492211028025.
11. O'Malley KJ, Roddey TS, Gartsman GM, et al. Outcome expectancies, functional outcomes, and expectancy fulfillment for patients with shoulder problems. Med Care 2004;42(2):139–46.
12. Henn RF 3rd, Kang L, Tashjian RZ, et al. Patients' preoperative expectations predict the outcome of rotator cuff repair. J Bone Joint Surg Am 2007;89(9):1913–9.
13. Cho CH, Seo HJ, Bae KC, et al. The impact of depression and anxiety on self-assessed pain, disability, and quality of life in patients scheduled for rotator cuff repair. J Shoulder Elbow Surg 2013;22(9):1160–6.
14. Roh YH, Lee BK, Noh JH, et al. Effect of depressive symptoms on perceived disability in patients with chronic shoulder pain. Arch Orthop Trauma Surg 2012;132(9):1251–7.
15. Porter A, Greiwe RM. Psychological disorders confer poor functional outcomes after reverse total shoulder arthroplasty. JSES Rev Rep Tech 2021;1(4):357–60.
16. Ling DI, Schneider B, Ode G, et al. The impact of Charlson and Elixhauser comorbidities on patient

outcomes following shoulder arthroplasty. Bone Joint J 2021;103-b(5):964–70.

17. Cheah JW, Sing DC, McLaughlin D, et al. The perioperative effects of chronic preoperative opioid use on shoulder arthroplasty outcomes. J Shoulder Elbow Surg 2017;26(11):1908–14.

18. Chuang MJ, Jancosko JJ, Mendoza V, et al. The Incidence of Propionibacterium acnes in Shoulder Arthroscopy. Arthroscopy 2015;31(9):1702–7.

19. Foster AL, Cutbush K, Ezure Y, et al. Cutibacterium acnes in shoulder surgery: a scoping review of strategies for prevention, diagnosis, and treatment. J Shoulder Elbow Surg 2021;30(6):1410–22.

20. Phadnis J, Gordon D, Krishnan J, et al. Frequent isolation of Propionibacterium acnes from the shoulder dermis despite skin preparation and prophylactic antibiotics. J Shoulder Elbow Surg 2016;25(2):304–10.

21. Boyle KK, Duquin TR. Antibiotic Prophylaxis and Prevention of Surgical Site Infection in Shoulder and Elbow Surgery. Orthop Clin North Am 2018;49(2):241–56.

22. Campbell KA, Stein S, Looze C, et al. Antibiotic stewardship in orthopaedic surgery: principles and practice. J Am Acad Orthop Surg 2014;22(12):772–81.

23. Neu HC. Cephalosporin antibiotics as applied in surgery of bones and joints. Clin Orthop Relat Res 1984;190:50–64.

24. Bratzler DW, Dellinger EP, Olsen KM, et al. Clinical practice guidelines for antimicrobial prophylaxis in surgery. Am J Health Syst Pharm 2013;70(3):195–283.

25. Kheir MM, Tan TL, Azboy I, et al. Vancomycin Prophylaxis for Total Joint Arthroplasty: Incorrectly Dosed and Has a Higher Rate of Periprosthetic Infection Than Cefazolin. Clin Orthop Relat Res 2017;475(7):1767–74.

26. Yian EH, Chan PH, Burfeind W, et al. Perioperative Clindamycin Use in Penicillin Allergic Patients Is Associated With a Higher Risk of Infection After Shoulder Arthroplasty. J Am Acad Orthop Surg 2020;28(6):e270–6.

27. Rao AJ, Chalmers PN, Cvetanovich GL, et al. Preoperative Doxycycline Does Not Reduce Propionibacterium acnes in Shoulder Arthroplasty. J Bone Joint Surg Am 2018;100(11):958–64.

28. Caroom C, Tullar JM, Benton EG Jr, et al. Intrawound vancomycin powder reduces surgical site infections in posterior cervical fusion. Spine (Phila Pa 1976) 2013;38(14):1183–7.

29. Evaniew N, Belley-Côté EP, Khan M, et al. Letter to the Editor Regarding The Use of Vancomycin Powder in Modern Spine Surgery: Systematic Review and Meta-Analysis of the Clinical Evidence. World Neurosurg 2016;88:675.

30. Kanj WW, Flynn JM, Spiegel DA, et al. Vancomycin prophylaxis of surgical site infection in clean orthopedic surgery. Orthopedics 2013;36(2):138–46.

31. Molinari RW, Khera OA, Molinari WJ 3rd. Prophylactic intraoperative powdered vancomycin and postoperative deep spinal wound infection: 1,512 consecutive surgical cases over a 6-year period. Eur Spine J 2012;21(Suppl 4):S476–82.

32. Hatch MD, Daniels SD, Glerum KM, et al. The cost effectiveness of vancomycin for preventing infections after shoulder arthroplasty: a break-even analysis. J Shoulder Elbow Surg 2017;26(3):472–7.

33. Miquel J, Huang TB, Athwal GS, et al. Vancomycin is effective in preventing Cutibacterium acnes growth in a mimetic shoulder arthroplasty. J Shoulder Elbow Surg 2022;31(1):159–64.

34. Matsen FA, Whitson AJ, Hsu JE. While home chlorhexidine washes prior to shoulder surgery lower skin loads of most bacteria, they are not effective against Cutibacterium (Propionibacterium). Int Orthop 2020;44(3):531–4.

35. Hancock DS, Rupasinghe SL, Elkinson I, et al. Benzoyl peroxide + chlorhexidine versus chlorhexidine alone skin preparation to reduce Propionibacterium acnes: a randomized controlled trial. ANZ J Surg 2018;88(11):1182–6.

36. Hsu JE, Whitson AJ, Woodhead BM, et al. Randomized controlled trial of chlorhexidine wash versus benzoyl peroxide soap for home surgical preparation: neither is effective in removing Cutibacterium from the skin of shoulder arthroplasty patients. Int Orthop 2020;44(7):1325–9.

37. Grewal G, Polisetty T, Boltuch A, et al. Does application of hydrogen peroxide to the dermis reduce incidence of Cutibacterium acnes during shoulder arthroplasty: a randomized controlled trial. J Shoulder Elbow Surg 2021;30(8):1827–33.

38. Chalmers PN, Beck L, Stertz I, et al. Hydrogen peroxide skin preparation reduces Cutibacterium acnes in shoulder arthroplasty: a prospective, blinded, controlled trial. J Shoulder Elbow Surg 2019;28(8):1554–61.

39. Symonds T, Grant A, Doma K, et al. The Efficacy of Topical Preparations in Reducing The Incidence of Cutibacterium Acnes at The Start and Conclusion of Total Shoulder Arthroplasty (TSA): A Randomized Controlled Trial. J Shoulder Elbow Surg 2022. https://doi.org/10.1016/j.jse.2022.01.133.

40. Fredrickson MJ, Krishnan S, Chen CY. Postoperative analgesia for shoulder surgery: a critical appraisal and review of current techniques. Anaesthesia 2010;65(6):608–24.

41. Warrender WJ, Syed UAM, Hammoud S, et al. Pain Management After Outpatient Shoulder Arthroscopy: A Systematic Review of Randomized Controlled Trials. Am J Sports Med 2017;45(7):1676–86.

42. Barnett ML. Opioid Prescribing in the Midst of Crisis — Myths and Realities. N Engl J Med 2020; 382(12):1086–8.

43. Busse JW, Wang L, Kamaleldin M, et al. Opioids for Chronic Noncancer Pain: A Systematic Review and Meta-analysis. JAMA 2018;320(23):2448–60.

44. Benyamin R, Trescot AM, Datta S, et al. Opioid complications and side effects. Pain Physician 2008;11(2 Suppl):S105–20.

45. Gray BM, Vandergrift JL, Weng W, et al. Clinical Knowledge and Trends in Physicians' Prescribing of Opioids for New Onset Back Pain, 2009-2017. JAMA Netw Open 2021;4(7):e2115328.

46. Kaidi AC, Lakra A, Jennings EL, et al. Opioid Prescription Consumption Patterns After Total Joint Arthroplasty in Chronic Opioid Users Versus Opioid Naive Patients. J Am Acad Orthop Surg Glob Res Rev 2020;4(6). e20.00066.

47. Morris BJ, Laughlin MS, Elkousy HA, et al. Preoperative opioid use and outcomes after reverse shoulder arthroplasty. J Shoulder Elbow Surg 2015;24(1): 11–6.

48. Williams BT, Redlich NJ, Mickschl DJ, et al. Influence of preoperative opioid use on postoperative outcomes and opioid use after arthroscopic rotator cuff repair. J Shoulder Elbow Surg 2019;28(3): 453–60.

49. Syed UAM, Aleem AW, Wowkanech C, et al. Neer Award 2018: the effect of preoperative education on opioid consumption in patients undergoing arthroscopic rotator cuff repair: a prospective, randomized clinical trial. J Shoulder Elbow Surg 2018; 27(6):962–7.

50. Patel MS, Abboud JA, Sethi PM. Perioperative pain management for shoulder surgery: evolving techniques. J Shoulder Elbow Surg 2020;29(11):e416–33.

51. Ding DY, Mahure SA, Mollon B, et al. Comparison of general versus isolated regional anesthesia in total shoulder arthroplasty: A retrospective propensity-matched cohort analysis. J Orthop 2017;14(4):417–24.

52. D'Alessio JG, Rosenblum M, Shea KP, et al. A retrospective comparison of interscalene block and general anesthesia for ambulatory surgery shoulder arthroscopy. Reg Anesth 1995;20(1):62–8.

53. Brown AR, Weiss R, Greenberg C, et al. Interscalene block for shoulder arthroscopy: comparison with general anesthesia. Arthroscopy 1993;9(3): 295–300.

54. Singh VK, Trehan R, Banerjee S, et al. Blood Loss and the Need for Transfusion after Shoulder Surface Replacement. Shoulder Elbow 2013;5(2):100–5.

55. Yim G, Lin Z, Shirley C, et al. The late diagnosis of nerve injuries following interscalene block and shoulder surgery. 01/01 2019;doi:10.4103/ jmsr.jmsr_65_18.

56. Borgeat A, Ekatodramis G, Kalberer F, et al. Acute and nonacute complications associated with interscalene block and shoulder surgery: a prospective study. Anesthesiology 2001;95(4):875–80.

57. Fredrickson MJ, Kilfoyle DH. Neurological complication analysis of 1000 ultrasound guided peripheral nerve blocks for elective orthopaedic surgery: a prospective study. Anaesthesia 2009;64(8): 836–44.

58. El-Boghdadly K, Chin KJ, Chan VWS. Phrenic Nerve Palsy and Regional Anesthesia for Shoulder Surgery: Anatomical, Physiologic, and Clinical Considerations. Anesthesiology 2017;127(1):173–91.

59. Riazi S, Carmichael N, Awad I, et al. Effect of local anaesthetic volume (20 vs 5 ml) on the efficacy and respiratory consequences of ultrasound-guided interscalene brachial plexus block. Br J Anaesth 2008;101(4):549–56.

60. Namdari S, Nicholson T, Abboud J, et al. Randomized Controlled Trial of Interscalene Block Compared with Injectable Liposomal Bupivacaine in Shoulder Arthroplasty. J Bone Joint Surg Am 2017;99(7):550–6.

61. Okoroha KR, Lynch JR, Keller RA, et al. Liposomal bupivacaine versus interscalene nerve block for pain control after shoulder arthroplasty: a prospective randomized trial. J Shoulder Elbow Surg 2016; 25(11):1742–8.

62. Shanthanna H, Ladha KS, Kehlet H, et al. Perioperative Opioid Administration. Anesthesiology 2021; 134(4):645–59.

63. McLaughlin DC, Cheah JW, Aleshi P, et al. Multimodal analgesia decreases opioid consumption after shoulder arthroplasty: a prospective cohort study. J Shoulder Elbow Surg 2018;27(4):686–91.

64. Elkassabany NM, Wang A, Ochroch J, et al. Improved Quality of Recovery from Ambulatory Shoulder Surgery After Implementation of a Multimodal Perioperative Pain Management Protocol. Pain Med 2019;20(5):1012–9.

65. Jin F, Chung F. Multimodal analgesia for postoperative pain control1 1This paper is partially sponsored by Pharmacia Corporation, Skokie, IL. J Clin Anesth 2001;13(7):524–39.

66. Updegrove GF, Stauch CM, Ponnuru P, et al. Efficacy of local infiltration anesthesia versus interscalene nerve blockade for total shoulder arthroplasty. JSES Int 2020;4(2):357–61.

67. Carling MS, Jeppsson A, Eriksson BI, et al. Transfusions and blood loss in total hip and knee arthroplasty: a prospective observational study. J Orthop Surg Res 2015;10(1):48.

68. White CCt, Eichinger JK, Friedman RJ. Minimizing Blood Loss and Transfusions in Total Knee Arthroplasty. J Knee Surg 2018;31(7):594–9.

69. Cunningham G, Hughes J, Borner B, et al. A single dose of tranexamic acid reduces blood loss after

reverse and anatomic shoulder arthroplasty: a randomized controlled trial. J Shoulder Elbow Surg 2021;30(7):1553–60.

70. Kuo LT, Hsu WH, Chi CC, et al. Tranexamic acid in total shoulder arthroplasty and reverse shoulder arthroplasty: a systematic review and meta-analysis. BMC Musculoskelet Disord 2018;19(1):60.

71. Carson JL, Grossman BJ, Kleinman S, et al. Red blood cell transfusion: a clinical practice guideline from the AABB. Ann Intern Med 2012;157(1):49–58.

72. Burns KA, Robbins LM, LeMarr AR, et al. Estimated blood loss and anemia predict transfusion after total shoulder arthroplasty: a retrospective cohort study. JSES Open Access 2019;3(4):311–5.

73. Fan D, Ma J, Zhang L. Tranexamic acid achieves less blood loss volume of in primary shoulder arthroplasty: a systematic review and meta-analysis of level I randomized controlled trials. JSES Rev Rep Tech 2021;1(4):344–52.

74. Reed MR, Woolley LT. Uses of tranexamic acid. Contin Educ Anaesth Crit Care Pain 2015;15(1):32–7.

75. Friedman RJ, Gordon E, Butler RB, et al. Tranexamic acid decreases blood loss after total shoulder arthroplasty. J Shoulder Elbow Surg 2016;25(4):614–8.

76. Kirsch JM, Bedi A, Horner N, et al. Tranexamic Acid in Shoulder Arthroplasty: A Systematic Review and Meta-Analysis. JBJS Rev 2017;5(9):e3.

77. Gillespie R, Shishani Y, Joseph S, et al. Neer Award 2015: A randomized, prospective evaluation on the effectiveness of tranexamic acid in reducing blood loss after total shoulder arthroplasty. J Shoulder Elbow Surg 2015;24(11):1679–84.

78. Vara AD, Koueiter DM, Pinkas DE, et al. Intravenous tranexamic acid reduces total blood loss in reverse total shoulder arthroplasty: a prospective, double-blinded, randomized, controlled trial. J Shoulder Elbow Surg 2017;26(8):1383–9.

79. Cvetanovich GL, Fillingham YA, O'Brien M, et al. Tranexamic acid reduces blood loss after primary shoulder arthroplasty: a double-blind, placebo-controlled, prospective, randomized controlled trial. JSES Open Access 2018;2(1):23–7.

80. Anthony SG, Patterson DC, Cagle PJ Jr, et al. Utilization and real-world effectiveness of tranexamic use in shoulder arthroplasty: a population-based study. J Am Acad Orthop Surg 2019;27(19):736–42.

81. Shin YS, Yoon JR, Lee HN, et al. Intravenous versus topical tranexamic acid administration in primary total knee arthroplasty: a meta-analysis. Knee Surg Sports Traumatol Arthrosc 2017;25(11):3585–95.

82. Liu X, Liu J, Sun G. A comparison of combined intravenous and topical administration of tranexamic acid with intravenous tranexamic acid alone for blood loss reduction after total hip arthroplasty: A meta-analysis. Int J Surg 2017;41:34–43.

83. Sun Q, Li J, Chen J, et al. Comparison of intravenous, topical or combined routes of tranexamic acid administration in patients undergoing total knee and hip arthroplasty: a meta-analysis of randomised controlled trials. BMJ Open 2019;9(1):e024350.

84. Yang Y, Lv YM, Ding PJ, et al. The reduction in blood loss with intra-articular injection of tranexamic acid in unilateral total knee arthroplasty without operative drains: a randomized controlled trial. Eur J Orthop Surg Traumatol 2015;25(1):135–9.

85. Gómez-Luque J, Cruz-Pardos A, Garabito-Cociña A, et al. Topical, intravenous tranexamic acid and their combined use are equivalent in reducing blood loss after primary total hip arthroplasty. Rev Esp Cir Ortop Traumatol (Engl Ed) 2021;65(5):349–54.

86. Belay ES, O'Donnell J, Flamant E, et al. Intravenous tranexamic acid vs. topical thrombin in total shoulder arthroplasty: a comparative study. J Shoulder Elbow Surg 2021;30(2):312–6.

87. Budge M. Topical and Intravenous Tranexamic Acid Are Equivalent in Decreasing Blood Loss in Total Shoulder Arthroplasty. J Shoulder Elbow arthroplasty 2019;3. 2471549218821181.

88. Koutserimpas C, Besiris GT, Giannoulis D, et al. Tranexamic Acid in Shoulder Arthroplasty. A Comprehensive Review. Maedica (Bucur) 2021;16(1):97–101.

89. Lei Y, Huang Q, Huang Z, et al. Multiple-Dose Intravenous Tranexamic Acid Further Reduces Hidden Blood Loss After Total Hip Arthroplasty: A Randomized Controlled Trial. J Arthroplasty 2018;33(9):2940–5.

90. Lei Y, Xie J, Xu B, et al. The efficacy and safety of multiple-dose intravenous tranexamic acid on blood loss following total knee arthroplasty: a randomized controlled trial. Int Orthop 2017;41(10):2053–9.

91. Goyal T, Choudhury AK, Gupta T. Are Three Doses of Intravenous Tranexamic Acid more Effective than Single Dose in Reducing Blood Loss During Bilateral Total Knee Arthroplasty? Indian J Orthop 2020;54(6):805–10.

92. Chalmers BP, Mishu M, Cushner FD, et al. Is There a Synergistic Effect of Topical Plus Intravenous Tranexamic Acid Versus Intravenous Administration Alone on Blood Loss and Transfusions in Primary Total Hip and Knee Arthroplasties? Arthroplast Today 2021;7:194–9.

93. Palija S, Bijeljac S, Manojlovic S, et al. Effectiveness of different doses and routes of administration of tranexamic acid for total hip replacement. Int Orthop 2021;45(4):865–70.

Foot and Ankle

Patient Complaints in Orthopedic Surgery: An Analysis Utilizing a Large National Database

Shumaila Sarfani, MD[a],*, Andrew Rees, BS[a],
Justin Vickery, MD[a], John E. Kuhn, MD, MS[a],
Mitchell B. Galloway, MS[b], Henry Domenico, MS[b],
James W. Pichert, PhD[b], William O. Cooper, MD, MPH[b,c]

KEYWORDS

- Unsolicited patient complaints • Orthopedic surgeons • Patient advocacy reporting system
- Malpractice

KEY POINTS

- Orthopedic surgeons are significantly more likley to receive unsolicited patient complaints than non surgeons or other surgeons.
- A small proportion of orthopedic surgeons make up a disproprtionate number of overall complaints.
- Certain subspecialties are at higher risk than others for receiving complaints.
- Primary complaint types are related to care and communication.

INTRODUCTION

Medical malpractice claims are an important challenge for orthopedic surgeons. Orthopedic surgeons practice in one of the top four medical subspecialties with regard to proportion of physicians facing malpractice claims.[1,2] Fourteen percent of orthopedic surgeons face malpractice claims annually, and 4% of those are associated with claim payments. This makes orthopedics a "high-risk" surgical specialty with malpractice risk that follows only neurosurgery, cardiothoracic surgery, and general surgery.[3,4] In addition to financial implications, malpractice claims have significant personal repercussions including increased rates of burnout and depression.[4–6] Understanding more about risk factors for malpractice claims, particularly to support prevention, would be valuable to orthopedics.

Although studies of procedure-specific risks for malpractice claims are known to vary,[1,2,7–9] much less is known about individual orthopedists' risk factors. Unsolicited patient complaints (UPCs) among surgeons have previously been linked to quality and outcomes of care, most notably in terms of medical malpractice claims and post-procedure complications, but have not been assessed in orthopedics to date.[10–12] The objectives of this study were to use a large national validated database of UPCs to (1) describe the distribution of UPCs among orthopedic surgeons; (2) assess for clinical characteristics that may be associated with UPCs about orthopedists; and (3) assess for differences in

[a] Department of Orthopaedic Surgery, Vanderbilt University Medical Center, 1215 21st Avenue South, Medical Center East South Tower, Suite 4200, Nashville, TN 37232, USA; [b] Vanderbilt University Medical Center, Center for Patient and Professional Advocacy, 1215 21st Avenue South, Medical Center East South Tower, Suite 4200, Nashville, TN 37232, USA; [c] Department of Pediatrics, Vanderbilt University Medical Center, 1215 21st Avenue South, Medical Center East South Tower, Suite 4200, Nashville, TN 37232, USA
* Corresponding author.
E-mail address: s.sarfani@ortho-sa.com

Orthop Clin N Am 53 (2022) 491–497
https://doi.org/10.1016/j.ocl.2022.05.004
0030-5898/22/© 2022 Elsevier Inc. All rights reserved.

number and types of complaints between orthopedists and other physicians who are not identified as orthopedists.

METHODS
Study Design

The Vanderbilt Center for Patient and Professional Advocacy (CPPA) developed the Patient Advocacy Reporting System (PARS), which includes a database containing UPC reports and medical/surgical specialty data for more than 66,000 physicians across 36 participating health care systems and physician group practices. As part of the PARS program, participating institutions create narrative electronic reports by collecting and recording patient and family reports of their health care experiences. Organizations securely forward these reports to CPPA for entry into the PARS database for coding and analysis. Trained coders review each report and categorize them into five types of complaints (care and treatment, communication, access and availability, concern for patient and family, and billing concerns). Inter-rater reliability is well established and ranges from 73% to 100%.[4,13] The database for this study was created by linking coded UPC data to unambiguously identified physicians in a de-identified manner using the same procedures applied in other studies.[6,14–16]

Study Population

All physicians in active practice in PARS participating medical centers or medical groups from January 1, 2015 to December 31, 2018 were included in the study. Excluded were orthopedists in training (residents and fellows), those who were double-boarded, and any without 4 consecutive years of UPC data or with insufficient demographic information publicly available online. Trainees and those double-boarded were excluded to ease analysis that would be done based on orthopedic subspecialty.

The covariates of interest included orthopedic subspecialty, US or non-US medical school or residency, practice setting type, board certification status, sex, region of practice, and allopathic versus osteopathic medical training. Information was obtained from publicly available online sources.

Statistical Analysis

Characteristics of the orthopedic surgeon population were summarized using medians and interquartile ranges for continuous variables or frequencies and proportions for categorical variables. Differences in these characteristics by

quartile of total complaints were tested for using a Kruskal–Wallis rank sum test for continuous variables or an uncorrected chi-square test for categorical variables. Differences in median UPC totals by physician type and orthopedic subspecialty were tested for using a Kruskal–Wallis rank sum test. Differences in UPC totals by orthopedic subspecialty were tested for using a Kruskal–Wallis rank sum test for each type of complaint. Ordinal regression was used to assess the adjusted effect of orthopedic surgeon characteristics on the odds of receiving higher number of total complaints compared with a reference category. Two-sided P-values of less than .05 were considered to be statistically significant. All analyses were performed using R statistical software version 3.6.1.

RESULTS

There were 53,123 physicians practicing in 36 PARS-affiliated institutions from 2015 to 2018. Of these, 33,208 had 4 consecutive years of data during the audit period and were included in the analysis. Among them were 1568 orthopedic surgeons, 6747 other surgeons, and 25,279 non-surgeons. Four hundred and twenty of the orthopedic surgeons were excluded due to trainee status, being double-boarded, or having insufficient information publicly available online. Therefore, a total of 1148 orthopedic surgeons' patient complaint data were analyzed. Table 1 presents the selected demographic characteristics of the sample. Counts were limited by what was publicly available. The most represented subspecialties were sports (23%) and adult reconstruction (17%), followed by hand/upper extremity (13%) and spine (13%); 92% were male, and 42% practiced in a Midwestern state.

Fig. 1 represents the cumulative distribution of UPCs across physician specialties. As with other surgeons and non-surgeons, a small percentage of orthopedic surgeons were associated with a disproportionate number of overall complaints. A smaller percentage of orthopedic surgeons were associated with few or no UPCs than other surgeons and non-surgeons (see Fig. 1). The median number of complaints differed significantly by physician type (orthopedic surgeon median UPCs = 5 [0–13 interquartile range (IQR)], other surgeons at 2 [0–8], and non-surgeons at 1 [0–5] (P <.001)).

In comparisons of the proportion of total complaints among orthopedic surgeons, a small proportion of orthopedic surgeons accounted for a disproportionate share of the total

Table 1 Demographic analysis	
	Orthopedic Surgeons (N = 1148)
Sex; N(%)	
F	87 (8%)
M	1061 (92%)
Subspeciality; N(%)	
Sports	265 (23%)
Adult Reconstruction	191 (17%)
Hand/UE	153 (13%)
Spine	152 (13%)
Pediatrics	93 (8%)
Trauma	86 (7%)
Foot and Ankle	83 (7%)
General	77 (7%)
Oncology	27 (2%)
Shoulder/Elbow	21 (2%)
Non-US Medical School; N (%)	
No	1095 (95%)
Yes	52 (5%)
Non-US Residency; N (%)	
No	1121 (98%)
Yes	24 (2%)
Academic vs Private; N (%)	
Private	554 (51%)
Academic	538 (49%)
Board-Certified in Specialty; N (%)	
No	71 (6%)
Yes	1077 (94%)
Medical School Grad. Year; Q1, Median, Q3	1984, 1993, 2002
Region; N (%)	
Midwest	485 (42%)
West	259 (23%)
South	268 (23%)
East	136 (12%)
MD or DO; N (%)	
DO	54 (5%)
MD	1091 (95%)

Abbreviations: DO, Doctor of Osteopathic Medicine; MD, Doctor of Medicine; UE, Upper Extremity.

complaints received by orthopedists in the study (Fig. 2). The top 20% were associated with half of all UPCs, and the top 50% were associated with 90% of total UPCs. A small proportion (~30%) had 0 UPCs. In comparisons of the type of UPCs by orthopedics subspecialties, complaints about care and treatment were consistently the most common, followed by complaints about communication (Fig. 3).

Associations between orthopedists' demographic variables and UPCs were assessed via ordinal regression (Fig. 4). Several subspecialties were associated with more UPCs compared with orthopedists in general practice, namely Foot and Ankle (odds ratio [OR] 2.6 [1.4–4.6], $P = .002$), followed by Adult Reconstruction (OR 2.2 [1.3–3.8], $P = .002$), Spine (OR 2.2 [1.3–3.8], $P = .005$), and Trauma (OR 2.2 [1.2–4.0], $P = .01$). Those who practiced in the Midwest were significantly less likely to receive UPCs (OR 0.4 [0.3–0.5], $P < .001$) compared with the reference group of orthopedists who practiced in the Northeast United States. Orthopedist sex was not a significant risk factor for UPCs (OR 1.0 [0.8–2.5], $P = .96$). Those who graduated from an allopathic medical school were significantly more likely than those who graduated from an osteopathic school to receive a patient complaint (OR 3.7 [1.2–11.1], $P = .02$).

DISCUSSION

In this study which compared orthopedists to other surgeons and non-surgeons, orthopedists were significantly more likely to receive UPCs, which are an important marker of risk for complications and malpractice claims. A small portion of orthopedists were associated with a large proportion of the UPCs: the top 20% of surgeons receiving the highest number of complaints made up 50% of all UPCs filed, and the top 50% of surgeons made up 90% of all UPCs. Prior studies in otorhinolaryngology, ophthalmology, urology, and general surgery report similar patterns.[12,14,15,17,18] However, orthopedists' distribution of complaints was shifted to the left when compared with physicians in other specialties, suggesting that fewer orthopedic surgeons receive zero UPCs. In fact, the median number of UPCs for orthopedic surgeons was five, compared with two for surgeons of other subspecialties and one for non-surgeons.

The orthopedic specialties associated with significantly greater number of UPCs (Foot and Ankle, Adult Reconstruction, Spine, and Trauma surgeons) also received more "care and

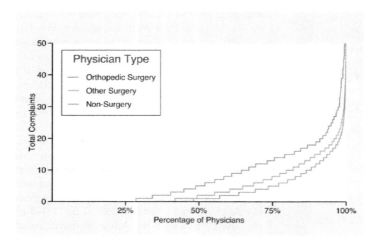

Fig. 1. Cumulative distribution of total unsolicited patient complaints by physician type, comparing orthopedists to other surgeon and non-surgeons.

treatment" UPCs than generalists. These findings mirror orthopedic malpractice research that shows the most commonly litigated areas in orthopedics by area of the body to be the hip, knee, and spine.[19] Fewer overall numbers of UPCs were reported for those practicing in the Midwest and more were reported for those

who trained at allopathic medical schools. Studies of other specialties have not demonstrated these differences, although they do reflect patterns of malpractice suits with the Northeast reporting highest rate of malpractice suits compared with other areas of the country. Similar to studies of UPCs in other specialties,

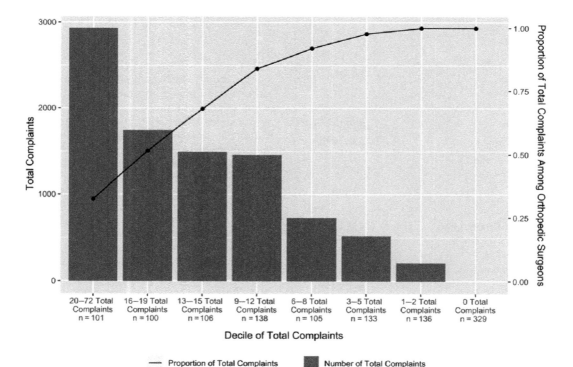

Fig. 2. Distribution of unsolicited patient complaints among orthopedic surgeons. Each bar represents the number and proportion of total complaints attributable to orthopedists within each decile of total complaints (n, b, "0 total complaints" groups first 3 deciles). For example, the top 20th percentile of surgeons received between 16 and 19 complaints and made up 50% of the total number of complaints.

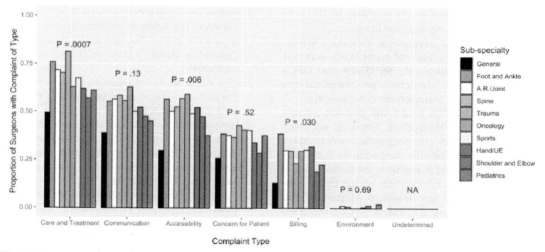

Fig. 3. Frequency of complaints by type and subspeciality.

no differences were found based on sex or practice setting. UPCs most commonly reflected concerns about aspects of care and treatment followed by communication and accessibility.[12,14,15,17,18]

With recent studies showing the association between UPCs and postoperative complications and increased malpractice risk, UPCs may become an increasingly important quality and a performance improvement metric.[12] A recent

study examining UPCs in otolaryngologists identified physicians who were in the top 5% of UPCs.[17] It is possible for surgeons to reduce their numbers of UPCs and overall risk. Following peer-to-peer interventions where physicians' UPC data and peer-comparative risk status were discussed, subsequent UPCs for the identified physicians significantly decreased, with 69% of the identified physicians having a

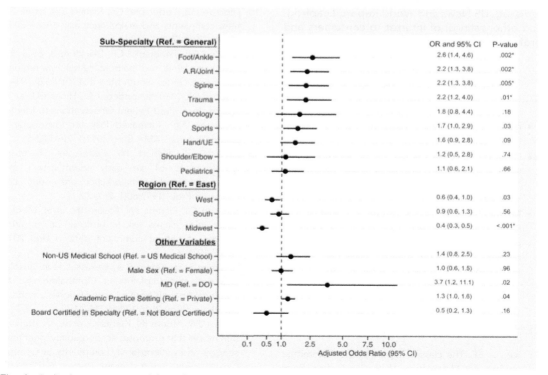

Fig. 4. Ordinal regression model predicting complaints.

45% mean decrease in the number of UPCs in the 2 years following interventions.[18]

This study does have some important limitations. First, the number of complaints was not controlled by patient volume. Given that UPCs are a significant predictor for complications and malpractice, independent of volume,[10,12] understanding UPCs could still provide important insight to orthopedists. Second, accuracy of specialty and demographic information collected for orthopedic surgeons in the study was limited to what is available on publicly available sites. Finally, information about those submitting UPC was not available as part of the database for review and could not be included in the analysis to describe characteristics of those who submit UPCs.

Understanding drivers of UPCs and why some orthopedists are associated with many more than peer subspecialists may not only help address patient dissatisfaction, but may positively impact surgical complications and malpractice claims. Prospective studies could investigate the effect of interventions on numbers and types of orthopedic physicians' subsequent UPCs and risk of adverse clinical, administrative, and personal outcomes. Future studies could also assess relationships between department-wide UPCs and elements of publicly reported safety/quality/reputation rating systems (eg, US News and World Report, Leapfrog, and other ratings) of interest to consumers and professionals alike.

CLINICS CARE POINTS

- Patient complaints correlate to medical malpractice suits and surgical complications.
- Orthopedic surgery is the 4th highest medical specialty for malpractice and is considered "high risk" with 14% of of surgeons facing claims annually.
- Most patient complaint types are related to communication errors.
- Identifying those surgeons at risk and allowing points of intervention can help to reduce risk of complaints in the future.

REFERENCES

1. Sanger EF. The classic: Report of the Committee on Suits for Malpractice. 1879. Clin Orthop Relat Res 2009;467(2):328–38.

2. Matsen FA 3rd, Stephens L, Jette JL, et al. Lessons regarding the safety of orthopaedic patient care: an analysis of four hundred and sixty-four closed malpractice claims. J Bone Joint Surg Am 2013; 95(4):e201–8.

3. Jena AB, Seabury S, Lakdawalla D, et al. Malpractice risk according to physician specialty. N Engl J Med 2011;365(7):629–36.

4. Hickson G, Pichert JW. Identifying and addressing physicians at high risk for medical malpractice claims. In: Youngberg B, editor. Principles of risk management and patient safety. Sudbury: Jones and Bartlett Publishers, Inc.; 2012. p. 347–68.

5. Balch CM, Oreskovich MR, Dyrbye LN, et al. Personal consequences of malpractice lawsuits on American surgeons. J Am Coll Surg 2011;213(5): 657–67.

6. Mukherjee K, Pichert JW, Cornett MB, et al. All trauma surgeons are not created equal: asymmetric distribution of malpractice claims risk. J Trauma 2010;69(3):549–54.

7. Higgins LD. Medicolegal aspects of the orthopaedic care for shoulder injuries. Clin Orthop Relat Res 2005;433:58–64.

8. Gould MT, Langworthy MJ, Santore R, et al. An analysis of orthopaedic liability in the acute care setting. Clin Orthop Relat Res 2003;407:59–66.

9. Bishop TF, Ryan AM, Casalino LP. Paid malpractice claims for adverse events in inpatient and outpatient settings. JAMA 2011;305(23):2427–31.

10. Hickson GB, Federspiel CF, Pichert JW, et al. Patient complaints and malpractice risk. JAMA 2002; 287(22):2951–7.

11. Hickson GB, Federspiel CF, Blackford J, et al. Patient complaints and malpractice risk in a regional healthcare center. South Med J 2007;100(8):791–6.

12. Cooper WO, Guillamondegui O, Hines OJ, et al. Use of Unsolicited Patient Observations to Identify Surgeons With Increased Risk for Postoperative Complications. JAMA Surg 2017;152(6):522–9.

13. Hickson GB, Pichert JW, Federspiel CF, et al. Development of an early identification and response model of malpractice prevention. Law Contemp Probl 1997;60(1–2):7–29.

14. Stimson CJ, Pichert JW, Moore IN, et al. Medical malpractice claims risk in urology: an empirical analysis of patient complaint data. J Urol 2010; 183(5):1971–6.

15. Kohanim S, Sternberg P Jr, Karrass J, et al. Unsolicited Patient Complaints in Ophthalmology: An Empirical Analysis from a Large National Database. Ophthalmology 2016;123(2):234–41.

16. Pichert JW, Moore IN, Karrass J, et al. An intervention model that promotes accountability: peer messengers and patient/family complaints. Jt Comm J Qual Patient Saf/Jt Comm Resour 2013;39(10): 435–46.

17. Nassiri AM, Pichert JW, Domenico HJ, et al. Unsolicited Patient Complaints among Otolaryngologists. Otolaryngol Head Neck Surg 2019;160(5):810–7.

18. Fathy C, Pichert J, Domenico H, et al. Association between ophthalmologist age and unsolicited patient complaints. JAMA Ophthalmol 2018;136(1): 1–7.

19. Atrey A, Gupte CM, Corbett SA. Review of successful litigation against english health trusts in the treatment of adults with orthopaedic pathology: clinical governance lessons learned. J Bone Joint Surg Am 2010;92(18):e36.

Modified Lapidus Procedure and Hallux Valgus

A Systematic Review and Update on Triplanar Correction

Dang-Huy Do, MD, Joshua Jian Sun, MD,
Dane K. Wukich, MD*

KEYWORDS

- Hallux valgus • Bunion • Lapidus • IMA • HVA • TSP • Triplanar correction

---

KEY POINTS

- Hallux valgus has traditionally been viewed as a biplanar deformity (transverse and sagittal); however, during the past 2 decades, the triplanar deformity has been increasingly recognized.
- Our systematic review with meta-analysis techniques demonstrates that historically, the Lapidus procedure results in significant improvement in the IMA, HVA, and TSP.
- Contemporary triplane correct with orthogonal biplanar plating has the potential to permit early weight bearing and sooner return to full activities, *without increasing the rate of mechanical complications and recurrence.*

INTRODUCTION

Hallux valgus is a common condition affecting nearly 25% of adults between the ages of 18 and 65 years and 33% of adults aged older than 65 years.[1] Surgical management was reported approximately 185 years ago, and since then more than 100 different procedures have been described.[2,3]

Dr Paul Lapidus originally reported on his method for the operative correction of the metatarsus primus varus in hallux valgus in 1934,[4] introducing subsequent updates in 1956 and 1960.[5,6] He addressed the increased intermetatarsal angle (IMA) by performing an arthrodesis of the first tarsometatarsal joint and creating a bone bridge between the base of the first and second metatarsals. In addition, he performed a distal lateral release and a Silver procedure. During the past 50 years, many surgeons have utilized the Lapidus procedure to treat hallux valgus successfully. Complications of the Lapidus procedure include painful hardware, nonunion, malunion, recurrence, hallux varus, transfer metatarsalgia, and sesamoiditis.

Hallux valgus has traditionally been viewed as a biplanar deformity (transverse and sagittal); however, during the past 2 decades, the triplanar deformity has been increasingly recognized. The concept of frontal plane rotation or torsion was reported in 1956 by Mizuno and colleagues.[7] The authors described a "detorsion osteotomy" of the hallux to correct this. Subsequently, many authors have contributed to the understanding of the relationship between metatarsal rotation in the axial plane and hallux valgus. Eustace and colleagues[8] demonstrated a significantly positive correlation between metatarsal pronation and the IMA (metatarsus primus varus) [r = 0.69, p < .001]. Okuda and colleagues[9] introduced the concept of the "round sign," utilizing a geometric Mose sphere to determine the best shape of the metatarsal head. The authors explained the "round sign"

Department of Orthopaedic Surgery, University of Texas Southwestern Medical Center, 1801 Inwood Road, Dallas, TX 75390-8883, USA
* Corresponding author.
E-mail address: Dane.Wukich@UTSouthwestern.edu

Orthop Clin N Am 53 (2022) 499–508
https://doi.org/10.1016/j.ocl.2022.05.005
0030-5898/22/

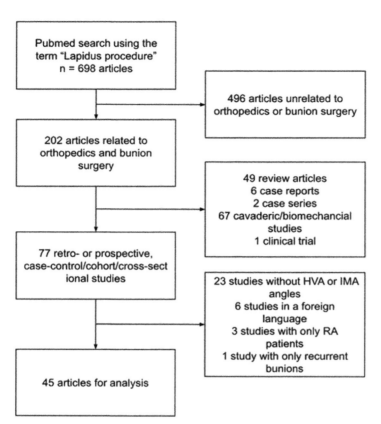

Fig. 1. Flowchart depicting search results and articles included in analysis.

as the lateral surface of the metatarsal head on the dorsoplantar radiograph because of pronation of the first metatarsal. The prevalence of a "round sign" was significantly higher in patients with hallux valgus compared with control patients (p < .0001), and the authors hypothesized that the persistence of a "round sign" postoperatively could increase the risk of recurrence.

Two years later, the same authors found a strong positive correlation (r = 0.708, p < .001) between the grade of tibial sesamoid displacement and the hallux valgus angle (HVA). From a pathoanatomic perspective, the authors noted that sesamoid position remained relatively unchanged but appeared laterally translated due to metatarsus primus varus. Because of medial deviation of the first metatarsal (metatarsus primus varus), the adductor hallucis and transverse metatarsal ligament acted as a restraint to maintain sesamoid position. Further progression of metatarsus primus varus and pronation results in dorsolateral sesamoid translation with respect to the distal metatarsal. This further contributes to deformity as the short and long hallux flexors become a lateralizing force driving the proximal phalanx laterally.

The aim of this review article is to examine a contemporary method of triplanar correction and historically assess both radiographic outcomes and postoperative complications following the modified Lapidus procedure utilizing a systematic review.

METHODS

We aimed to review current literature on the modified Lapidus technique and associated procedures in describing its utility for the surgical correction of hallux valgus. In doing so, we analyzed preoperative and postoperative radiographic parameters (IMA, HVA, tibial sesamoid position [TSP]) along with complication rates in patients undergoing modified Lapidus procedures for symptomatic hallux valgus.

We searched PubMed using the term "Lapidus procedure" and found 698 results between 1950 and 2022. Of these articles, we excluded 496 articles unrelated to orthopedics or foot deformity, 49 review articles, 6 case reports, 2 case series and 67 articles of cadaveric or biomechanical relevance, and one clinical trial (Fig. 1). We also excluded 23 articles that did not include IMA and HVA angles, 6 studies in a foreign

Table 1
Median preoperative and postoperative radiographic values

Radiographic Measurement	N	Preoperative (IQR)	Postoperative (IQR)	Correction (%)	P-Value
IMA	2231	15.8 (14.2–17.0)	6.5 (5.5–8.2)	58.9	P<.001[a]
HVA	1598	32.7 (29.9–35.3)	12.5 (9.7–16)	61.8	P<.001[a]
TSP	865	5 (3–5.3)	2 (1–2.8)	60	P<.001[a]

Abbreviations: HVA, hallux valgus angle; IMA, intermetatarsal angle; TSP, tibial sesamoid position.
[a] P-value <.05 considered statistically significant.

language, 3 articles that studied only rheumatoid arthritis patients, and 1 study that only examined patients with recurrent bunions. There remained 45 articles of retrospective, prospective, or cross-sectional study design for analysis (Table 1).[10–52] We collected demographic data on each study including the number of patients, number of feet treated, sex, age, follow-up period, and body mass index (BMI). Outcomes included pre-op and post-op IMA, pre-op and post-op HVA, pre-op and post-op TSP, types of complications, and reasons for unexpected return to the operating room.

Median and interquartile range were used to describe continuous variables. A Mann-Whitney U parametric test was used to compare preoperative and postoperative IMA, HVA, and TSP across all included articles. All statistical significance was set at $p < .05$. Statistical analyses were performed using GraphPad Prism 9.0 (GraphPad, San Diego, California, USA).

RESULTS

Among the 45 articles retrieved in the review, there were 2231 patients (2344 feet) that underwent a modified Lapidus procedure. Of these, 1763 patients were women (79%). The median age was 51.5 years (Interquartile Range [IQR] 44.4–54.7 years). The median follow-up period was 17.5 months (IQR 11.38–38.5). The median BMI was 26.4 (IQR 26.4–27.05). Additionally, in several studies, patients underwent additional procedures, which included modified McBride, Akin, gastrocnemius recession, tendo-Achilles lengthening, Weil osteotomy, and lesser toe procedures including hammer-toe correction.

Of 45 articles totaling 2231 Lapidus procedures reviewed, 33 articles with 1823 Lapidus procedures presented postoperative complications (see Table 1). In 1823 Lapidus procedures performed, there were 305 complications for an overall complication rate of 16.7%. Specific complications related to the Lapidus procedures are listed in Table 2 (see Table 2). The most complication was hardware pain in 51 patients (2.8%), followed by nonunion in 50 patients (2.7%), recurrence in 36 patients (2.0%), delayed union in 31 patients (1.7%), hallux varus in 25 patients (1.4%), transfer metatarsalgia in 20 patients (1.1%), neuritis in 16 patients (0.9%), sesamoiditis in 12 patients (0.7%), and wound complications in 24 patients (1.4%). The following complications had less than 10 patients each: deep vein thrombosis (7 patients, 0.4%), first ray elevation (3 patients, 0.2%), hyperkeratosis (3 patients, 0.2%), suture reaction (5 patients, 0.3%), persistent first ray instability (3 patients, 0.2%), uncomfortable shoe wear (2 patients, 0.1%), hallux limitus (2 patients, 0.1%), mild residual pain (6 patients, 0.3%), hallux supination (2 patients, 0.1%), cuneiform widening (1 patient, 0.1%), first metatarsal fracture (1 patient, 0.1%), adjacent metatarsal stress fracture (1 patient, 0.1%), tibialis anterior rupture (1 patient, 0.1%), undercorrection (1 patient, 0.1%), and painful exostosis (1 patient, 0.1%). In addition to complication data, 26 out of 45 articles (1604 of 2231 procedures) provided data on unexpected return to the operating room. Review

Table 2
Complications

Variable	n (%)
Articles with complications	33/45 (73.3)
Complication rate	305/1823 (16.7)
Hardware pain	51 (2.8)
Nonunion/delayed union	81 (4.4)
Recurrence	36 (2)
Hallux varus	25 (1.4)
Transfer metatarsalgia	20(1.1)
Neuritis/sesamoiditis	28 (1.6)
Wound	24 (1.3)
Other[a]	40 (2.5)

[a] Less frequent complications (n < 10) were categorized for presentation purposes. See appendix for specific data regarding these grouped variables.

Table 3
Indications for return to operating room

Variable	n (%)
Articles	26/45 (57.8)
Reoperation rate	96/1604(6)
Painful hardware	44(2.7)
Nonunion	24 (1.5)
Hallux varus	8 (0.5)
Recurrence	9 (0.6)
Broken hardware	3 (0.2)
Lesser toe pain	3 (0.2)
Infection/wound dehiscence	2 (0.1)
Other	3 (0.2)

Less frequent indications for reoperation (n < 2) were categorized as "Other" for presentation purposes. See appendix for specific date regarding these grouped variables.

of these studies reveals 96 unexpected returns to the operating room for a reoperation rate of 6% (96/1604). Indications for reoperation can be found in Table 3 (see Table 3). Notably, the most common complication and indication for reoperation was symptomatic hardware (2.8% and 2.7%, respectively).

All 45 articles included preoperative and postoperative IMA angles. The median preoperative IMA was 15.8° (IQR 14.2–17.0) and the median postoperative IMA was 6.5° (IQR 5.5–8.2). There was a significant reduction in the IMA angle of 9.3° (p < .001). Only 35 of 45 articles (78%) included HVA angles, consisting of 1598 feet. The median preoperative HVA was 32.7° (IQR 29.9–35.3) and the median postoperative HVA was 12.5° (IQR 9.7–16). There was a

significant reduction the HVA angle of 20.2° (p < .001). Fifteen of 45 articles (33%) included the TSP, consistent of 865 feet. The median preoperative TSP was 5 (IQR 3–5.3) and the median postoperative TSP was 2 (IQR 1–2.8). There was a significant reduction in TSP for 3 positions (p < .001).

CASE A: PRIMARY BUNION TRIPLANAR CORRECTION WITH BIPLANAR PLATING

A novel technique known as The Lapiplasty System (Treace Medical Concepts, Inc., Ponte Vedra, FL) performs triplanar correction of the first tarsometatarsal joint, correcting hallux valgus in all 3 anatomical planes. This technique is illustrated by the case of a 62-year-old woman with osteoporosis who has had a long history of severe hallux valgus. For many years, she had significant difficulty with balance and pain due to her bilateral bunions. Despite activity modification and more comfortable wide-toed shoes, her pain has limited her from performing her daily routine activities. Her pain was worse on the right than left. On examination of her right foot, she had some imbalance with push off. There was tenderness to palpation over the medial eminence and no pain with range of motion of the first metatarsophalangeal joint. The hallux abutted the second toe, the HVA deformity was reducible, and there was sagittal plane hypermobility to the first tarsometatarsal joint. Preoperative IMA was 20.3°, HVA was 42.5°, and TSP was 6 (Fig. 2).

A modified Lapidus procedure was performed on the right foot with a modified McBride procedure. An incision was made over the dorsal aspect of the first tarsometatarsal

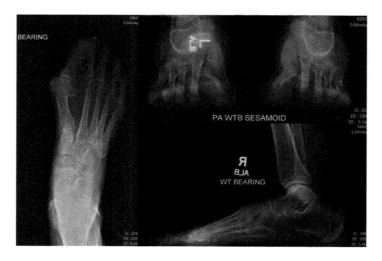

Fig. 2. Standing anteroposterior and lateral radiographs of 65-year-old woman with symptomatic right hallux valgus. Preoperative IMA was 20.3°, HVA was 42.5°, and tibial sesamoid position was 6.

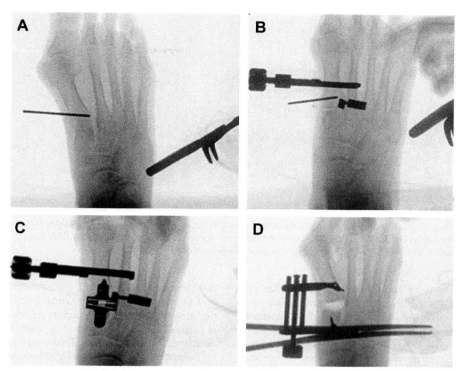

Fig. 3. Intraoperative fluoroscopic images of the patient illustrated in Fig. 2. (A) (top left), (B) (top right), (C) (bottom left), and (D) (bottom right).

joint, and dissection procedure while the extensor tendons were retracted. The first tarsometatarsal joint was identified and mobilized initially using a sagittal saw, without removing the articular surface at this stage. A joystick pin was placed about one cm distal to the joint to allow for correction of first metatarsal rotation (Fig. 3A). Next, a lateral release at the first metatarsophalangeal joint was performed to improve the position of the hallux. The medial eminence was not removed at this time. A small incision was made over the lateral aspect of second metatarsal to place the C-shaped reduction clamp, which is tightened down. Although correcting metatarsal rotation using the joystick, fluoroscopy was used to confirm adequate rotational reduction and correction of the IMA and a k-wire is inserted through the cannulated reduction clamp and across both the distal aspects of the first and second metatarsal bones (Fig. 3B). Because the first tarsometatarsal joint had been mobilized, the cutting guide was inserted into the joint and proper positioning confirmed under fluoroscopy (Fig. 3C). A sagittal saw was used to resect the first tarsometatarsal articular surfaces, with reduction occurring mostly from resection of lateral cuneiform (Fig. 3D). Using the pins of the cutting guide, a distractor was

placed to permit the removal of the resected articular surfaces and perform subchondral drilling to aid in fusion. The deformity was reduced by tightening the distractor. At our institution, temporary fixation is held into place with a guide wire that will ultimately be used to place a cannulated headless screw that spans the first tarsometatarsal joint. The system comes with 2 4-hole locking plates, which are placed orthogonally to each other on the medial and dorsal aspect of the joint.

Postoperative radiographs demonstrated reduction of the IMA from 20.3 to 6.4°, HVA correction from 42.5 to 14.1°, and TSP improved from 6 to 1 (Fig. 4). Postoperatively, weight-bearing as tolerated was permitted after the first week in a controlled ankle motion boot. The patient did well and their daily function improved. By the 3-month postoperative visit, she had requested to have the same procedure done on her contralateral side.

CASE B: RECURRENT BUNION CORRECTION USING LAPIPLASTY SYSTEM

The triplanar correction is also a powerful procedure to correct recurrent hallux valgus. We describe the case of a healthy 46-year-old

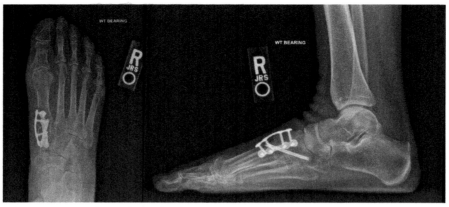

Fig. 4. Standing anteroposterior and lateral radiographs the patient illustrated in Fig. 2, taken 10 weeks postoperative. The fusion has healed. Postoperative radiographs demonstrate reduction of the IMA from 20.3 to 6.4°, HVA correction from 42.5 to 14.1°, and tibial sesamoid improved from 6 to 1.

woman was referred with left foot pain after undergoing a left bunionectomy 2 years prior. It is unknown what her initial IMA and HVA measurements were before the index procedure but she underwent a proximal opening wedge metatarsal osteotomy with plate-and-screw fixation. The patient developed recurrence and has been unable to return to her presurgery level of activity, despite wearing more comfortable shoes. Her symptoms include foot pain, lesser toe discomfort, cramping, generalized stiffness, and numbness over the surgical incision site, all negatively affecting her quality of life. She had a reducible bunion deformity with the hallux abutting the second toe. There was tenderness to palpation over the medial eminence but no pain with range of motion of the first metatarsophalangeal joint or the sesamoids. Despite a proximal metatarsal osteotomy, hypermobility in the sagittal and transverse planes were

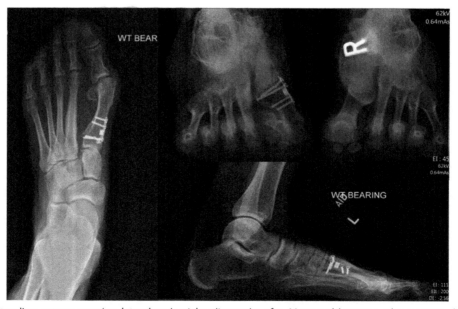

Fig. 5. Standing anteroposterior, lateral and axial radiographs of a 46-year-old woman who presented with left foot pain after undergoing a left bunionectomy utilizing a proximal medial opening wedge osteotomy 2 years prior. Notice the residual metatarsus primus varus, hallux valgus, and abnormal tibial sesamoid position. The axial view demonstrates severe pronation on the left compared with the right hallux. Preoperative IMA was 15°, HVA was 34°, and tibial sesamoid position was 6.

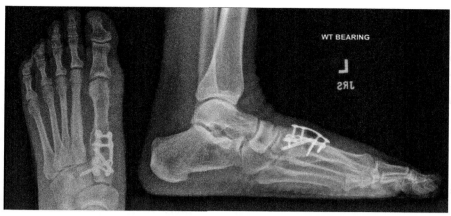

Fig. 6. Postoperative standing radiographs at 6 weeks of patient illustrated in Fig. 5. The postoperative IMA improved from 15 to 2°, HVA improved from 34 to 5°, and tibial sesamoid position improved from 6 to 2.

observed at the first tarsometatarsal joint. Preoperative IMA was 15°, HVA was 34°, and TSP was 6 (Fig. 5).

Based on the clinical and radiographic findings, the decision was made for hardware removal, open lateral release, and modified Lapidus procedure using triplanar first tarsometatarsal (TMT) arthrodesis with biplanar plating system. Due to the significant tarsometatarsal joint hypermobility, a modification was planned in the form of additional fixation from the metatarsal base into the middle cuneiform to improve stability and prevent recurrence.

Upon removal of the hardware from the index surgery, one of the screws was found to be broken and remained deep within the bone. Using the same technique described with case A, the first metatarsal was corrected in a triplanar fashion and a distal lateral release. No additional medial eminence was resected. The tarsometatarsal joint was fused using 2 headless screws and 2 orthogonal plates. One screw spanned the base of the first metatarsal and the medial cuneiform while other screw spanned the medial cuneiform and second cuneiform. A small area of cortical defect where her prior hardware was removed was packed with autogenous bone from the arthrodesis resection and supplemental demineralized bone graft.

The postoperative IMA improved from 15 to 2°, HVA improved from 34 to 5°, and TSP improved from 6 to 2 (Fig. 6). The patient's postoperative regimen consisted of weight-bearing as tolerated after the first week, followed by weight-bearing as tolerated with physical therapy. The patient did well and returned to normal levels of activity by 12 weeks.

DISCUSSION

The prevalence of hallux valgus has been estimated to be as high as 34% in the general population.[1] Furthermore, there have been more than 100 surgical options reported when it comes to correcting this pathologic condition.[2] These include soft tissue procedures, various distal, middle, and proximal osteotomies of the first metatarsal different biomechanical patterns, and a wide array of first tarsometatarsal joint arthrodesis techniques that differ in the screw/plate number, screw/plate orientation, and even external fixation. Currently, there is no consensus on the surgical management of hallux valgus. During the past few decades, our understanding of hallux valgus has advanced, and the "multiplanar" nature of the deformity has assumed an important role in planning surgical correction.

Our systematic review with meta-analysis techniques demonstrates that historically, the Lapidus procedure results in significant improvement in the IMA, HVA, and TSP. In general, previous reports have focused on sagittal and transverse plane correction. More recently, the rotational component with the metatarsal pronated has become an area of keen interest. Clinically, this often manifests as a pinch callus medially and plantar to the hallux IP joint. Ongoing prospective studies will provide additional evidence on the relative importance of multiplanar correction in preventing recurrence. As demonstrated in the systematic review, the quality of the studies reporting on outcomes of Lapidus procedures creates opportunities in the future. Surprisingly, only 78% of the studies assessed for this review reported on the HVA and only 33% reported on TSP. Contemporary triplane correct with orthogonal biplanar plating has the potential to permit early weight bearing and sooner return to full activities, *without increasing the rate of mechanical complications and recurrence. An ongoing prospective study will determine if this technique maintains the optimistic results of interim analysis.*

CLINICS CARE POINTS

- Hallux valgus is a triplanar deformity.
- The most common complications after the Lapidus procedure are non-union/delayed union (4.4%), hardware related pain (2.8%), recurrence (2%), hallux varus (1.4%), postoperative wound complications (1.3%) and transfer metatarsalgia (1.1%).

ACKNOWLEDGMENTS

The authors would like to acknowledge that Treace Medical Concepts, Inc., Ponte Vedra Beach, FL provided institutional research support to the authors' institution. D.K. Wukich is the principal investigator of an ongoing prospective that is funded by Treace Medical Concepts, Inc., Ponte Vedra Beach, FL.

DISCLOSURE

The authors would like to acknowledge that Treace Medical Concepts, Inc., Ponte Vedra Beach, FL provided institutional research support to the authors' institution. D.H. Do, J.J. Sun, and D.K. Wukich certify that neither they nor any member of their immediate family has funding or commercial associations (consultancies, stock ownership, equity interest, patent/licensing arrangements, and so forth) that might pose a conflict of interest in connection with the submitted article. DKW is the principal investigator of an ongoing prospective that is funded by Treace Medical Concepts, Inc., Ponte Vedra Beach, FL. Each author certifies that his or her institution approved the human protocol for this investigation and that all investigations were conducted in conformity with ethical principles of research.

REFERENCES

1. Nix S, Smith M, Vicenzino B. Prevalence of hallux valgus in the general population: a systematic review and meta-analysis. J Foot Ankle Res 2010;3:21.
2. Easley ME, Trnka HJ. Current concepts review: hallux valgus part II: operative treatment. Foot Ankle Int 2007;28(6):748–58.
3. Smyth NA, Aiyer AA. Introduction: why are there so many different surgeries for hallux valgus? Foot Ankle Clin 2018;23(2):171–82.
4. Lapidus PW. Operative correction of the metatarsus primus varus in hallux valgus. Surg Gynecol Obstet 1934;58:183–91.
5. Lapidus PW. The author's bunion operation from 1931 to 1959. Clin Orthop 1960;16:119–35.
6. Lapidus PW. A quarter of a century of experience with the operative correction of the metatarsus varus primus in hallux valgus. Bull Hosp Joint Dis 1956;17(2):404–21.
7. Mizuno SSY, Yamazaki K. Detorsion osteotomy of the first metatarsal bone in hallux valgus. J Jpn Orthop Assoc 1956;30:813–9.
8. Eustace S, Byrne JO, Beausang O, et al. Hallux valgus, first metatarsal pronation and collapse of the medial longitudinal arch–a radiological correlation. Skeletal Radiol 1994;23(3):191–4.
9. Okuda R, Kinoshita M, Yasuda T, et al. The shape of the lateral edge of the first metatarsal head as a risk factor for recurrence of hallux valgus. J Bone Joint Surg Am 2007;89(10):2163–72.
10. Bednarz PA, Manoli A 2nd. Modified lapidus procedure for the treatment of hypermobile hallux valgus. Foot Ankle Int 2000;21(10):816–21.
11. Boffeli TJ, Hyllengren SB. Can we abandon saw wedge resection in lapidus fusion? A Comparative study of joint preparation techniques regarding correction of deformity, union rate, and preservation of first ray length. J Foot Ankle Surg 2019; 58(6):1118–24.
12. Catanzariti AR, Mendicino RW, Lee MS, et al. The modified Lapidus arthrodesis: a retrospective analysis. J Foot Ankle Surg 1999;38(5):322–32.
13. Chopra S, Moerenhout K, Crevoisier X. Subjective versus objective assessment in early clinical outcome of modified Lapidus procedure for hallux valgus deformity. Clin Biomech (Bristol, Avon) 2016; 32:187–93.
14. Coetzee JC, Resig SG, Kuskowski M, et al. The Lapidus procedure as salvage after failed surgical treatment of hallux valgus. Surgical technique. J Bone Joint Surg Am 2004;86-A(Suppl 1):30–6.
15. Coetzee JC, Wickum D. The Lapidus procedure: a prospective cohort outcome study. Foot Ankle Int 2004;25(8):526–31.
16. Conti MS, MacMahon A, Ellis SJ, et al. Effect of the modified lapidus procedure for hallux valgus on foot width. Foot Ankle Int 2020;41(2): 154–9.
17. Conti MS, Patel TJ, Zhu J, et al. Association of first metatarsal pronation correction with patient-reported outcomes and recurrence rates in hallux valgus. Foot Ankle Int 2022;43(3):309–20.
18. Conti MS, Willett JF, Garfinkel JH, et al. Effect of the modified lapidus procedure on pronation of

the first ray in hallux valgus. Foot Ankle Int 2020; 41(2):125–32.

19. Cottom JM, Vora AM. Fixation of lapidus arthrodesis with a plantar interfragmentary screw and medial locking plate: a report of 88 cases. J Foot Ankle Surg 2013;52(4):465–9.

20. Dayton P, Feilmeier M. Comparison of tibial sesamoid position on anteroposterior and axial radiographs before and after triplane tarsal metatarsal joint arthrodesis. J Foot Ankle Surg 2017;56(5): 1041–6.

21. Faber FW, Mulder PG, Verhaar JA. Role of first ray hypermobility in the outcome of the Hohmann and the Lapidus procedure. A prospective, randomized trial involving one hundred and one feet. J Bone Joint Surg Am 2004;86(3):486–95.

22. Faber FW, van Kampen PM, Bloembergen MW. Long-term results of the Hohmann and Lapidus procedure for the correction of hallux valgus: a prospective, randomised trial with eight- to 11-year follow-up involving 101 feet. Bone Joint J 2013; 95-b(9):1222–6.

23. Ferreyra M, Viladot Pericé R, Nuñez-Samper M, et al. Can we correct first metatarsal rotation and sesamoid position with the 3D Lapidus procedure? Foot Ankle Surg 2021. https://doi.org/10.1016/j.fas. 2021.04.001.

24. Fleming JJ, Kwaadu KY, Brinkley JC, et al. Intraoperative evaluation of medial intercuneiform instability after Lapidus arthrodesis: intercuneiform hook test. J Foot Ankle Surg 2015;54(3):464–72.

25. Foran IM, Mehraban N, Jacobsen SK, et al. Radiographic impact of lapidus, proximal lateral closing wedge osteotomy, and suture button procedures on first ray length and dorsiflexion for hallux valgus. Foot Ankle Int 2020;41(8):964–71.

26. Grace D, Delmonte R, Catanzariti AR, et al. Modified lapidus arthrodesis for adolescent hallux abducto valgus. J Foot Ankle Surg 1999;38(1):8–13.

27. Greeff W, Strydom A, Saragas NP, et al. Radiographic assessment of relative first metatarsal length following modified lapidus procedure. Foot Ankle Int 2020;41(8):972–7.

28. Gutteck N, Wohlrab D, Zeh A, et al. Comparative study of Lapidus bunionectomy using different osteosynthesis methods. Foot Ankle Surg 2013; 19(4):218–21.

29. Haas Z, Hamilton G, Sundstrom D, et al. Maintenance of correction of first metatarsal closing base wedge osteotomies versus modified Lapidus arthrodesis for moderate to severe hallux valgus deformity. J Foot Ankle Surg 2007;46(5):358–65.

30. Jagadale VS, Thomas RL. A clinicoradiological and functional evaluation of lapidus surgery for moderate to severe bunion deformity shows excellent stable correction and high long-term patient satisfaction. Foot Ankle Spec 2020;13(6):488–93.

31. King CM, Richey J, Patel S, et al. Modified lapidus arthrodesis with crossed screw fixation: early weightbearing in 136 patients. J Foot Ankle Surg 2015;54(1):69–75.

32. King CM, Hamilton GA, Ford LA. Effects of the lapidus arthrodesis and chevron bunionectomy on plantar forefoot pressures. J Foot Ankle Surg 2014;53(4):415–9.

33. Klos K, Wilde CH, Lange A, et al. Modified Lapidus arthrodesis with plantar plate and compression screw for treatment of hallux valgus with hypermobility of the first ray: a preliminary report. Foot Ankle Surg 2013;19(4):239–44.

34. Klouda J, Hromádka R, Šoffová S, et al. The change of first metatarsal head articular surface position after Lapidus arthrodesis. BMC Musculoskelet Disord 2018;19(1):347. https://doi.org/10.1186/s12891-018-2262-9.

35. Kopp FJ, Patel MM, Levine DS, et al. The modified Lapidus procedure for hallux valgus: a clinical and radiographic analysis. Foot Ankle Int 2005;26(11): 913–7.

36. Lamm BM, Wynes J. Immediate weightbearing after Lapidus arthrodesis with external fixation. J Foot Ankle Surg 2014;53(5):577–83.

37. Langan TM, Greschner JM, Brandão RA, et al. Maintenance of correction of the modified lapidus procedure with a first metatarsal to intermediate cuneiform cross-screw technique. Foot Ankle Int 2020;41(4):428–36.

38. Long J, Lauf JA, Whitehead B, et al. Recurrence of hallux valgus after modified lapidus procedure with successful fusion of the intermetatarsal and intercuneiform joints. Cureus 2021;13(6):e15418.

39. Manchanda K, Chang A, Wallace B, et al. Short term radiographic and patient outcomes of a biplanar plating system for triplanar hallux valgus correction. J Foot Ankle Surg 2021;60(3):461–5.

40. McAlister JE, Peterson KS, Hyer CF. Corrective realignment arthrodesis of the first tarsometatarsal joint without wedge resection. Foot Ankle Spec 2015;8(4):284–8.

41. McCabe FJ, McQuail PM, Turley L, et al. Anatomical reconstruction of first ray instability hallux valgus with a medial anatomical TMTJ1 plate. Foot Ankle Surg 2021;27(8):869–73.

42. McInnes BD, Bouché RT. Critical evaluation of the modified Lapidus procedure. J Foot Ankle Surg 2001;40(2):71–90.

43. Michels F, Guillo S, de Lavigne C, et al. The arthroscopic Lapidus procedure. Foot Ankle Surg 2011; 17(1):25–8.

44. Nishikawa DRC, Duarte FA, Saito GH, et al. Correlation of first metatarsal sagittal alignment with clinical and functional outcomes following the Lapidus procedure. Foot Ankle Surg 2021. https://doi.org/ 10.1016/j.fas.2021.08.009.

45. Nishikawa DRC, Duarte FA, Saito GH, et al. Is first metatarsal shortening correlated with clinical and functional outcomes following the Lapidus procedure? Int Orthop 2021;45(11):2927–31.

46. Ravenell RA, Camasta CA, Powell DR. The unreliability of the intermetatarsal angle in choosing a hallux abducto valgus surgical procedure. J Foot Ankle Surg 2011;50(3):287–92.

47. Ray JJ, Koay J, Dayton PD, et al. Multicenter early radiographic outcomes of triplanar tarsometatarsal arthrodesis with early weightbearing. Foot Ankle Int 2019;40(8):955–60.

48. Reilly ME, Conti MS, Day J, et al. Modified lapidus vs scarf osteotomy outcomes for treatment of hallux valgus deformity. Foot Ankle Int 2021; 42(11):1454–62.

49. Rink-Brüne O. Lapidus arthrodesis for management of hallux valgus–a retrospective review of 106 cases. J Foot Ankle Surg 2004;43(5):290–5.

50. Rippstein PF, Park YU, Naal FD. Combination of first metatarsophalangeal joint arthrodesis and proximal correction for severe hallux valgus deformity. Foot Ankle Int 2012;33(5):400–5.

51. Saxena A, Nguyen A, Nelsen E. Lapidus bunionectomy: early evaluation of crossed lag screws versus locking plate with plantar lag screw. J Foot Ankle Surg 2009;48(2):170–9.

52. Unangst AM, Ryan PM. Return to run rates following hallux valgus correction: a retrospective comparison of metatarsal shaft osteotomies versus the modified lapidus procedure. Foot Ankle Surg 2021;27(8):892–6.

Spine

Degenerative Cervical Myelopathy
Evaluation and Management

Jestin Williams, MD*, Peter D'Amore, MD,
Nathan Redlich, MD, Matthew Darlow, MD,
Patrik Suwak, DO, Stefan Sarkovich, BS,
Amit K. Bhandutia, MD

KEYWORDS

- Cervical myelopathy • Cervical spondylotic myelopathy • Degenerative cervical myelopathy
- Cervical myelopathy treatment

KEY POINTS

- Degenerative cervical myelopathy causes chronic compression of the spinal cord resulting in myelopathic symptoms.
- The natural history of disease is well understood to be a stepwise decline.
- Gait dysfunction and hand impairment are hallmark symptoms.
- Recent data shows favorable outcomes with surgical intervention.
- Decompression surgery can proceed from an anterior, posterior, or combined approach depending on patient and pathologic condition characteristics, with similar outcomes.

INTRODUCTION

Degenerative cervical myelopathy (DCM) is a condition of the cervical spine involving progressive degenerative changes that result in chronic compression and dysfunction of the spinal cord. Although it is understood that DCM is the most common cause of spinal cord impairment worldwide because it is a broadened term for many complementary degenerative processes, literature has been unable to accurately report incidence or prevalence.[1] In a cohort of 2104 patients with nontraumatic spastic paraparesis or tetraparesis, Moore and Blumhardt demonstrated that DCM was the most common diagnosis (23.6%).[2] An observational study found DCM to be more common in men (2.7:1) with an average diagnosis of 63.8 years.[3] The natural history of DCM is that of a stepwise deterioration and proven resistance to nonoperative treatments. Given this natural history, treatment strategy favors surgical intervention. su.

ANATOMY

Knowledge of cervical spine anatomy (Figs. 1 and 2) allows for understanding of DCM pathophysiology and facilitates surgical planning. The cardinal elements of a typical cervical vertebra include the vertebral body and 2 articular pillars, each with a corresponding transverse process. The 2 pillars are united posteriorly by laminae, which support a midline spinous process. Adjacent articular pillars are united by the zygapophyseal joints, comprising superior and inferior articular facets. Adjacent vertebral bodies are united by intervertebral discs, and the anterior and posterior longitudinal ligaments. Uncinate processes are found along the superolateral border of each vertebral body.

The authors have nothing to disclose.
LSUHSC Orthoapedic Surgery, 1542 Tulane Avenue Box T6-7, New Orleans, LA 70112, USA
* Corresponding author.
E-mail address: jwil68@lsuhsc.edu

Orthop Clin N Am 53 (2022) 509–521
https://doi.org/10.1016/j.ocl.2022.05.007
0030-5898/22/Published by Elsevier Inc.

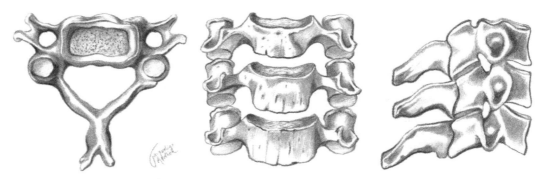

Fig. 1. The typical cervical vertebrae (C3-C5).

NATURAL HISTORY

DCM has classically been described as a step-wise decline with periods of stability interrupted by exacerbations; approximately, 20% to 60% of patients diagnosed will experience neurological deterioration.[4] Prolonged periods of moderate-to-severe neurologic symptoms portend a poor prognosis and will typically continue to progress without surgical intervention.[5] Thus, early diagnosis and treatment of this disease is prudent and advantageous.

PATHOGENESIS

The neurological sequelae of progressive spinal cord compression can result in a constellation of symptoms including gait abnormalities, difficulty with fine motor coordination, and motor/sensory deficits. Severity and symptoms depend on duration and degree of stenosis, and the level of involvement, with C5-C6 being the most common.[6] Cervical stenosis is often multifactorial; age-related degeneration, congenital stenosis, or a combination of both contributes to a reduction of the spinal canal volume.

Cervical spondylosis is the most common pathological process resulting in DCM. It encompasses a collection of pathophysiologic changes that can cause cord compression. Anterior cord compression may result from degenerative disk disease, disk-osteophyte complexes, and/or hypertrophic osseous changes at the uncovertebral joints. Posterior spinal compression may result from hypertrophic zygapophyseal joints and hypertrophic/buckled ligamentum flavum. Cervical kyphosis with

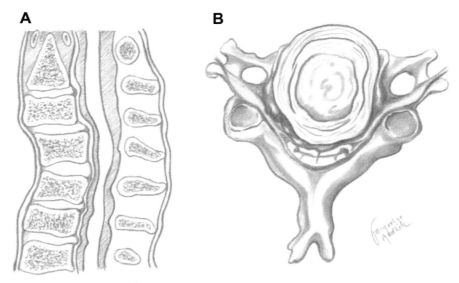

Fig. 2. (A) A sagittal cross-section of the cervical spine demonstrating various pathologies that contribute to cervical stenosis including spondylolisthesis, degenerative kyphosis, and disc degeneration/herniation. (B) An axial cross-section of a degenerative cervical vertebrae demonstrating cervical and neuroforaminal stenosis resulting from disc herniation, uncinate process hypertrophy, and facet arthropathy.

significant spondylosis will result in draping of the spinal cord over the kyphosis and aggravate the degree of cervical stenosis. Instability (anterolisthesis/retrolisthesis) may impinge the spinal cord and further exacerbate existing stenosis.

Genetic factors may influence specific pathologic condition that lowers the degree of degeneration needed to cause spinal cord compression. Minor pathologic condition (eg, disc protrusion) carries a higher risk of causing myelopathy in patients with congenital stenosis. Patients with Klippel-Feil syndrome, congenital fusion of cervical vertebrae, may have abnormal motion resulting in dynamic spinal cord compression. In contrast to the standard degenerative population, patients who may be predisposed to cord compression often present with myelopathic symptoms at a younger age (30–40 years).[7] Bajwa and colleagues,[8] through a cadaveric study, established parameters for the presence of congenital stenosis at levels C3-C7; a spinal sagittal canal diameter less than 13 mm and interpedicular distance less than 23 mm. Ossification of the posterior longitudinal ligament (OPLL), characterized by ectopic bone formation in the posterior longitudinal ligament, may also cause cord compression and myelopathy.

There are secondary effects seen at the cellular level from spinal cord compression. Dynamic and chronic compression causes ischemia and cellular injury: repetitive microtrauma causes an inflammatory cascade that induces apoptosis of neuronal cells and chronic hypoxic ischemic injury.[4,9] Eventually, atrophy develops throughout the gray matter and damaged white matter undergoes demyelination,[10] resulting in the neuropathological sequelae of deterioration.

PATIENT PRESENTATION

DCM can present with a broad spectrum of signs and symptoms. Diagnosis relies on the presence of symptoms such as upper extremity weakness/paresthesia, decreased dexterity, gait abnormalities, or neck pain.[11] Onset is typically insidious with subtle clinical findings. Altered gait and balance is often the initial presenting complaint.[12] Diminished proprioception and gait impairment from dorsal column involvement may manifest as an increasing need of assistive ambulatory devices. Difficulty with fine motor tasks may manifest as trouble with buttoning shirts or writing/typing. Lower extremities are typically more affected by advanced disease, with more commonly proximal leg weakness, resulting in

difficulty climbing stairs or rising out of chair. Autonomic symptoms such as bowel or bladder incontinence may be present in severe cases. Symptoms may be acutely worsened by trauma (eg, fall). Difficulty with speech or swallowing, breathing, or neck extensor weakness should prompt referral to neurology or consideration of electromyography (EMG)/nerve conduction study. Given variability in cause and severity of symptoms, a thorough history is required for early and accurate diagnosis.

PHYSICAL EXAMINATION

A complete spine and full neurologic examination are essential for evaluating and detecting fine motor or sensory abnormalities. C-spine range of motion may show limited and painful neck extension from underlying spondylosis. Findings may include upper extremity muscle wasting, with particular attention to the intrinsic hand musculature, and spasticity. "Myelopathy hand" has been described as the loss of adduction and extension of the ulnar 2 digits; it is associated with the "finger escape sign" (abduction and flexion drift of ulnar 2 digits).[13] The "grip and release test" may aid in quantifying the severity of cervical myelopathy.[14] Patients may exhibit pinprick and vibratory sensory abnormalities. Reflex examination may show increased or decreased upper limb reflexes and increased lower limb reflexes. A hallmark of DCM is the presence of long tract signs: clonus, Hoffman sign, Babinski sign, and inverted radial reflexes. Balance and gait are examined by tandem walking, heel/toe walking, and the Romberg test.[15] A broad-based or unstable gait may be observed in more advanced cases.

Gait and hand impairment are often the presenting symptoms of DCM. A retrospective review of 40 patients assessed by spinal surgeons found upper limb paresthesia (65%) and limb pain (53%) as the most common presenting symptoms of DCM.[16] They also demonstrated hyperreflexia to be the most common physical examination finding (80%), followed by Hoffman sign (47%), Babinski sign (47%), and gait abnormality (28%). Nemani and colleagues[17] conducted a retrospective review examining 43 patients with spinal cord changes on imaging, finding 67% with a Hoffman sign, 60% with gait abnormality, and 44% with a Romberg sign. A comparative study investigated abnormal long tract signs as a screening tool for spinal cord compression; they demonstrated a high sensitivity (91.7%) and specificity (87.5%) when an abnormal finger flexor reflex, Hoffman sign,

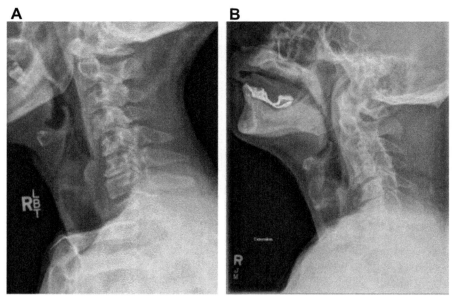

Fig. 3. (A) Lateral radiograph showing anterolisthesis at C4-C5 and degenerative disc disease most prominent at C6-C7 with loss of disc height and osteophytosis. (B) Lateral extension-view radiograph showing anterolisthesis at C4-C5, multilevel degenerative disc disease, kyphosis, and inability to extend past neutral.

and Babinski sign were present on physical examination.[18]

It is important to distinguish between pathologic conditions of the cervical cord and the brain because symptoms may overlap. The presence of a jaw jerk reflex (hyperactive jaw reflex when tapping the mandible at the chin) may indicate cranial pathologic condition and warrant further work-up.

IMAGING

Imaging of DCM begins with plain radiographs of the cervical spine in the AP and lateral projections, with flexion/extension (Fig. 3). This initial assessment allows for evaluation of cervical spinal alignment, disk height, end plate abnormalities, uncovertebral and facet joints, osteophytosis, translational deformity, spinal instability, and spinal canal dimension (see Fig. 3).

Traditionally, the Torg-Pavlov ratio has been used to assess developmental narrowing (anterior–posterior canal diameter divided by vertebral body width; <0.8 is considered stenotic).[19] Further investigation has suggested a poor correlation with actual canal diameter.[20] More recently, a rapid visual assessment of the cervical canal was evaluated based on visual characterization of the percentage of the spinal canal overlay by facet articulation on lateral cervical

radiographs. Greater than 80% facet: canal overlap was shown to be a valid screening tool in identifying potential canal narrowing.[21]

MRI is the gold standard for assessment of spinal cord compression. It allows for the evaluation of both soft tissues and osseous structures. Presence of cerebrospinal fluid (CSF) surrounding an "oval" cord indicates a patent spinal canal and is best viewed on T2 imaging. Lack of the hyperintense signal circumferentially surrounding the cord indicates some degree of cervical stenosis, which studies have shown to be a common finding in the general population (Fig. 4).[22] Cord deformation due to compression takes on a flattened or "kidney bean" shape (see Fig. 4). Hyperintense signal within the cord on T2, believed to represent myelomalacia, has historically been associated with increased disease severity and worse prognosis (Fig. 5), with more recent evidence demonstrating a higher specificity with concomitant hypo-intense T1 signal, believed to represent secondary cavitation or necrosis.[23,24]

Computed tomography (CT) scanning may be used for complex pathologic condition that requires a more comprehensive illustration of the bony anatomy. CT scans are helpful to fully evaluate spondylotic bars, disc-osteophyte complexes, and OPLL (Fig. 6). CT myelography is useful for patients who are unable to undergo an MRI or those with prior instrumentation.

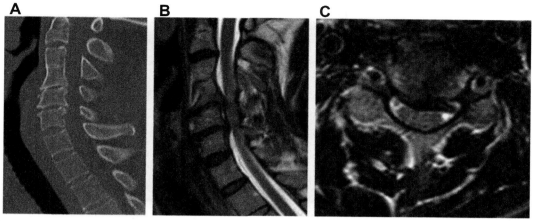

Fig. 4. (A) Sagittal CT showing congenital fusion of C3-C4 and degenerative disc disease of C4-C6 with the loss of disc height and osteophytosis. (B) Sagittal T2 MRI demonstrating C3-C4 fusion and moderate-to-severe central canal stenosis of C4-C5 and C5-C6 due to disc herniation and ligamentum flavum thickening. (C) Axial T2 MRI demonstrating C4-C5 disc herniation with associated central canal stenosis and spinal cord compression resulting in "kidney bean" cord.

Compression is characterized by a disruption of contrast in the spinal canal. Myelography poses risks with its invasive procedural nature and possible reaction to contrast.

CLASSIFICATION

The modified Japanese Orthopedic Association Scale (mJOA) and the Nurick grading scale (NGS) are 2 common classification systems used to stratify disease severity (Box 1, Table 1). Historically the NGS was used: it focused on symptoms of radiculopathy/myelopathy, gait dysfunction, and employment status. The mJOA encompasses upper and lower extremity motor dysfunction, upper extremity sensory dysfunction, and micturition. Clinically, most practitioners subgroup patients into mild, moderate, and severe, which correspond to an mJOA score of 15-17, 12-14, and 0-11, respectively.[25]

NONOPERATIVE TREATMENT

Nonoperative treatment may be offered to patients who are asymptomatic with radiographic evidence of cord compression and those with mild symptoms but there is bias toward surgical treatment. A systematic review analyzing patients with DCM who were treated

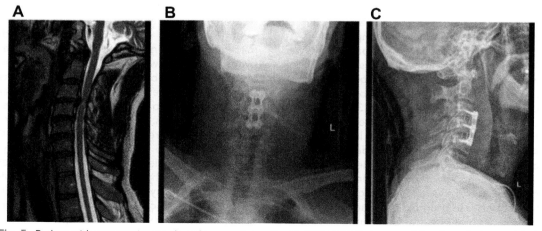

Fig. 5. Patient with progressive myelopathic symptoms. Sagittal T2 MRI (A) shows multilevel cervical spondylosis with central canal stenosis at C3-C5 and hyperintensity consistent with myelomalacia C3-C4. AP (B) and lateral (C) X-ray after C3-C5 anterior cervical discectomy and fusion (ACDF).

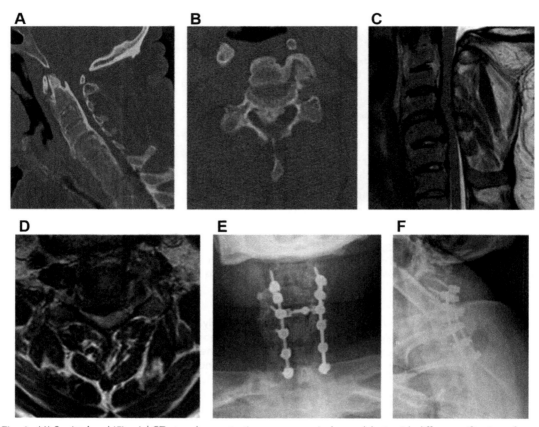

Fig. 6. (A) Sagittal and (B) axial CT scan demonstrating severe cervical spondylosis with diffuse ossification of anterior and posterior longitudinal ligaments and resulting central stenosis involving C2-C6. (C, D) MRI redemonstrating severe multilevel central stenosis with severe cord compression and intramedullary T2 hyperintense signal within the right hemicord of C4-C5. (E, F) Postoperative X-rays: C2-C7 posterior cervical fusion and laminectomy.

nonoperatively found that 20% to 60% of patients had neurological deterioration within 3 to 6 months.[4] Yoshimatsu and colleagues conducted a prospective cohort analyzing the effectiveness of nonoperative treatment in 69 patients; 16 patients showed improvement, 10 patients had no change, and 43 patients showed worsening of symptoms.[26] Those who underwent a rigorous treatment protocol were likely to do better. Rigorous protocol consisted of continuous cervical traction for 3 to 4 hours a day, anti-inflammatory drug therapy, exercise therapy, and cervical orthotic immobilization. All study patients eventually underwent surgery due to no improvement or worsening of symptoms. Patients treated nonoperatively should be thoroughly counseled on signs and symptoms of disease progression. Many patients are offered surgical treatment as an "elective-urgency" given favorable outcomes in those who underwent decompression early rather than late.[27]

Recent Clinical Practice Guidelines in addition to a recent systematic review demonstrated strong evidence supporting the surgical treatment of moderate and severe disease but weaker evidence for mild disease.[28,29] Surgical treatment can be considered in patients with mild disease. Alternatively, a trial of conservative management with structured rehabilitation. Surgery should be considered in patients experiencing deterioration, whereas surgery can be offered in patients with lack of improvement in symptoms. In patients with asymptomatic cord compression on imaging, it is recommended to follow patients clinically. In contrast, patients demonstrating either clinical or electrophysiologic evidence of radiculopathy without myelopathic symptoms should be more strongly considered for surgical intervention because cervical radiculopathy in patients with cord compression have a higher rate of developing myelopathic signs and symptoms.[30]

Box 1
Modified Japanese Orthopedic Association scale

Motor dysfunction–Upper extremities

  0 Unable to move hands

  1 Unable to eat with a spoon but able to move hands

  2 Unable to button shirt but able to eat with a spoon

  3 Able to button shirt with great difficulty

  4 Able to button shirt with slight difficulty

  5 No dysfunction

Motor dysfunction–Lower extremities

  0 Complete loss of motor and sensory function

  1 Sensory preservation without ability to move legs

  2 Able to move legs but unable to walk

  3 Able to walk on flat floor with a walking aid (cane or crutch)

  4 Able to walk upstairs and/or downstairs with aid of a handrail

  5 Moderate-to-significant lack of stability but able to walk upstairs and/or downstairs without handrail

  6 Mild lack of stability but able to walk unaided with smooth reciprocation

  7 No dysfunction

Sensory dysfunction–Upper extremities

  0 Complete loss of hand sensation

  1 Severe sensory loss or pain

  2 Mild sensory loss

  3 No sensory loss

Sphincter dysfunction

  0 Unable to micturate voluntarily

  1 Marked difficulty in micturition

  2 Mild-to-moderate difficulty in micturition

  3 Normal micturition

SURGICAL TREATMENT PRE-OP CONSIDERATIONS

Surgery has inherent risks, particularly in the elderly and those with multiple comorbidities.[31] The most prevalent were found to be hypertension, lung disease, and diabetes.[31]

Patients with 3 or more comorbidites had a 2-fold increase in complication and mortality rates compared with patients without comorbid conditions.[31]

Neck hyperextension can put the spinal cord at risk, due to decreased canal volume and space for the spinal cord.[32] Thus, fiber-optic intubation may be advantageous, allowing safe intubation with the neck in a neutral position. Intraoperative neuromonitoring (IONM) including somatosensory-evoked potentials, transcranial motor-evoked potentials, and EMG have been routinely used in spinal surgery to monitor neurological changes. IONM can assist the surgeon in evaluation and treatment of intraoperative neurologic deficits and ensure meaningful intervention can be carried out by the surgeon and anesthesiologist, including blood pressure maintenance, administration of steroids, fluid resuscitation, blood transfusion, and reversal of deformity correction as needed. However, a higher rate of false-positive alerts, especially with motor-evoked potentials can increase stress to the surgeon and operating room personnel and should be used judiciously in concert with patient pathologic condition.[33]

SURGICAL APPROACHES

Goals of surgery include decompression of the neural elements, avoidance of deformity and/or correction of deformity, and maintaining a stable spinal column while minimizing complications to the patient. These goals can be achieved from an anterior, posterior, or combined approach. A systematic review showed comparable results in effectiveness of treatment and safety with either approach.[34] Considerations for surgical approach include patient characteristics including age of the patient, obesity, barrel chest, Klippel-Feil syndrome, previous cervical surgery, previous radiation, anterior or posterior location of pathologic condition, number of involved levels, sagittal alignment, and axial neck pain. Specific considerations for anterior approach are postoperative dysphagia, and potential difficulty in surgical exposure of the C3-C4 level or C7-T1 levels. In the posterior approach, patients have a higher incidence of postoperative infection, pain, and risk of injury to posterior musculature and ligamentous stabilizers of the cervical spine.

ANTERIOR APPROACH

An anterior approach permits direct decompression of anterior compressive pathologic conditions it is favored for pathologic condition that

Table 1
Nurick grades

0	Signs or symptoms of root involvement but without evidence of spinal cord disease
1	Signs of spinal cord disease but no difficulty in walking
2	Slight difficulty in walking that did not prevent a full-time employment
3	Difficulty in walking that prevented a full-time employment or the ability to do all housework but that was not so severe as to require someone else's help to walk
4	Able to walk only with someone else's help or with the aid of a frame
5	Chair bound or bedridden

is ventral to the spinal cord in either a retrodiscal or retrovertebral location. Dysphagia is the most common complication.[35] Multiple studies have shown female gender, older age, longer surgery time, and multiple levels fused as risk factors for dysphagia.[36,37] The use of steroids has been proven to decrease the risk of dysphagia particular in those undergoing multilevel fusion.[38] Anterior structures such as the esophagus, trachea, carotid artery, and carotid sheath contents are typically at risk. In addition, the recurrent laryngeal nerve, as well as the superior laryngeal nerve in high cervical approaches are at risk. Anterior approaches are preferred in up to 3 levels. An anterior approach is favorable in a kyphotic cervical spine when applicable because it better addresses cervical kyphosis. Anterior corpectomy and fusion may be considered with retrovertebral pathologic condition to allow decompression behind a vertebral body. In the setting OPLL an anterior approach with a "floating technique" may be acceptable but there is an increased risk of dural tears approaching anteriorly.[39]

In revision anterior cervical spine surgery, there is an increased risk of injuring surrounding structures as normal tissue planes have been disrupted; and risk of scar tissue tethering the esophagus, trachea, or laryngeal neurovascular structures increases the risk of injury. Before revision anterior cervical approach, Otolaryngology evaluation with laryngoscopic evaluation to assess the status of the vocal cords should be performed to allow for a contralateral approach to avoid scar tissue. If unilateral vocal cord dysfunction is present, surgical approach should be performed on the ipsilateral side to avoid

further injury to vocal cord innervation from the contralateral side.

POSTERIOR APPROACH

Posterior decompression relies on "drift back" of the spinal cord away from anterior compressive pathologic condition, allowing for an indirect decompression. Taniyama and colleagues[40] proposed the "modified K-Line," a line connecting the midpoints of the spinal cord at C2 and C7, as a preoperative assessment of the potential "drift back" position and adequacy of posterior decompression. The posterior approach is considered in patients with 3 or more levels of pathologic condition, when the compressive pathologic condition is posteriorly based (buckling of the ligamentum flavum or shingling of the laminae), OPLL, or as an adjunct fixation. Anterior resection of OPLL has a higher risk of intraoperative durotomy; posterior approach allows for avoidance of this complication and has become more popular in those with neutral to lordotic alignment.[39] Posterior-only approach is contraindicated in a fixed kyphotic spine, correlating with worse outcomes compared with an anterior approach, due to the draping of the spinal cord over the kyphotic segments. Suitability for posterior approach is typically determined through the lateral extension film and ability of the cervical spine to extend to a neutral position.

COMBINED APPROACHES

In certain patients, a combined anterior and posterior approaches may be utilized, either during the same operative setting or in a staged fashion. Combined approaches are considered in patient with significant deformity or multilevel diseases (>3 levels) to optimize fusion rates, prevent implant failure, and maintain deformity correction. In addition, this method can be useful in patients with postlaminectomy kyphosis to restore sagittal alignment with an anterior approach and additional stability with supplemental posterior fixation.

SURGICAL TREATMENTS BASED ON APPROACH

Anterior Surgery

Anterior surgery entails the use of ACDF, anterior cervical corpectomy and fusion (ACCF), or in select circumstances motion-sparing total disc arthroplasty. Multiple treatment variations exist for the treatment of multilevel cervical myelopathy. A systematic review gathered results from 10 studies comparing multilevel ACDF, multilevel corpectomy, and hybrid procedures for cervical myelopathy.[41] Results demonstrated favorable improvements in clinical outcome scores for all procedures (Visual Analog Score [VAS], Neck Disabilty Index [NDI], Japanese Orthopedic Association [JOA]). Moreover, data supported greater improvements with multilevel ACDF compared with both multilevel corpectomy and hybrid procedures. Based on this systemic review, results advocate for multilevel ACDF above other anterior-based procedures under the correct indications.

POSTERIOR SURGERY

Posterior-based techniques including decompression and fusion or laminoplasty are utilized for patients with multilevel disease and well-maintained cervical lordosis. Prospective results of laminoplasty with 20-year patient follow-up demonstrated stability in JOA and neurologic recovery scores at 10 years.[42] Although there was a decline in scores after 10 years, these often were secondary to nonspinal pathologic condition. Thus, long-term results support the efficacy of laminoplasty for cervical myelopathy.

Systematic literature review comparing laminoplasty and laminectomy plus fusion found equal efficacy in the treatment of cervical myelopathy.[43] Recent systematic review and meta-analysis of laminectomy and fusion versus laminoplasty for multilevel cervical myelopathy demonstrated similar clinical improvements and loss of cervical lordosis.[44] Results found no statistical difference in JOA, VAS, cervical curvature index, reoperation rate, or Nurick grade between groups. Higher total complication rate and pooled rate of nerve palsies in the laminectomy and fusion cohort was noted. These results showed similar clinical improvements in both groups and cannot support either procedure over the other for cervical myelopathy.

ANTERIOR VERSUS POSTERIOR

Systematic review of retrospective cohort studies comparing anterior versus posterior approach for cervical myelopathy found no difference in JOA and neck pain scores.[34] Moreover, complication rates between the 2 approaches were similar. Additional systemic review and meta-analysis of 8 nonrandomized retrospective/prospective cohort studies demonstrated no significant difference in neural recovery between anterior and posterior approaches.[45] Complication and reoperation rates

were significantly higher in the anterior group compared with the posterior group due to higher rates of pseudoarthrosis/nonunion, adjacent segment disease, and fixation loosening.

SURGICAL COMPLICATIONS

The natural history and favorable surgical outcomes in DCM have led to an increase in surgical intervention; however, risk still needs to be considered. The AOSpine group published a prospective study with an overall complication rate of 18.7% at one year.[35] Dysphagia was the most common complication, followed by superficial infection and cardiopulmonary events.

INTRAOPERATIVE COMPLICATIONS

Limited data is available on intraoperative complications, due to the heterogeneity in reporting. In a prospective observational study of surgically treated patients for DCM, intraoperative adverse event rate of 13.5% was shown, with the most common adverse event of malpositioned hardware, followed by CSF leak.[46]

POSTOPERATIVE COMPLICATIONS

DCM has a 37.5% late post-op complication rate.[46] The most common complications were dysphagia (13.5%), neuropathic pain (7.7%), neurologic deterioration (4.8%), and wound complications (3.9%).[46] A population-based cohort with 4 years of follow-up found the revision rate for anterior surgery, posterior laminoplasty, and posterior laminectomy and fusion were 2.5%, 7.9%, and 12.5%, respectively.[47] A reoperation rate of 3% was noted with an increased risk in men, diabetics, and those with associated comorbidities.

Pseudoarthrosis leads to 7% of revisions in single level ACDF as seen in a prospective trial.[48] In multilevel anterior procedures, smoking had a significant effect on fusion rates with a study demonstrating 81% of nonsmokers and 62% of smokers obtaining a stable fusion.[35] Although smoking has an influence on anterior surgery, literature has not shown a significant effect of fusion rates for posterior surgery.[49]

Postoperative kyphosis can affect surgical outcomes. A study assessing different interbody graft morphologies in ACDF, inadvertently found that patients with improved or maintained sagittal alignment had significant improvements in SF-36 physical component summary and NDI scores.[50] In a retrospective analysis of patients undergoing either expansive laminoplasty, laminectomy alone, or laminectomy and fusion for cervical OPLL the incidence of postoperative kyphosis was 20%; patients with laminectomy alone had the highest progression of deformity at 62.5%, followed by laminoplasty at 45.5% and laminectomy with fusion at 30%.[51]

Cervical nerve root palsy is a complication that can occur with anterior or posterior procedures. A meta-analysis demonstrated a 4.6% incidence of C5 nerve palsy, with no statistical differences in approach, procedure, or cause of myelopathy.[52]

Postoperative infection rates after spinal fusion vary from 2% to 13% but there is a significant risk with posterior procedures.[47,52] Risk factors for developing an infection after posterior surgery are active smoking, rheumatoid arthritis, and obesity.[53]

SURGICAL OUTCOMES

A large multicenter multinational prospective trial was conducted to evaluate outcomes for patients undergoing surgery for DCM, representing the best dataset on surgical intervention to date. The study was developed to evaluate patients who were able to achieve an mJOA of 16 or greater to indicate minimal impairment compared with those who were not able to achieve this outcome. Patients were treated with all potential approaches, anterior with either ACDF or ACCF, posteriorly through laminectomy/fusion or laminoplasty, or combined approach. At 1 year follow-up, mean mJOA score improved from 12.5 to 15.2, with surgical intervention demonstrating meaningful improvement among all patients. Notably, although the majority (90%) of patients improved to an mJOA of 12 or greater, 10% were not able to improve past severe myelopathy. Those who were able to achieve an mJOA of 16 or greater were younger, shorter duration of preoperative symptoms, had milder myelopathy, were nonsmokers, had less comorbid conditions, and did not have gait dysfunction on presentation.[54] Although patients with severe nonambulatory myelopathy may not improve to minimal impairment, recent data demonstrates there is still a significant improvement in both Nurick and mJOA scores with potential to regain the ability to ambulate without use of a walker,[55] although with a potential for higher risk of perioperative complications.[56] Notably, patients with milder myelopathy will make most improvement in the first 3 months, whereas patients with more severe myelopathy will take more time to recover, continuing to demonstrate recovery through the 12-month period compared with those with milder symptoms.[57]

SUMMARY

DCM is typically caused by cervical spondylosis resulting in narrowing of the spinal canal and spinal cord compression. Its symptoms are characterized by upper extremity weakness or paresthesia, clumsiness of hands, and gait abnormalities. The natural history of DCM is that of a stepwise deterioration. Nonoperative treatment can be attempted in asymptomatic patients and potentially those with mild symptoms but clinical follow-up is recommended to monitor for deterioration. Otherwise, surgical intervention is recommended either through an anterior, posterior, or combined approach while considering patient and pathologic condition characteristics to minimize complications. Outcome measures have proven significant improvement is gained with surgical intervention regardless of approach. Better outcomes are seen in younger, nonsmoking, less comorbid patients, with shorter duration of symptoms, and those presenting without gait dysfunction.

CLINICS CARE POINTS

- Degenerative cervical myelopathy involves degenerative changes that result in compression of the spinal cord.
- Natural history usually involves slow stepwise progressive process.
- Patients can present with gait dysfunction, coordination difficulty, problems with fine motor tasks, and weakness.
- Plain radiographs, and advanced imaging, with either MRI or computed tomography myelogram are diagnostic of spinal cord compression.
- Nonoperative management can be considered in asymptomatic patients with spinal cord compression or those with mild symptoms.
- Patients with moderate-to-severe symptoms will require surgical intervention through anterior, posterior, or combined approaches.
- Surgical outcomes demonstrate clinically significant improvement for a majority of myelopathic patients.

REFERENCES

1. Kalsi-Ryan S, Karadimas SK, Fehlings MG. Cervical spondylotic myelopathy: the clinical phenomenon

and the current pathobiology of an increasingly prevalent and devastating disorder. Neuroscientist 2013;19(4):409–21.

2. Moore AP, Blumhardt LD. A prospective survey of the causes of non-traumatic spastic paraparesis and tetraparesis in 585 patients. Spinal Cord 1997;35(6):361–7.

3. Northover J, Wild J, Braybrooke J, et al. The epidemiology of cervical spondylotic myelopathy. Skeletal Radiol 2012;41(12):1543–6.

4. Karadimas SK, Erwin WM, Ely CG, et al. Pathophysiology and natural history of cervical spondylotic myelopathy. Spine 2013;38(22S):S21–36.

5. Matz PG, Anderson PA, Holly LT, et al. The natural history of cervical spondylotic myelopathy. J Neurosurg Spine 2009;11(2):104–11.

6. Matsumoto M, Fujimura Y, Suzuki N, et al. MRI of cervical intervertebral discs in asymptomatic subjects. J Bone Joint Surg Br 1998;80(1):19–24.

7. Guille JT, Miller A, Bowen JR, et al. The natural history of Klippel-Feil syndrome: clinical, roentgenographic, and magnetic resonance imaging findings at adulthood. J Pediatr Orthop 1995; 15(5):617–26.

8. Bajwa NS, Toy JO, Young EY, et al. Establishment of parameters for congenital stenosis of the cervical spine: an anatomic descriptive analysis of 1,066 cadaveric specimens. Eur Spine J 2012; 21(12):2467–74.

9. Breig A, Turnbull I, Hassler O. Effects of mechanical stresses on the spinal cord in cervical spondylosis: A study on fresh cadaver material. J Neurosurg 1966;25:45–56.

10. Ito T, Oyanagi K, Takahashi H, et al. Cervical spondylotic myelopathy. Clinicopathologic study on the progression pattern and thin myelinated fibers of the lesions of seven patients examined during complete autopsy. Spine (Phila Pa 1976) 1996;21(7):827–33.

11. Tracy JA, Bartleson JD. Cervical spondylotic myelopathy. Neurologist 2010;16(3):176–87.

12. Bohlman HH. Cervical Spondylosis with Moderate to Severe Myelopathy. Spine 1977;2(2):151–62.

13. Ono K, Ebara S, Fuji T, et al. Myelopathy hand. New clinical signs of cervical cord damage. J Bone Joint Surg Br 1987;69(2):215–9.

14. Hosono N, Sakaura H, Mukai Y, et al. A simple performance test for quantifying the severity of cervical myelopathy. J Bone Joint Surg Br 2008;90-B(9): 1210–3.

15. Hassanzadeh H, Bell J, Dooley E, et al. Evaluation of gait and functional stability in preoperative cervical spondylotic myelopathy patients. Spine 2022; 47(4):317–23.

16. Hilton B, Tempest-Mitchell J, Davies B, et al. Assessment of degenerative cervical myelopathy differs between specialists and may influence time to diagnosis and clinical outcomes. PLoS One 2018;13(12):e0207709.

17. Nemani VM, Kim HJ, Piyaskulkaew C, et al. Correlation of cord signal change with physical examination findings in patients with cervical myelopathy. Spine (Phila Pa 1976) 2015;40(1):6–10.

18. Tejus MN, Singh V, Ramesh A, et al. An evaluation of the finger flexion, Hoffman's and plantar reflexes as markers of cervical spinal cord compression - A comparative clinical study. Clin Neurol Neurosurg 2015;134:12–6.

19. Pavlov H, Torg JS, Robie B, et al. Cervical spinal stenosis: determination with vertebral body ratio method. Radiology 1987;164(3):771–5.

20. Blackley HR, Plank LD, Robertson PA. Determining the sagittal dimensions of the canal of the cervical spine: the reliability of ratios of anatomical measurements. J Bone Joint Surg Br 1999;81(1):110–2.

21. Iclal ET, Lomasney LM, Jones NS, et al. A practical radiographic visual estimation technique for the prediction of developmental narrowing of cervical spinal canal. Br J Radiol 2017;90(1078):20170286.

22. Boden SD, McCowin PR, Davis DO, et al. Abnormal magnetic-resonance scans of the cervical spine in asymptomatic subjects: A prospective investigation. J Bone Joint Surg Am 1990;72(8):1178–84.

23. Fernández de Rota JJ, Meschian S, Fernández de Rota A, et al. Cervical spondylotic myelopathy due to chronic compression: the role of signal intensity changes in magnetic resonance images. J Neurosurg Spine 2007;6(1):17–22.

24. Mastronardi L, Elsawaf A, Roperto R, et al. Prognostic relevance of the postoperative evolution of intramedullary spinal cord changes in signal intensity on magnetic resonance imaging after anterior decompression for cervical spondylotic myelopathy. J Neurosurg Spine 2007;7(6):615–22.

25. Tetreault L, Kopjar B, Nouri A, et al. The modified Japanese Orthopaedic Association scale: establishing criteria for mild, moderate and severe impairment in patients with degenerative cervical myelopathy. Eur Spine J 2017;26(1):78–84.

26. Yoshimatsu H, Nagata K, Goto H, et al. Conservative treatment for cervical spondylotic myelopathy. prediction of treatment effects by multivariate analysis. Spine J 2001;1(4):269–73.

27. Lee TT, Manzano GR, Green BA. Modified open-door cervical expansive laminoplasty for spondylotic myelopathy: operative technique, outcome, and predictors for gait improvement. J Neurosurg 1997;86(1):64–8.

28. Fehlings MG, Tetreault LA, Riew KD, et al. A clinical practice guideline for the management of degenerative cervical myelopathy: introduction, rationale, and scope. Glob Spine J 2017;7(Supplement 3): 21S–7S.

29. Rhee JM, Shamji MF, Erwin WM, et al. Nonoperative management of cervical myelopathy. Spine 2013;38(22S):S55–67.
30. Bednarik J, Kadanka Z, Vohanka S, et al. Presymptomatic spondylotic cervical myelopathy: an updated predictive model. Eur Spine J 2008;17(3):421–31.
31. Kawaguchi Y, Kanamori M, Ishihara H, et al. Pathomechanism of myelopathy and surgical results of laminoplasty in elderly patients with cervical spondylosis. Spine 2003;28(19):2209.
32. Dalbayrak S, Yaman O, Firidin MN, et al. The contribution of cervical dynamic magnetic resonance imaging to the surgical treatment of cervical spondylotic myelopathy. Turk Neurosurg 2015;25(1):36–42.
33. Lall RR, Lall RR, Hauptman JS, et al. Intraoperative neurophysiological monitoring in spine surgery: indications, efficacy, and role of the preoperative checklist. Neurosurg Focus 2012;33(5):E10.
34. Lawrence BD, Jacobs WB, Norvell DC, et al. Anterior versus posterior approach for treatment of cervical spondylotic myelopathy a systematic review. Spine 2013;38(22, Suppl. 1):S173–82.
35. Fehlings MG, Wilson JR, Kopjar B, et al. Efficacy and safety of surgical decompression in patients with cervical spondylotic myelopathy: results of the aospine north america prospective multicenter study. J Bone Joint Surg 2013;95(18):1651–8.
36. Kalb S, Reis MT, Cowperthwaite MC, et al. Dysphagia after anterior cervical spine surgery: incidence and risk factors. World Neurosurg 2012;77(1):183–7.
37. Bazaz R, Lee MJ, Yoo JU. MD incidence of dysphagia after anterior cervical spine surgery. Spine 2002;27(22):2453–8.
38. Cui S, Daffner SD, France JC, et al. The effects of perioperative corticosteroids on dysphagia following surgical procedures involving the anterior cervical spine: a prospective, randomized, controlled, double-blinded clinical trial. J Bone Joint Surg 2019;101(22):2007–14.
39. ONeill KR, Neuman BJ, Peters C, et al. Risk factors for dural tears in the cervical spine. Spine 2014;39(17):E1015–20.
40. Taniyama T, Hirai T, Yoshii T, et al. Modified k-line in magnetic resonance imaging predicts clinical outcome in patients with nonlordotic alignment after laminoplasty for cervical spondylotic myelopathy. Spine 2014;39(21):E1261–8.
41. Shamji MF, Massicotte EM, Traynelis VC, et al. Comparison of anterior surgical options for the treatment of multilevel cervical spondylotic myelopathy: a systematic review. Spine (Phila Pa 1976) 2013;38(22suppl 1):S195–209.
42. Kawaguchi Y, Nakano M, Yasuda T, et al. More than 20 years follow-up after en bloc cervical laminoplasty. Spine (Phila Pa 1976) 2016;41(20):1570–9.
43. Yoon ST, Hashimoto RE, Raich A, et al. Outcomes after laminoplasty compared with laminectomy and fusion in patients with cervical myelopathy: A systematic review. Spine (Phila Pa 1976) 2013;38(22suppl 1):S183–94.
44. Phan K, Scherman DB, Xu J, et al. Laminectomy and fusion vs laminoplasty for multi-level cervical myelopathy: a systematic review and meta-analysis. Eur Spine J 2017;26(1):94–103.
45. Zhu B, Xu Y, Liu X, et al. Anterior approach versus posterior approach for the treatment of multilevel cervical spondylotic myelopathy: a systemic review and meta- analysis. Eur Spine J 2013;22(7):1583–93.
46. Hartig D, Dea N, Kelly A, et al. Adverse events in surgically treated cervical spondylopathic myelopathy: a prospective validatedobservational study. Spine 2015;40(5):292–8.
47. Park MS, Kim T-H, Ju Y-S, et al. Reoperation rates after surgery for degenerative cervical spine disease according to different surgical procedures: National population-based cohort study. Spine 2016;41(19):1484–92.
48. Van Eck CF, Regan C, Donaldson WF, et al. The revision rate and occurrence of adjacent segment disease after anterior cervical discectomy and fusion: a study of 672 consecutive patients. Spine 2014;39(26):2143–7.
49. Eubanks JD, Thorpe SW, Cheruvu VK, et al. Does smoking influence fusion rates in posterior cervical arthrodesis with lateral mass instrumentation? Clin Orthopaedics Relat Research 2011;469(3):696–701.
50. Villavicencio AT, Ashton A, Busch E, et al. Prospective, randomized, double-blind clinical study evaluating the correlation of clinical outcomes and cervical sagittal alignment. Neurosurgery 2011;68(5):1309–16.
51. Lee C-H, Jahng T-A, Hyun S-J, et al. Expansive laminoplasty versus laminectomy alone versus laminectomy and fusion for cervical ossification of the posterior longitudinal ligament. J Spinal Disord Tech 2016;29(1):E9–15.
52. Sakaura H, Hosono N, Mukai Y, et al. C5 palsy after decompression surgery for cervical myelopathy: review of the literature. Spine 2003;28(21):2447–51.
53. Pahys JM, Pahys JR, Cho SK, et al. Methods to decrease postoperative infections following posterior cervical spine surgery. J Bone Joint Surg 2013;95-A(6):549–54.
54. Tetreault L, Kopjar B, Côté P, et al. A clinical prediction rule for functional outcomes in patients undergoing surgery for degenerative cervical myelopathy. J Bone Joint Surg 2015;97(24):2038–46.

55. Boehm BA, Njoku I, Furey CG. Single-site retrospective assessment of surgical outcomes in nonambulatory patients with degenerative cervical myelopathy. Spine (Phila Pa 1976) 2022;47(4):331–6.

56. Kopjar B, Bohm PE, Arnold JH, et al. Outcomes of Surgical decompression in patients with very severe degenerative cervical myelopathy. Spine (Phila Pa 1976) 2018;43(16):1102–9.

57. Khan I, Archer KR, Wanner JP, et al. Trajectory of improvement in myelopathic symptoms from 3 to 12 months following surgery for degenerative cervical myelopathy. Neurosurgery 2020;86(6):763–8.

A Pathway for the Diagnosis and Treatment of Lumbar Spinal Stenosis

Matthew Darlow, MD*, Patrik Suwak, DO,
Stefan Sarkovich, BS, Jestin Williams, MD,
Nathan Redlich, MD, Peter D'Amore, MD,
Amit K. Bhandutia, MD

KEYWORDS

- Lumbar • Stenosis • DDD • Decompression • Laminectomy • Neurogenic claudication

---

KEY POINTS

- Lumbar spinal stenosis most commonly occurs due to degenerative spinal changes in the elderly population, and presentation can range from asymptomatic to severely disabled.
- Imaging findings, in conjunction with symptoms, can help guide treatment and inform surgical versus nonsurgical shared decision making.
- Recent data have shown that surgical intervention can lead to improved functional outcomes and decreased pain compared with nonsurgical management.

INTRODUCTION

Lumbar spinal stenosis (LSS) is defined as the narrowing of the lumbar spinal canal with subsequent compression of neural elements. The cause of the disease and its associated pathology is varied. Although some symptoms may be dismissed as part of the normal aging process by patients and physicians alike, LSS can be debilitating and take a significant toll on the patients and their families.[1] The exact prevalence of LSS is unknown, and furthermore, the proportion of those who are asymptomatic versus symptomatic is similarly imprecise. The Framingham study, a cross-sectional observation study, attempted to quantify this information. Of their 191 study participants, who had a mean age of 52.6 years, the prevalence of LSS was 23.6%. Not surprisingly, as age increased, the percentage of patients with LSS increased.[2] Other research estimates that LSS affects more than 200,000 patients in the United States[3] and that approximately 6 of 100 patients diagnosed with degenerative lumbar conditions will require lumbar fusion within 1 year of diagnosis.[4] In another study, the estimated prevalence of symptomatic LSS was around 10%.[5] Although the exact magnitude of LSS is uncertain, what is clear is the staggering toll LSS exacts on the health care system. A retrospective cohort analysis of Medicare claims looking at surgical intervention for LSS from 2002 to 2007 demonstrated that mean hospital charges for decompression compared with complex fusion procedures were US $23,724 and $80,888, respectively.[6]

Anatomy

To fully understand the pathology of LSS, functional knowledge of the normal anatomy of the lumbar spine and its contribution to pathology is necessary. The anterior border of the spinal canal is composed of the vertebral body, the intervertebral disk, and the posterior longitudinal ligament. The lateral border is formed by the pedicles, the lateral ligamentum flavum, and the neural foramen. The posterior border is formed by the facet joints, lamina, and ligamentum flavum (Fig. 1). The paired nerve roots

---

LSU-Orthopaedics, 1542 Tulane Avenue, Box T6-7, New Orleans, LA 70112, USA
* Corresponding author.
E-mail address: mdarlo@lsuhsc.edu

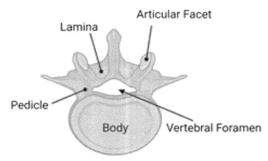

Fig. 1. Anatomy of lumbar vertebrae.

travel through the spinal canal before exiting at each respective neural foramen below the pedicle (right L4 nerve root exits below the right L4 pedicle above the L4-5 disk).

Pathophysiology

As individuals age, the intervertebral disk undergoes a process of degeneration. Within the disk, the annulus undergoes a transformation in which the level of type I collagen increases, subsequently leading to decreased hydration of the gelatinous nucleus pulposus. This decreased hydration causes the disk to desiccate, hindering its ability to handle a mechanical load. As the disk further degenerates, disk height is lost and the disk may begin to bulge and impinge on the spinal canal as well as causing the ligamentum flavum to buckle and the facet joints to settle. The facet joints, which help produce the smooth gliding motion necessary for movement in the lumbar spine, begin to see increased stress across the joint, which leads to further joint degeneration, hypertrophy, and osteophyte formation. These osteophytes can impinge on the thecal sac as well as the nerve root in the neural foramen. The intervertebral foramen, the space in which the nerve root exists, becomes tighter secondary to these degenerative changes, further compressing neural elements. This cascade, known as degenerative spondylosis, is one of the most common causes of LSS[7] (Figs. 2, 3, and 4).

The degenerative changes thus far described can be worsened by dynamic factors such as segmental instability. Instability can be in the form of translational or rotational abnormality. A translational abnormality is most often seen as an anterior slippage of one vertebral body on top of the next vertebral segment (typically L4-on-L5) resulting in substantially decreased room for the neural elements; this is known as degenerative spondylolisthesis. In scoliosis, a rotational instability is seen that leads to altered spine biomechanics and further narrowing of the central canal, lateral recess, and the intervertebral foramen, in addition to potential coronal or sagittal imbalance.

Classification

Stenosis can be anatomically classified as central, lateral recess, or foraminal based on the location of neural compression. Central stenosis is usually caused by a combination of disk bulging, hypertrophied ligamentum flavum, and facet joint overgrowth. Lateral recess stenosis is due to facet joint osteophytes as well as disk protrusion. Foraminal stenosis causes compression of the exiting nerve root and dorsal root ganglion due to loss of disk height, foraminal disk protrusion, or osteophyte formation. Finally, extraforaminal stenosis is usually due to far lateral disk herniation with resultant exiting nerve root compression.

Other acquired conditions, although less common, should be considered when attempting to determine the cause of LSS. These conditions can include space-occupying masses, postsurgical fibrosis, rheumatologic conditions such as ankylosing spondylitis or diffuse idiopathic skeletal hyperostosis, or congenital conditions such as achondroplasia or congenital stenosis.[8]

ASSESSMENT AND EVALUATION

Clinical Presentation

The diagnosis of LSS is becoming increasingly common, which may be due in part to increased access to advanced imaging and an aging patient population. A distinguishing feature of LSS is the association of pain with postural changes. Lumbar extension decreases cross-sectional spinal canal volume, which corresponds with increased pain associated with lumbar stenosis, compared with lumbar flexion, which results in the opposite effect. These symptoms are referred to as neurogenic claudication or pseudoclaudication, which consists of pain in the buttock, groin, and thigh regions. However, patients often present with additional symptoms such as heaviness, fatigue, burning, aching, dysesthesia, and rarely weakness in the buttock, groin, and thigh regions. Symptoms are typically bilateral but can affect one extremity more than the other.[9] Pain is thus exacerbated by walking, going up stairs, or standing and relieved by sitting down or leaning forward, sometimes referred to as the "shopping cart sign." Patients should be followed subjectively based on their walking tolerance in terms of time or distance.

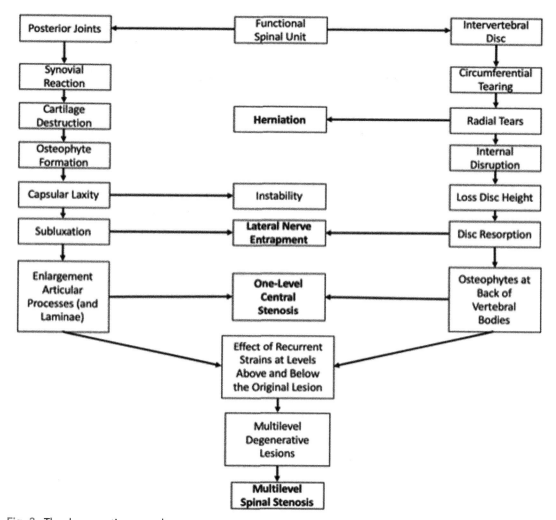

Fig. 2. The degenerative cascade.

Neurogenic claudication should not be confused with vascular claudication or other forms of nonspecific lower back pain. Vascular claudication is pain caused by peripheral arterial disease leading to insufficient blood flow to the extremity. The symptoms of vascular claudication occur more distally in the extremity, most commonly calf pain, contrary to neurogenic claudication that primarily occurs more proximal in the buttocks and thigh regions. Vascular claudication is commonly aggravated by increased movement and activity in a distance-related fashion, meaning that a patient typically can walk a certain distance until pain arises and requires rest to alleviate the pain[10]; this is in stark contrast to neurogenic claudication in that it is not the amount of activity that causes the pain but the type of activity, typically involving lumbar extension.

Patients with LSS may also present with radicular leg pain in addition to neurogenic claudication. Neurogenic claudication results from compression of the thecal sac, whereas radicular pain or radiculopathy is due to compression of a nerve root or dorsal root ganglion in the lateral recess or the neural foramen, respectively. This leg pain occurs in a dermatomal distribution. Most commonly, a patient may present with numbness and weakness in the extensor hallucis longus and tibialis anterior group due to compression of the L4 or L5 nerve root within the lateral recess.

Low back pain involvement with spinal stenosis varies, likely due to variable presentation of degenerative disk disease and facetogenic disease resulting in neural compression. Neurogenic claudication differs from other forms of nonspecific low back pain in that sitting typically

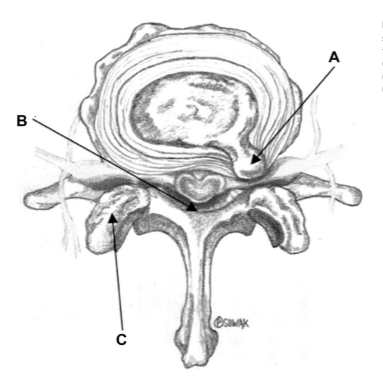

Fig. 3. Axial cross section demonstrating areas of stenosis secondary to intervertebral disk desiccation (A), thickened ligamentum flavum (B), and hypertrophied facet capsules (C).

brings relief for patients with LSS, whereas nonspecific low back pain is typically worsened from prolonged periods of sitting. However, back pain is much less of a reliable finding in terms of both diagnosis and outcomes compared with the presence of neurogenic claudication.

In addition, other common maladies plaguing older populations that can lead to back and leg pain include osteoarthritis of the spine or hip, peripheral arterial disease, and greater trochanteric pain syndrome. These conditions may lead to symptoms that mimic the pseudoclaudication of LSS and may warrant further evaluation and management. Symptoms of bowel or bladder incontinence are atypical for spinal stenosis, and a careful history must be elucidated because various causes of genitourinary dysfunction are common in older patient populations.

Physical Examination

The physical examination of patients with LSS is often equivocal. It is important to note a patient's body position during standing and ambulation because forward flexion of the trunk is how a patient with LSS will decrease their symptoms. In addition, the neurologic examination is commonly normal with patients not demonstrating any evidence of weakness or sensory

deficit. Decreased deep tendon reflexes are typical in older patients, and provocative maneuvers, such as the straight leg raise test, may not elicit a clear response. Hyperreflexia in the lower extremities or proximal thigh weakness should prompt an evaluation for the remainder of the neural axis to evaluate for myelopathy. The hip is frequently confused for spinal pathology, and care should be taken to examine the hip in addition to obtaining a lower extremity vascular examination to avoid misdiagnosis of the patient's condition.

Radiology

Diagnostic testing of LSS typically starts with plain radiographs, including anteroposterior and lateral views, with consideration of flexion and extension lateral views. Because most patients with LSS are elderly, there will likely be a variety of spondylotic or degenerative changes. In fact, even severe degenerative spine changes can be seen in asymptomatic patients. In addition, particular attention should be paid to evaluate for coronal and sagittal deformity, which is best evaluated with full-length standing films. The gold standard of radiologic diagnosis of LSS remains MRI. Dural sac cross-sectional area is used to measure the degree of stenosis. An area between 76 and 100 mm indicates relative

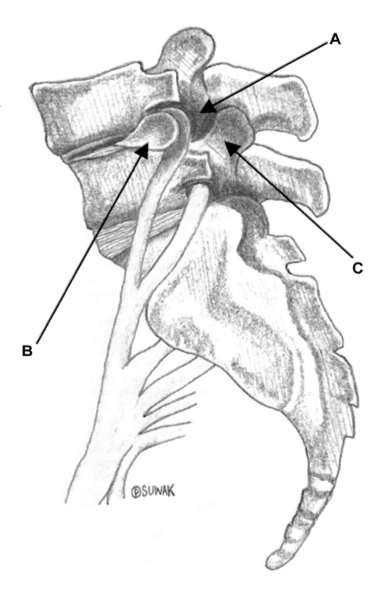

Fig. 4. Sagittal view demonstrating foraminal stenosis (A) secondary to disk degeneration and collapse (B) as well as facet osteophytes (C).

stenosis, whereas less than 75 mm indicates substantial stenosis.[11] Another morphologic classification system exists that grades stenosis, A (no or minor stenosis) through D (extreme stenosis), based on the nerve rootlet/cerebrospinal fluid (CSF) ratio on axial T2 images[12] (Table 1). In patients who are unable to tolerate an MRI or have previous spinal instrumentation, a computed tomographic (CT) myelogram, a study in which dye is injected into the CSF, allows for evaluation of the thecal sac and the surrounding soft tissue and bony pathology. Typically, workup for lumbar spinal stenosis does not require electromyography or nerve conduction velocity studies,

but may be helpful when diagnostic imaging is equivocal or for evaluation of demyelinating disease, peripheral neuropathy, or peripheral nerve compression.

DISCUSSION

Once clinical diagnosis of LSS has been reached, and both the severity of symptoms and the degree of compression on imaging has been assessed, a meaningful discussion regarding the management of LSS between patient and physician should be undertaken. The goal in managing LSS is to restore function and reduce

Table 1 Classification of spinal stenosis based on morphology of the dural sac on MRI		
Grade	**Description**	**Image**
A	CSF present in dural sac with heterogeneous distribution. This is true for A1-A4. If not true, then it is grade B, C, or D.	
A1	Nerve rootlets are dorsal and CSF occupies >50% of the dural sac.	
A2	Rootlets remain dorsal and in contact with the dura, but they are in a horseshoe pattern.	
A3	Rootlets are dorsal and occupy >50% of the dural sac area.	
A4	Rootlets are central and occupy >50% of the dural sac area.	
B	Rootlets can be individually identified, but they occupy the entire dural sac area.	
C	Rootlets cannot be individually identified; entire dural sac area is a homogeneous gray signal	

(continued on next page)

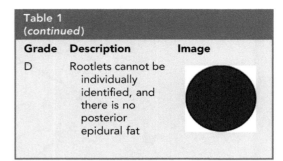

Table 1 (continued)		
Grade	**Description**	**Image**
D	Rootlets cannot be individually identified, and there is no posterior epidural fat	

From Schizas C, Theumann N, Burn A, et al. Qualitative Grading of Severity of Lumbar Spinal Stenosis Based on the Morphology of the Dural Sac on Magnetic Resonance Images. *Spine.* 2010;35(21):1919-1924.

pain; this can be achieved through both medical treatments and surgical interventions. Typically, conservative management is the first-line treatment; this includes lifestyle changes, oral antiinflammatory medications, physical therapy, and epidural corticosteroid injections.

Nonoperative Management

Although widely used and often efficacious, there are no formal studies evaluating the use of analgesics or nonsteroidal anti-inflammatory drugs in patients with LSS. Studies looking into the use of acetaminophen in the treatment of spinal pain have shown the drug to be ineffective.[13] In addition, because the patient population with LSS is typically older and as a result, often has multiple comorbidities including hypertension, cardiovascular disease, and diabetes, nonsteroidal anti-inflammatory drugs may actually do more harm than good by negatively impacting a patient's cardiovascular, renal, and gastrointestinal systems.[14,15] Opioids, although pure analgesics, have not been shown to improve functional outcomes when combined with therapy, and in fact, the adverse effects including cognitive impairment and sedation can be dangerous and lead to increased risk of falls in older populations.[16] Gabapentin, which is effective in the treatment of different neuropathic pain syndromes, has been shown in small studies to improve pain scores, lead to increased walking distances, and improve sleep.[17] However, careful attention must be paid to the side effects of gabapentin including lethargy and dizziness, which could be detrimental to older populations.

There is no standardized physical therapy regimen to treat LSS. Traditional exercise programs focus on decreasing lumbar lordosis and extension forces while improving core strength. It is not uncommon for patients with LSS to be deconditioned as a result of their symptoms and other age-related comorbidities. Aerobic training including stationary biking, ellipticals, treadmills, or aquatic programs can lead to improved walking tolerance and pain scores.[18] The efficacy of other modalities including ultrasonography, transcutaneous electrical nerve stimulation, and heat packs in addition to physical therapy are inconclusive.[19] Lumbar corsets, which maintain a small degree of lumbar flexion, may offer some benefit and have been shown to decrease pain and increase walking distance.[20] Ultimately, a physical therapy program must be tailored to the individual.

The purpose of epidural steroid injections (ESIs) is to reduce inflammation and edema at the stenotic segment. Fluoroscopy is typically used for caudal, interlaminar, or transforaminal ESIs. It is unclear whether ESIs result in long-term improvement in patients with LSS. Several studies have shown no differences in functional outcomes at either 6 or 12 weeks.[21] However, some case series using multiple injection protocols have led to long-term improvements up to 2 years in some patients.[22] A transient headache is a common adverse effect but more rare complications including epidural abscess, meningitis, and spinal hematomas have been noted.

If symptoms persist or progressively worsen after using conservative treatment modalities, surgical management can be considered. Ultimately, it is the patient's desire combined with failure of nonoperative management that will drive the decision for surgical intervention. Proper patient selection is critical to achieving successful outcomes with spinal stenosis surgery. Ideally, the patient will exhibit symptoms of neurogenic claudication including pain, numbness, and paresthesias in the posterolateral legs and thighs associated with prolonged walking, standing, or extension-type activities and relieved with forward flexion. In fact, one of the most common reasons for early failure after LSS surgery was absence of neurogenic symptoms coupled with nonsevere stenosis on imaging.[23]

Data have shown that certain patient variables are associated with better outcomes after surgical management compared with conservative management including male sex, shorter duration of systems, higher income levels, higher levels of education, better overall mental health, no diabetes mellitus, and few medical comorbidites.[24] In addition, it appears that baseline Oswestry Disability Index, a validated measurement of a patient's permanent functional disability, and smoking had the greatest effect on LSS surgical outcomes.[24] Typically, surgical decompression is performed on an elective basis unless there is a rapidly progressive neurologic decline or bowel/bladder dysfunction. It is imperative that before proceeding with any surgical management, the patient is medically optimized and understands the risks and associated complications of any surgical procedure.

Surgical Management

There are several surgical techniques that can be used in the treatment of LSS surgery. The most common is a decompressive laminectomy. The purpose of decompressive laminectomy is to relieve the pressure at a specific level of the spinal cord and its respective nerve roots. Other possible surgical techniques include laminotomy, minimally invasive decompression, and indirect decompression through the use of an interbody device. Among the available surgical options, there is currently no evidence to support superiority of one technique over the others.[25] Nonetheless, preferences among these surgical techniques exist.

Decompressive laminectomy is the most common technique used and serves as the gold standard for LSS surgical treatment.[26] The procedure involves removal of the lamina in its near entirety and any thickened ligaments to allow for sufficient decompression (Fig. 5). It is essential during this procedure to maintain and preserve most of the facet joints and the pars interarticularis. Loss of anatomic landmarks and overzealous resection can lead to pars fracture and iatrogenic spondylolisthesis. Several studies have demonstrated that patients undergoing surgical management have had significant improvement in primary outcomes compared with nonsurgical management.[27]

One of the largest studies focusing on the topic is the Spine Patient Outcomes Research Trial (SPORT), a multicenter prospective study that evaluated patients undergoing operative compared with nonoperative treatment. More than 650 patients with at least 12 weeks of symptoms were separated into 2 cohorts—a prospective observational cohort and a randomized control cohort—and both groups were further split into an operative and a nonoperative group. Patients with lumbar instability (defined by greater than 4 mm translation or 10° of angular motion) were excluded. Notably, nonoperative treatment was not standardized. In addition, the study was impacted by a high rate of crossover (approximately 40%) between nonoperative and operative groups. Nonetheless, the data from the SPORT study generally represents

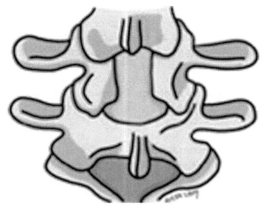

Fig. 5. In a laminectomy, the lamina is removed to decompress the spinal cord.

the highest level of evidence to date. In an as-treated analysis, decompressive laminectomy for symptomatic degenerative spinal stenosis provided significant improvements in function, pain, and disability compared with nonoperative treatment for both short term (3 month) and 4-year follow-up.[28]

The SPORT trial also investigated long-term outcomes at 8 years follow-up. The as-treated analysis demonstrated that the surgical group in the randomized control cohort had diminished benefits in surgical treatment after 4 years, specifically showing no significant effect of surgery between 6 and 8 years follow-up. It should be noted that 52% of the patients randomized to the nonoperative treatment eventually underwent surgery during the 8-year period. However, in the observational study group, surgical intervention demonstrated a consistent improvement in primary outcomes maintained across the 8-year follow-up period.[29]

Additional studies have shown the significant benefit of surgical management for LSS in both short- and long-term outcomes. At 1-year follow-up, patients with LSS treated surgically demonstrated significantly better and improved patient-reported outcomes than patients treated nonsurgically.[30] The same Maine Lumbar Spine Study group showed in their prospective observational cohort similar improved patient-reported outcomes in long-term follow-up of 8 to 10 years. Specifically, patients who underwent surgical management were more active and had significantly less severe leg pain than patients who underwent nonsurgical management at 8 to 10 years' follow-up.[24] Other randomized controlled trials have investigated patient-reported outcomes of decompressive surgical management versus nonsurgical management

in patients with LSS and demonstrated similar favorable results for surgical management. Patients who underwent decompressive surgery experienced significantly greater improvement in overall disability, leg pain, and back pain at all follow-up examinations during the 2-year study period.[31] Taken into consideration, the various published findings indicate that surgical management of LSS provides a reliable and effective benefit for patients up to 4 years follow-up compared with nonsurgical management.

A laminotomy procedure is an alternative approach to a decompressive laminectomy, especially in the circumstances of primarily lateral recess stenosis. In a laminotomy, only a portion of the vertebral lamina is removed, which allows for decompression of the nerve root (Fig. 6). Some propose that by maintaining the midline structures, namely, the spinous process and interspinous and supraspinous ligaments, as opposed to removing them during a laminectomy, there is a decreased possibility of iatrogenic instability and postoperative lumbar back pain.[32] Studies comparing unilateral or bilateral laminotomy to laminectomy in patients with lateral recess LSS without significant central stenosis demonstrated that laminotomy resulted in better perceived recovery at final follow-up visits as well as lower rates of iatrogenic instability and less postoperative back pain.[33–35]

Minimally invasive surgeries have been increasing since the introduction of laparoscopic instruments. Microendoscopic decompression of LSS provides small incisions that preserve the surrounding soft tissue structures while providing equivalent resection to that of open laminectomy. Compared with open decompressive laminectomy, studies have shown that microendoscopic decompressive laminectomy has been proved to yield significantly less operative blood loss, shorter time to mobilization and length of hospital stay, less muscle destruction, less low back and leg pain at final follow-up, as well as less probability of requiring opioids for postoperative pain.[36,37]

Interbody fusion, a surgical technique in which the intervertebral disk is removed and replaced with a metal, plastic, or bone spacer, is also used in the management of lumbar degenerative conditions. Although more commonly used for the treatment of spondylolisthesis, the placement of an interbody device can provide indirect decompression of the lumbar spine by increasing disk height, foraminal height, foraminal area, and spinal canal diameter[38,39] (Fig. 7). By decompressing the neural elements

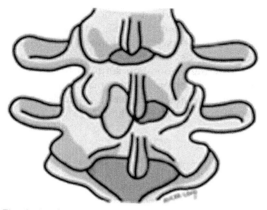

Fig. 6. In a laminotomy, as opposed to a laminectomy, only a portion of the lamina is removed.

in a minimally disruptive way, the surgeon avoids direct resection of posterior structures and its associated morbidities. However, the addition of an interbody increases both the cost and time of surgery and may increase the complication rate.

Postoperatively, patients are encouraged to get out of bed with physical therapy and ambulate as soon as possible. Patients are advised to avoid bending, lifting, and twisting for 6 to 12 weeks. Typically, patients are seen in the office 2 to 3 weeks after surgery for an assessment of the surgical incision and radiographs and are given a prescription for outpatient physical therapy. In the event of a fusion procedure, flexion-extension radiographs are obtained at each subsequent clinic visit to ensure no further instability

has occurred. Long-term follow-up is necessary to confirm that a solid fusion has occurred and there are no hardware-related complications. Absence of bridging bone on radiographs or continued symptoms should warrant a CT scan to assess for pseudoarthrosis of the fusion mass. Follow-up at regular intervals can proceed as per patient needs.

Complications

As with all surgical procedures, potential complications are ever present, including infection, CSF leaks, nerve root injuries, vascular sequelae, nonunion or hardware failure, instability, and adjacent segment disease. CSF leaks are one of the most common complications following LSS surgery with rates ranging from 1.8% to 17.4%.[40,41] Management of these tears varies by surgeon but are generally managed by repair ± spinal sealant ± closed-suction drainage. Vascular complications following LSS surgery including deep vein thrombosis, pulmonary embolism, postoperative hematoma, and rarely, vascular catastrophe lead to unexplained hypotension. Typical postoperative prophylaxis includes compression socks and pneumatic sequential compression devices, thromboembolic prophylaxis, and early ambulation. When postsurgical infections occur, they usually occur in the early postoperative period (<3 months). It is important to diagnose infections early and obtain C-reactive protein measurements as an adjunct to the physical examination. If infection is suspected, irrigation and debridement with retention of intact hardware, if present, as well

A
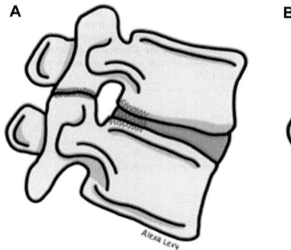

B
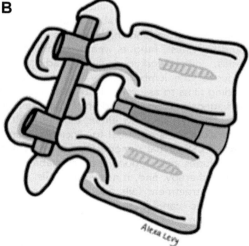

Fig. 7. By replacing the degenerative disk (A) with a spacer (B), the interbody fusion technique indirectly decompresses the lumbar spine by restoring spine biomechanics.

as long-term intravenous antibiotics are required. During LSS surgery, despite adequate decompression, overresection of the lumbar facets can lead to iatrogenic spondylolisthesis and subsequent long-term instability requiring further surgeries. Adjacent-segment disease, a condition in which adjacent levels further degenerate causing debilitating symptoms, can be a potential issue after lumbar fusion. However, although the rate of radiographic adjacent-level degeneration is high, clinically symptomatic patients only make up a small subset of the overall group. Although LSS is typically a condition of older patients with greater comorbidities, studies have shown that morbidity rates associated with decompression and/or fusion are comparable to that in young populations undergoing similar procedures.[42] In addition, in patients older than 80 years with LSS and degenerative spondylolisthesis, operative treatment produced significant benefit over nonoperative management and they experienced no significant increases in complications or mortality rates after surgery compared with younger patients.[43] However, other studies have shown that although older patients may actually experience significantly greater relief of pain, there were more postoperative adverse complications in the older group including cardiac and respiratory events and infections.

SUMMARY

LSS is typically an age-associated degenerative condition characterized by a narrowing of the spinal canal, resulting in nerve root compression. Although asymptomatic disease is common, symptoms can often be debilitating and patients may present with unilateral or bilateral pain in the buttock, groin, and thigh regions with associated heaviness, fatigue, weakness, and paresthesias. Initial workup includes radiographic images of the lumbar spine, including lateral standing films to assess for instability. Although the diagnosis of LSS is based on clinical examination, advanced imaging either through MRI or CT myelogram is essential for accurate assessment of LSS. Initial nonoperative treatment of LSS includes medication, such as gabapentin, physical therapy, and, if necessary, ESIs. If conservative treatment fails and the patient is an appropriate candidate for surgery, operative intervention can be initiated. The type of lumbar decompressive surgery is based on symptoms, levels involved, and whether there is evidence of instability. A decompressive laminectomy is the most common procedure. Recent literature supports operative intervention over nonoperative management for LSS in appropriately selected patients. Postoperatively, the patient will quickly be mobilized and regularly monitored by their operating surgeon to assess for any possible complications including infection, adjacent segment disease, instability, and nonunion or hardware failure.

CLINICS CARE POINTS

- Lumbar disk degeneration is nearly ubiquitous in elderly patients.
- The diagnosis of LSS is based on the clinical presentation. Many patients with radiographic stenosis do not exhibit symptoms of neurogenic claudication. In addition, one should be wary of mimickers of LSS such as hip disease and peripheral arterial disease.
- Initial radiographic images are necessary to obtain to evaluate for instability. MRI is the preferred radiologic study in assessing spinal stenosis.
- Conservative management with medications and physical therapy are first line for the treatment of LSS. ESIs can be considered as a potential option. Most patients will do well with nonoperative care.
- Patients with neurogenic claudication with correlating radiographic findings of LSS who fail nonoperative care are the ideal surgical candidates.
- Open decompressive laminectomy is the gold standard of treatment of LSS without instability.
- An as-treated analysis performed in the SPORT study, a large multicenter level 1 prospective randomized controlled trial, demonstrates the efficacy of operative intervention over nonoperative management for LSS.

DISCLOSURE

The authors have nothing to disclose.

REFERENCES

1. Chad DA. Lumbar spinal stenosis. Neurol Clin 2007;25(2):407–18.
2. Kalichman L, Cole R, Kim DH, et al. Spinal stenosis prevalence and association with symptoms: the Framingham Study. Spine J 2009;9(7):545–50.

3. Lurie J, Tomkins-Lane C. Management of lumbar spinal stenosis. BMJ 2016;h6234.

4. Buser Z, Ortega B, D'Oro A, et al. Spine degenerative conditions and their treatments: national trends in the United States of America. Glob Spine J 2017;8(1):57–67.

5. Ishimoto Y, Yoshimura N, Muraki S, et al. Prevalence of symptomatic lumbar spinal stenosis and its association with physical performance in a population-based cohort in Japan: the Wakayama Spine Study. Osteoarthritis Cartilage 2012;20(10):1103–8.

6. Deyo RA. Trends, major medical complications, and charges associated with surgery for lumbar spinal stenosis in older adults. JAMA 2010;303(13):1259.

7. Yong-Hing K, Kirkaldy-Willis WH. The Pathophysiology of degenerative disease of the lumbar spine. Orthop Clin North Am 1983;14(3):491–504.

8. Verbiest H. Pathomorphologic aspects of developmental lumbar stenosis. Orthop Clin North Am 1975;6(1):177–96.

9. Genevay S, Atlas SJ. Lumbar spinal stenosis. Best Pract Res Clin Rheumatol 2010;24(2):253–65.

10. Nadeau M, Rosas-Arellano MP, Gurr KR, et al. The reliability of differentiating neurogenic claudication from vascular claudication based on symptomatic presentation. Can J Surg 2013;56(6):372–7.

11. Lønne G, Ødegård B, Johnsen LG, et al. MRI evaluation of lumbar spinal stenosis: is a rapid visual assessment as good as area measurement? Eur Spine J 2014;23(6):1320–4.

12. Schizas C, Theumann N, Burn A, et al. Qualitative grading of severity of lumbar spinal stenosis based on the morphology of the dural sac on magnetic resonance images. Spine 2010;35(21):1919–24.

13. Machado GC, Maher CG, Ferreira PH, et al. Efficacy and safety of paracetamol for spinal pain and osteoarthritis: systematic review and meta-analysis of randomised placebo controlled trials. BMJ 2015;350(mar31 2):h1225.

14. Gutthann SP, GarcíaRodríguez LA, Raiford DS. Individual nonsteroidal antiinflammatory drugs and other risk factors for upper gastrointestinal bleeding and perforation. Epidemiology 1997;8(1):18–24.

15. Griffin MR, Yared A, Ray WA. Nonsteroidal antiinflammatory drugs and acute renal failure in elderly persons. Am J Epidemiol 2000;151(5):488–96.

16. Schofferman J, Mazanec D. Evidence-informed management of chronic low back pain with opioid analgesics. Spine J 2008;8(1):185–94.

17. Yaksi A, Özgönenel L, Özgönenel B. The efficiency of gabapentin therapy in patients with lumbar spinal stenosis. Spine 2007;32(9):939–42.

18. Whitman JM, Flynn TW, Childs JD, et al. A comparison between two physical therapy treatment programs for patients with lumbar spinal stenosis. Spine 2006;31(22):2541–9.

19. Macedo LG, Hum A, Kuleba L, et al. Physical therapy interventions for degenerative lumbar spinal stenosis: a systematic review. Phys Ther 2013;93(12):1646–60.

20. Prateepavanich P, Thanapipatsiri S, Santisatisakul P, et al. The effectiveness of lumbosacral corset in symptomatic degenerative lumbar spinal stenosis. J Med Assoc Thai 2001;84(4):572–6.

21. A randomized trial of epidural glucocorticoid injections for spinal stenosis. N Engl J Med 2014;371(4):390.

22. Botwin KP, Gruber RD, Bouchlas CG, et al. Fluoroscopically guided lumbar transformational epidural steroid injections in degenerative lumbar stenosis. Am J Phys Med Rehabil 2002;81(12):898–905.

23. Deen HG Jr, Zimmerman RS, Lyons MK, et al. Analysis of early failures after lumbar decompressive laminectomy for spinal stenosis. Mayo Clin Proc 1995;70(1):33–6.

24. Atlas SJ, Keller RB, Wu YA, et al. Long-term outcomes of surgical and nonsurgical management of lumbar spinal stenosis: 8 to 10 year results from the maine lumbar spine study. Spine 2005;30(8):936–43.

25. Overdevest GM, Jacobs W, Vleggeert-Lankamp C, et al. Effectiveness of posterior decompression techniques compared with conventional laminectomy for lumbar stenosis. Cochrane Database Syst Rev 2015;(3):CD010036. doi:10.1002/14651858.CD010036.pub2. PMID: 25760812.

26. Su BW, Rihn J, Byers R, et al. Surgical management of lumbar spinal stenosis. In: Bono CN, Fischgrund JS, editors. Rothman simeone the spine. Philadelphia, PA: Elsevier; 2011. p. 1083–100.

27. Weinstein JN, Tosteson TD, Lurie JD, et al. Surgical versus nonsurgical therapy for lumbar spinal stenosis. N Engl J Med 2008;358(8):794–810.

28. Weinstein JN, Tosteson TD, Lurie JD, et al. Surgical versus nonoperative treatment for lumbar spinal stenosis four-year results of the spine patient outcomes research trial. Spine 2010;35(14):1329–38.

29. Lurie JD, Tosteson TD, Tosteson A, et al. Long-term outcomes of lumbar spinal stenosis. Spine 2015;40(2):63–76.

30. Atlas SJ, Deyo RA, Keller RB, et al. The maine lumbar spine study, part III. Spine 1996;21(15):1787–94.

31. Malmivaara A, Slätis P, Heliövaara M, et al. Surgical or nonoperative treatment for lumbar spinal stenosis? Spine 2007;32(1):1–8.

32. Bresnahan L, Ogden AT, Natarajan RN, et al. A biomechanical evaluation of graded posterior element removal for treatment of lumbar stenosis. Spine 2009;34(1):17–23.

33. Gurelik M, Bozkina C, Kars Z. Unilateral laminotomy for decompression of lumbar stenosis is effective

and safe: a prospective randomized comparative study. J Neurol Sci 2012;29(4):744–53.

34. Thomé C, Zevgaridis D, Leheta O, et al. Outcome after less-invasive decompression of lumbar spinal stenosis: a randomized comparison of unilateral laminotomy, bilateral laminotomy, and laminectomy. J Neurosurg Spine 2005;3(2):129–41.

35. Çelik SE, Çelik S, Göksu K, et al. Microdecompressive laminatomy with a 5-year follow-up period for severe lumbar spinal stenosis. J Spinal Disord Tech 2010;23(4):229–35.

36. Yagi M, Okada E, Ninomiya K, et al. Postoperative outcome after modified unilateral-approach microendoscopic midline decompression for degenerative spinal stenosis. J Neurosurg Spine 2009;10(4):293–9.

37. Mobbs RJ, Li J, Sivabalan P, et al. Outcomes after decompressive laminectomy for lumbar spinal stenosis: comparison between minimally invasive unilateral laminectomy for bilateral decompression and open laminectomy. J Neurosurg Spine 2014;21(2):179–86.

38. Sato J, Ohtori S, Orita S, et al. Radiographic evaluation of indirect decompression of mini-open anterior retroperitoneal lumbar interbody fusion: oblique lateral interbody fusion for degenerated lumbar spondylolisthesis. Eur Spine J 2015;26(3):671–8.

39. Oliveira L, Marchi L, Coutinho E, et al. A radiographic assessment of the ability of the extreme lateral interbody fusion procedure to indirectly decompress the neural elements. Spine 2010;35(Supplement):S331–7.

40. Wang JC, Bohlman HH, Riew KD. Dural tears secondary to operations on the lumbar spine. management and results after a two-year-minimum follow-up of eighty-eight patients*. J Bone Joint Surg 1998;80(12):1728–32.

41. Stolke D, Sollmann W-P, Seifert V. Intra- and postoperative complications in lumbar disc surgery. Spine 1989;14(1):56–9.

42. Ragab AA, Fye MA, Bohlman HH. Surgery of the lumbar spine for spinal stenosis in 118 patients 70 years of age or older. Spine 2003;28(4):348–53.

43. Rihn JA, Hilibrand AS, Zhao W, et al. Effectiveness of surgery for lumbar stenosis and degenerative spondylolisthesis in the octogenarian population. J Bone Joint Surg Am 2015;97(3):177–85.

UNITED STATES POSTAL SERVICE®

Statement of Ownership, Management, and Circulation (All Periodicals Publications Except Requester Publications)

1. Publication Title	2. Publication Number		3. Filing Date
ORTHOPEDIC CLINICS OF NORTH AMERICA	950 – 920		9/18/2022

4. Issue Frequency	5. Number of Issues Published Annually	6. Annual Subscription Price
JAN, APR, JUL, OCT	4	$354.00

7. Complete Mailing Address of Known Office of Publication (Not printer) (Street, city, county, state, and ZIP+4®)

ELSEVIER INC.
230 Park Avenue, Suite 800
New York, NY 10169

Contact Person
Malathi Samayan

Telephone (Include area code)
91-44-4299-4507

8. Complete Mailing Address of Headquarters or General Business Office of Publisher (Not printer)

ELSEVIER INC.
230 Park Avenue, Suite 800
New York, NY 10169

9. Full Names and Complete Mailing Addresses of Publisher, Editor, and Managing Editor (Do not leave blank)

Publisher (Name and complete mailing address)

DOLORES MELONI, ELSEVIER INC.
1600 JOHN F KENNEDY BLVD. SUITE 1800
PHILADELPHIA, PA 19103-2899

Editor (Name and complete mailing address)

MEGAN ASHDOWN, ELSEVIER INC.
1600 JOHN F KENNEDY BLVD. SUITE 1800
PHILADELPHIA, PA 19103-2899

Managing Editor (Name and complete mailing address)

PATRICK MANLEY, ELSEVIER INC.
1600 JOHN F KENNEDY BLVD. SUITE 1800
PHILADELPHIA, PA 19103-2899

10. Owner (Do not leave blank. If the publication is owned by a corporation, give the name and address of the corporation immediately followed by the names and addresses of all stockholders owning or holding 1 percent or more of the total amount of stock. If not owned by a corporation, give the names and addresses of the individual owners. If owned by a partnership or other unincorporated firm, give its name and address as well as those of each individual owner. If the publication is published by a nonprofit organization, give its name and address.)

Full Name	Complete Mailing Address
WHOLLY OWNED SUBSIDIARY OF REED/ELSEVIER, US HOLDINGS	1600 JOHN F KENNEDY BLVD. SUITE 1800 PHILADELPHIA, PA 19103-2899

11. Known Bondholders, Mortgagees, and Other Security Holders Owning or Holding 1 Percent or More of Total Amount of Bonds, Mortgages, or Other Securities. If none, check box. ▶ ☐ None

Full Name	Complete Mailing Address
N/A	

12. Tax Status (For completion by nonprofit organizations authorized to mail at nonprofit rates) (Check one)
The purpose, function, and nonprofit status of this organization and the exempt status for federal income tax purposes:

☒ Has Not Changed During Preceding 12 Months
☐ Has Changed During Preceding 12 Months (Publisher must submit explanation of change with this statement)

PS Form **3526**, July 2014 [Page 1 of 4 (see instructions page 4)] PSN: 7530-01-000-9931 PRIVACY NOTICE: See our privacy policy on www.usps.com.

---

13. Publication Title			14. Issue Date for Circulation Data Below
ORTHOPEDIC CLINICS OF NORTH AMERICA			JULY 2022

15. Extent and Nature of Circulation			Average No. Copies Each Issue During Preceding 12 Months	No. Copies of Single Issue Published Nearest to Filing Date
a. Total Number of Copies (Net press run)			201	175
b. Paid Circulation (By Mail and Outside the Mail)	(1)	Mailed Outside-County Paid Subscriptions Stated on PS Form 3541 (Include paid distribution above nominal rate, advertiser's proof copies, and exchange copies)	64	53
	(2)	Mailed In-County Paid Subscriptions Stated on PS Form 3541 (Include paid distribution above nominal rate, advertiser's proof copies, and exchange copies)	0	0
	(3)	Paid Distribution Outside the Mails Including Sales Through Dealers and Carriers, Street Vendors, Counter Sales, and Other Paid Distribution Outside USPS®	98	93
	(4)	Paid Distribution by Other Classes of Mail Through the USPS (e.g., First-Class Mail®)	0	0
c. Total Paid Distribution [Sum of 15b (1), (2), (3), and (4)]		▶	162	146
d. Free or Nominal Rate Distribution (By Mail and Outside the Mail)	(1)	Free or Nominal Rate Outside-County Copies included on PS Form 3541	22	16
	(2)	Free or Nominal Rate In-County Copies Included on PS Form 3541	0	0
	(3)	Free or Nominal Rate Copies Mailed at Other Classes Through the USPS (e.g., First-Class Mail)	0	0
	(4)	Free or Nominal Rate Distribution Outside the Mail (Carriers or other means)	0	0
e. Total Free or Nominal Rate Distribution (Sum of 15d (1), (2), (3) and (4))		▶	22	16
f. Total Distribution (Sum of 15c and 15e)		▶	184	162
g. Copies not Distributed (See Instructions to Publishers #4 (page #3))		▶	17	13
h. Total (Sum of 15f and g)		▶	201	175
i. Percent Paid (15c divided by 15f times 100)			88.04%	90.12%

* If you are claiming electronic copies, go to line 16 on page 3. If you are not claiming electronic copies, skip to line 17 on page 3.

16. Electronic Copy Circulation		Average No. Copies Each Issue During Preceding 12 Months	No. Copies of Single Issue Published Nearest to Filing Date
a. Paid Electronic Copies	▶		
b. Total Paid Print Copies (Line 15c) + Paid Electronic Copies (Line 16a)	▶		
c. Total Print Distribution (Line 15f) + Paid Electronic Copies (Line 16a)	▶		
d. Percent Paid (Both Print & Electronic Copies) (16b divided by 16c × 100)	▶		

☒ I certify that 50% of all my distributed copies (electronic and print) are paid above a nominal price.

17. Publication of Statement of Ownership

☒ If the publication is a general publication, publication of this statement is required. Will be printed in the OCTOBER 2022 issue of this publication.

☐ Publication not required.

18. Signature and Title of Editor, Publisher, Business Manager, or Owner	Date
Malathi Samayan - Distribution Controller *Malathi Samayan*	9/18/2022

I certify that all information furnished on this form is true and complete. I understand that anyone who furnishes false or misleading information on this form or who omits material or information requested on the form may be subject to criminal sanctions (including fines and imprisonment) and/or civil sanctions (including civil penalties).

PS Form **3526**, July 2014 (Page 3 of 4) PRIVACY NOTICE: See our privacy policy on www.usps.com.

Moving?

Make sure your subscription moves with you!

To notify us of your new address, find your **Clinics Account Number** (located on your mailing label above your name), and contact customer service at:

Email: journalscustomerservice-usa@elsevier.com

800-654-2452 (subscribers in the U.S. & Canada)
314-447-8871 (subscribers outside of the U.S. & Canada)

Fax number: 314-447-8029

Elsevier Health Sciences Division
Subscription Customer Service
3251 Riverport Lane
Maryland Heights, MO 63043

*To ensure uninterrupted delivery of your subscription, please notify us at least 4 weeks in advance of move.

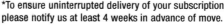

9780323961950